The Politics of Mental Health and Illness

Series Editor
Bruce M. Z. Cohen
Sociology
University of Auckland
Auckland, New Zealand

The Politics of Mental Health and Illness conceptualises the western mental health system as a social, economic, political, and cultural project which cannot be adequately theorised without considering wider societal and structural issues such as professional power, labelling and deviance, ideological and social control, consumption, capital, and self-governance. Engaging with both social theory and empirical evidence, and situated at the intersections of critical psychiatry, sociology, anthropology, social psychology, social work, history, media studies, and the health and education sciences, the series offers academics, researchers, postgraduate students, and practitioners new and innovative monographs and edited collections with which to contest and challenge the taken-for-granted understandings of psychiatry and the mental health system currently progressed in western society. Research topics for the collection may include: aspects of the medicalisation and/or pharmaceuticalisation of everyday life; psy-professional power and knowledge production; psychopolitics and the expansion of talk therapies; the biomedical model and the future of psychiatric nosology; the marketisation of mental health discourse; social media and self-diagnosing behaviour; capitalism and psychiatric violence; and specific analyses of psy-professionals and their practices from a variety of locations (including prisons, workplaces, addiction clinics, the military, schools, the home, and general hospitals). As the first book series to explicitly encourage critical contributions in the area of mental health and illness, we welcome scholarship from a wide range of different theoretical and empirical perspectives.

If you would like to discuss a book idea prior to submitting a proposal please contact the Series Editor, Dr Bruce M. Z. Cohen, via the Commissioning Editor, Beth Farrow (beth.farrow@palgrave.com).

Alison Fixsen

The Construction of Eating Disorders

Psychiatry, Politics and Cultural Representations of Disordered Eating

palgrave
macmillan

Alison Fixsen
Psychology
University of Westminster
LONDON, UK

ISSN 2731-5266 ISSN 2731-5274 (electronic)
The Politics of Mental Health and Illness
ISBN 978-3-031-70317-1 ISBN 978-3-031-70318-8 (eBook)
https://doi.org/10.1007/978-3-031-70318-8

Cover credit : Malte Mueller/Getty Images

This Palgrave Macmillan imprint is published by the registered company Springer Nature Switzerland AG.
The registered company address is: Gewerbestrasse 11, 6330 Cham, Switzerland

To my family who have supported me through some truly challenging times. May we continue to enjoy many happy adventures together. To my teachers, spiritual and intellectual, whose wisdom and inspiration has helped with me in some form through decades of living and writing.

Acknowledgments

No project is a lone endeavor. Both the genesis and writing of this book were made possible through collaborations and discussion of emerging ideas with colleagues, family, and my students who chose to investigate topics relating to mental health, bodies in contemporary society and disordered eating over several years.

I especially want to thank the following people for their contributions to this work and their help in undertaking this project:

Dr Anna Cheshire, Research Fellow in Psychology, University of Westminster, whose invitation to collaborate on a project on orthorexia nervosa began what became an in-depth exploration of contemporary eating disorders.

Damien Ridge, Professor of Health Studies, University of Westminster, without whose encouragement I might never have carried on with my work as qualitative researcher.

Alan Porter, Head of School of Social Sciences, University of Westminster, for being the most supportive line manager I have known in my long career.

The following co-authors of studies and articles cited in this book: Dr Panagiota Tragantzopoulou (perspectives on extreme heathy eating and eating disorder forums); Michelle Berry (perspectives on extreme heathy eating); Magdalena Kossewska and Dr Bardey Aurore (lived experiences of models); Mesha Holder, Olivia Ponsford, and Gurjeet Saran (experiences of health professionals working with eating disorder patients).

The following alumni from the University of Westminster, whose project data was used for secondary analysis: Qai Zhao who investigated experiences of health practitioners working with eating disorder patients on mainland China; Francesca Licciolo, who investigated the perspectives of professionals working in the eating disorder field in Italy; Jessica Smith who investigated experiences the eating choices of male body builders; Anna Britton who investigated the perspectives of fitness instructors and personal trainers concerning eating disorders; Bethany Shaw for her work on YouTube videos of anorexia nervosa.

Finally, a huge thanks to Chris, for your love and patience, for exchanging ideas, and for reading the work in its various stages. To Louis, for your astute comments, and to Alex, for your gentle encouragement.

Third Party Statement

Funding Acknowledgments

The original orthorexia study was aided by seed funding from the Centre for Psychological Medicine, Perdana University, Kuala Lumpur, Malaysia.

Contents

Abbreviations

AI	Artificial Intelligence
AN	Anorexia Nervosa
ARFID	Avoidant Restrictive Food Intake Disorder
BEAT	UK eating disorder charity
BED	Binge Eating Disorder
BMI	Body Mass Index
BN	Bulimia Nervosa
CBS	Culture Bound Syndrome
CDA	Critical Discourse Analysis
DSM	Diagnostic and Statistical Manual of Mental Disorders
EDNOS	Eating Disorder Not Otherwise Specified
EDs	Eating Disorders
FAO	Food and Agriculture Organization of the United Nations
HE Websites	Healthy Eating Websites
IBS	Irritable Bowel Syndrome
ICD	International Classification of Diseases
IPA	Interpretative Phenomenological Analysis
NEDA	National Eating Disorders Association
NHS	National Health Service
NICE	National Institute for Health and Care Excellence
OCD	Obsessive-Compulsive Disorder
OFED	Other Feeding or Eating Disorder
ON	Orthorexia Nervosa

OSFED	Other Specified Feeding or Eating Disorder
Pro-Ana	Pro-anorexia
Pro-ED Websites	Pro-Eating Disorder Websites
Pro-Mia	Pro-bulimia
UFED	Unspecified Feeding or Eating Disorder
UK	United Kingdom
US	United States
WHO	World Health Organisation

1

How We Became Disordered Eaters

The Business of Eating

It is difficult nowadays to go anywhere without coming across messages about eating and its consequences. Media and public health messages are constantly reinforcing the importance of making the right food and diet choices. Warnings to stay alert to the signs of an eating disorder (ED) feature not just in health and educational establishments but in advertising campaigns such Dove's *Cost of Beauty* video, in which a series of "selfie" shots reveal the downward spiral of one young girl into rapid weight loss.[1] By displaying the word "self-esteem" alongside the brand-name, the advert's message concerning how women should nurture their bodies is ambiguous. These types of strategies can be justified by emerging evidence that mental disorders[2] and disordered eating have reached epidemic proportions, suggesting that the culpable beauty market should campaign to protect its more vulnerable customers. They are part of a

[1] The video can be found on https://realcostofbeauty.dove.com.

[2] The World Health Organization (2022) estimates that around a billion people now suffer from a diagnosable mental disorder, a number that increased by around a quarter in the first year of the pandemic.

A. Fixsen, *The Construction of Eating Disorders*, The Politics of Mental Health and Illness, https://doi.org/10.1007/978-3-031-70318-8_1

diffuse system of governmentality over individuals' mental health and eating practices which has accompanied the increasing pathologization of eating, to the extent that around 9 percent of the United States (US) population are predicted to develop a clinically recognized eating disorder in their lifetime, with the number of females affected double that of males.[3] This book invites the reader to reflect on the forces that shape disordered eating, on food landscapes and policies, on market forces and technological developments, on cultural representations of ideal and disordered bodies, and on the politics of the body which defines or challenges definitions of normality.

How did we humans reach the point that eating, something vital and inherently sustaining and pleasurable, became so disordered as to now be viewed as one of the biggest psychiatric and medical problems in contemporary society? At its core, eating is a biological imperative intricately tied to survival. Our entire human journey has been shaped by our relationship with food. From an adaptive perspective, we can exploit a wide range of sources of nutrition. This allows for seasonal variation but requires cooperation and ingenuity to gather and process less palatable foodstuffs. We have had to find ways to distinguish between foods that are safe and health promoting and those which should be avoided. Since humans exist as social animals, our feeding processes are social constructions. As intelligent, but less agile mammals, we rely on our collective efforts to find, collect, store, test out, prepare, and cook available food items to render them digestible and palatable. Food provisions must then be divided up and safeguarded; war and famine ensue over the production and distribution of food. Food and eating are also imbued with cultural meaning. Social, religious, and other institutions of governance have constructed complex rules, rituals, and norms around food, informing people not only about what is good to eat but when to consume food and where. Growing up we come to adopt culturally accepted eating practices and preferences by copying from and listening to others; later this happens through a process of social and self-censure. In this sense, eating is a social performance, beset by rules of etiquette and constraints. Yet the

[3] For more statistics on the social and economic costs of eating disorders in the US, see: https://www.hsph.harvard.edu/striped/report-economic-costs-of-eating-disorders/

rituals of eating are not always followed, for various reasons people decide to deviate and transgress accepted norms—and it is at this point that we enter the territory of disordered eating and eating disorders.

For the modern consumer, working out how to eat well is a complicated process. Many of the traditional discourses and rules around eating practices have broken down or been subsumed into more commercialized ways of obtaining and consuming food. Urbanization has made it difficult to appreciate how profoundly food production shapes our lives (Steel, 2021). It is now almost impossible to consider eating and diet along the lines of a single culture or tradition because the various directives on health, eating, and body shaping are so changeable. Contradictions also exist between how we are expected to respond to messages about healthy foods and those advertising luxury foods accompanied by displays of bliss or affection (Graham et al., 2022). Often these messages are combined, as in "creamy low-fat desert." Food (as a pleasure) is highly amenable to moralization. Media and public health messages constantly reinforce the importance of making "good" as opposed to "bad" food and diet choices (Coveney, 2006; Ross Arguedas, 2020). Yet the freedom of choice supposedly enjoyed by consumers in the developed world is largely illusory. Powerful market forces determine most people's eating preferences and the selections they make. We have become less beings of place and culture and more faceless consumers of branding. Even in a vast shopping mall, with its mind-boggling variety of edible products, real food choice is surprisingly limited. Only a few companies control the production of raw food materials, and the branding and marketing of foods. Disruptions in food distribution systems, such as happened during Covid, bring home the message of the fragility of these systems and our reliance on food monopolies. When consumer choices move (or are moved) in new directions, such as toward meat-free products, these huge corporations then become the vegan brand-leaders.

Food and eating have also become thoroughly medicalized, not just in the sense of being "good" or "bad" for health (Eriksson & Machin, 2020), but in the way that pathological and psychiatric categories are applied to those who regularly transgress dietary norms or who try too hard to achieve them. Yet, the idea of eating disorders (ED) as psychiatric illnesses is relatively recent. For example, anorexia nervosa (AN) as a medical condition was first proposed in the 1870s but was still considered a rare disease a century later, while bulimia nervosa (BN) as a mental disorder only gained official recognition in 1980.[4] Even after experts such as Hilda Bruch (1978, 1982) brought anorexia nervosa to prominence, it was regarded as an affliction of the young, rich, and attractive. According to Bruch, anorexia nervosa (AN) was not a new disease, but its rapid increase in women from the 1960s was linked with the unhealthy pursuit of excessive thinness in modern society. Middle-class girls were seen as particularly vulnerable as they wanted to look slim for the modern workplace (Bruch, 1978). Nowadays eating disorders (EDs) are believed to have reached epidemic proportions and to cross social, ethnic, and gender divides.

The biopolitical "war on fat" has also been gaining momentum. Beginning its life as a nineteenth-century North American crusade, the fear of fat and its moral, physical, and medical consequences are deeply intertwined with capitalist economics. Fatness has shifted from a matter of individual discipline to a perceived societal burden linked to chronic disease (Williams, 2014). Directives toward weight loss now dominate governmental campaigns and advertising, leading to the daily touting of miracle cures for obesity in media (Shanouda & Orsini, 2023). The push to combat obesity is so entwined with markets that GOV.UK has a dedicated page on *Wegovy,* the NHS' slimming drug of choice.[5] While the messages of restrictive eating disorder and obesity campaigns appear to differ, both tap into the "pedagogies of self-fulfillment" (Rose, 1998) which are central to the neoliberal regime of self. They highlight the paradoxes of a society that simultaneously promotes and stigmatizes certain body types, sending mixed messages about which bodies and eating habits are desirable or undesirable, and who should purchase which products to achieve body norms. The present focus on marketing strategies and biotechnical developments has obscured wider socioeconomic issues

[4] Bulimia nervosa was added to DSM-III in 1980.

[5] *Wegovy* and *Ozempic* are part of a new class of weight-loss and diabetes drugs known as Glucagon-like peptide 1 receptor antagonists (GLP-1) which suppress people's appetite. Novo Nordisk, the manufacturers of the drug, is now Europe's most valuable company (Das & Ungoed-Thomas, 2023), with academics and experts backing the "skinny jab" *Wegovy* said to have been paid millions of dollars aby the company.

underlying much of what counts as disordered eating (Puhl & Suh, 2015). For example, in the UK, children living in the most deprived areas are more than twice as likely to be living with obesity than those in the least deprived areas (Children's Commissioner, 2024).

The marketing regulations around lucrative weight-loss products have yet to address the attractions and dangers for people engaging in restrictive eating practices, with the possibility that common side effects of slimming drugs such as nausea and vomiting could further contribute to the development of eating disorders in vulnerable persons (BEAT, 2023). An allied concern for the eating disorder sector is that well known celebrities have been publicising their use of drugs such as Ozempic, making skinniness again highly fashionable. The new advances in pharmacology, biotechnology, genetics, and surgery promising rapid solutions to disordered eating have been accompanied by the development of numerous therapeutic and beauty professions, now visible in every shopping mall and outlet. The collusion of the beauty world with the biotech industries marketing solutions aimed at tackling overweight and disordered eating has given birth to one of the most lucrative of contemporary market sectors. A multi-billion-dollar a year eating disorder industry has emerged to combat what is widely conceived of as the "global burden" of obesity and eating disorders (Erskine et al., 2016; Santomauro et al., 2021). Also now operating in this neoliberal marketplace[6] are the hugely influential media platforms which, alongside the commodification of ideal or modified bodies (via fashion, advertising, "selfies," social media videos, etc.), employ both fictitious and real-life stories about eating disorders and disordered bodies containing messages of personal failure, family dysfunction, self-care, and recovery.

A trim body has not always been a mark of social status, however for much of the last hundred years, it has been, not just medically, but socially and economically desirable—for those with the resources to eat well—to be slim. For those who are classed as overweight, the social and economic consequences can be grave. While obesity is not strictly classified as an

---

[6] The term neoliberalism has been differently interpreted. According to Boltanski and Chiapello (2005), neoliberalism has encouraged a free-market economy in which safety nets have been dismantled and people are viewed either as commodities or producers and consumers of them.

eating disorder, there are clearly overlaps between the two, both in terms of diagnosis and associations with socioeconomic status (SES). Research has long shown that working people defined as having a larger body mass index (BMI) (sometimes set at over 30) are significantly less likely to achieve as highly in economic terms as their slimmer counterparts. A recent study by the Economist (2023) analyzing data from twenty-three thousand workers confirmed that being classified obese continued to negatively impact the earnings of both men and women. Surprising to some, the higher the level of education, the greater the penalty in terms of earnings. Such studies appear to confirm that the aggregate costs of discrimination borne by overweight workers are substantial. Social and economic disruption, as occurred during the Covid pandemic, has also brought to light the intersectional nature of financial and environmental stress on mental health and obesity risk (Fixsen et al., 2022; Melamed et al., 2022). Pharmacological solutions to distress are no simple answer: a common side effect of many psychiatric medications—prescribed for depression, anxiety, psychosis, and sleep problems—is weight gain, and a potential worsening of obesity-related diseases (Anekwe, 2020).[7]

All this is happening at a time when human existence appears to be at its most disconnected from nature. Capitalism[8] promises prosperity, and yet by making the principal precept of contemporary society that of production and consumption, it has created ideas, conditions, and environments which are unequal; hidden the real costs of consumerism to people, animals, and the environment; and led to a situation in which both poverty and obesity abound. Hunger and food insecurity trends are, according-

---

[7] Among the antidepressants with the high risk of causing weight gain are *amitriptyline, citalopram, mirtazapine,* and *paroxetine.* Antipsychotics such as *olanzapine, risperidone,* and *quetiapine* are associated with impaired glucose metabolism and increased cholesterol and triglyceride levels. Hence, those taking multiple psychiatric medications are considered at high risk for obesity, high blood pressure, and metabolic syndrome (Anekwe, 2020).

[8] There are many definitions of capitalism. Here it refers to an economic system in which private actors own and control property in accordance with their own interests, where demand and supply freely sets the prices of labor and goods, markets compete with one another, and instability is the only constant. Due to their inherent instability and inequities, markets and capital must usually coexist alongside public institutions which operate on more than just profit-seeking lines, but in countries such as the US public welfare is very limited. To cite Michel Albert (1993), "since capitalism no longer has any real challengers, it has no mirror in which to examine itself, no alter ego against which to measure its performance."

ing to the Food and Agriculture Organisation of the United Nations (FAO, 2024), not yet moving in the right direction to see any end to them, as billions of people still lack access to nutritious safe and sufficient food. In the western hemisphere and now beyond, neoliberal capitalism,[9] with its emphasis on personal branding, has made the body the conduit for a large array of individual psychosocial symbols which require an endless supply of consumable products to sustain them. For those who can afford to buy based on "quality," food has become less about such things as satiation and companionship, and more about status and achieving a particular lifestyle.

Psychiatry and Eating Disorders

The genesis of eating disorders as psychiatric entities begins with the American Psychiatric Association and its ever-expanding volume, *The Diagnostic and Statistical Manual of Mental Disorders* (DSM). Along with its sister volume, *The International Classification of Diseases* or ICD (WHO, 2019),[10] DSM-V (the fifth edition) (APA, 2013) is widely considered the principle taxonomic system of mental disorders, including eating disorders. These volumes define which mental disorders are considered legitimate, how patients perceive their problems, who receives medical help and government benefits, which conditions are targeted by psychotropic drugs, and what illnesses insurance companies or health authorities will pay to treat (Horwitz, 2021). First appearing in 1952 as DSM-1, the third edition DSM-III (1980) was regarded as a turning point in medical history, as it marked psychiatry's rejection of psychoanalysis and its return to descriptive diagnosis (Wilson, 1993). DSM-III was swiftly hailed in popular science books as progressive, scientific, and

[9] I use this term to describe a recent form of capitalism associated with a more radical change of subjectivity, still founded on individual responsibility, accountability, but also alertness to entrepreneurial possibilities founded on creative risk, made more possible through biotechnology and digital marketing.

[10] Originating in the nineteenth century, the latest version of the ICD came into effect on January 1st, 2022 (World Health Organization, 2022). Developed as a variant of ICD-6 in 1952, the most recent version of the Diagnostic and Statistical Manual of Mental Disorders, DSM-V, was published in 2013 (APA, 2020).

revolutionary and a welcome transition to a scientific form psychiatry (Horwitz, 2021). Translated into many languages, the manual has had enormous international impact on the shaping of social thought and practice. Psychiatric drug regulation agencies, health insurance companies, policymakers, pharmaceutical companies, the legal system, charities, and researchers all refer to the criteria of the DSM in their planning and decision-making.

Despite its ubiquity, the DSM has garnered criticism, not least for its links to a phenomenally lucrative biomedical industry. Since psychiatric diagnosis cannot rely on biomarkers or lab tests, the manual has had to focus on observable or assumed symptoms when revising or adding new disorders (Horwitz & Grob, 2016). The APA describes its taxonomy as "a work in progress," responding to findings from diverse sources as well as demands from national government agencies, insurance companies, and the pharmaceutical industry. Critics of the DSM (some of them psychiatrists) have been scathing about its seemingly endless accumulation of mental disorders, which threaten to make us all "crazy" through pathologizing everyday behavior (Kutchins & Kirk, 2003; Brinkmann, 2016). Regardless of the efforts of DSM-V to establish greater validity by using complex psychological rating scales, the whole process became rife with accusations of secrecy, institutional corruption, and industrial colonization on the part of the APA (Angell, 2009; Cosgrove & Wheeler, 2013; Whitaker & Cosgrove, 2015).[11] Concerns were also expressed about its definition of mental disorder and poor methodology (Welch et al., 2013). In a special issue of the *Journal of Psychological Injury and Law*, DSM-V was declared, "rife with utility and scientific difficulties" (Young, 2013). Also in 2013, the National Institute of Mental Health (NIMH) announced it would no longer require researchers to use the DSM and would instead use its own classification system built for research, rather than clinical diagnosis (Freeborn, 2022). DSM-V (APA, 2013) was so

[11] Many books have been written on this topic, some of which became best sellers. They follow an anti-psychiatry and medical reform tradition which emerged in the 1960s, largely through the work of psychiatrists themselves such as R.D. Laing (1927–1989) and Thomas Szasz (1920–2012). The fact that de-institutionalization in the US resulted in people in serious distress being virtually dumped on the streets is evidence that simply changing a policy without tackling structural social and economic inequalities is likely to result in more disaster.

fraught with controversy that some within psychiatry itself claimed that it terminally undermined the scientific status of the APA's psychiatric bible (Frances, 2013).

A further critique pertaining to both the DSM and ICD concerns a lack of cultural and ethnic sensitivity within their criteria (Claudino et al., 2019; Sweet & Decoteau, 2018). DSM-V has been accused of creating a dividing line in psychiatry by making sociocultural context relevant only for some patients (Bredström, 2019). Psychiatry's exclusion of social, political, and economic issues underlying mental distress has seriously called into question its application in a complex world (Horwitz, 2012; Jackson & Rizq, 2019, Welch et al., 2013). In answer to these criticisms, psychologists and others were invited to respond during DSM-V-TR's (2022) minor revision process. The latest edition prides itself as being the first to include "a comprehensive review of the impact of racism and discrimination on the diagnosis and manifestations of mental disorders" (APA, 2022). Clearly, the APA have made efforts to align its much-used volume with contemporary issues and sensitivities, and in the process to render more non-psychiatric professionals familiar with its taxonomy.

Other criticisms of psychiatry touch on the very nature of medicalization as a means of social governance. Medical historians point out that the existence of psychiatric disorders themselves must not be taken for granted, since different explanations for what counts as a "madness" or "mental illness" have existed (Scull, 2022). The western medical approach has seen a progressive dismissal of lay explanations relating to distress in favor of themes considered objective and neutral but "descriptive of mechanical objects or human machines" (Mezzich, 2002, p. 5). While it is acknowledged that many people are made miserable by mental illness, the DSM is considered to overstep its boundaries by defining how people should think about themselves, how they should respond to stress, how much anxiety or sadness they should feel, and how and when they should eat and sleep (Kutchins & Kirk, 2003). Voicing these criticisms is not to suggest that psychiatry, as a discipline, has lost its power. Indeed, the language of psychiatry has become social new-speak, with labels such "OCD," "ADHD," and "bulimia" now absorbed into everyday talk. Paradoxically, the popular anti-psychiatry literature may have furthered this process by bringing these matters to public attention.

The Eating Disorder Epidemic

Regardless of all the knowledge about disordered eating and its different manifestations, the number of reported cases of EDs in western and non-western societies continues to grow. Statistical studies suggest that rates of anorexia nervosa (AN)[12] and bulimia nervosa (BN)[13] have not altered significantly in recent years, but there has been a substantial increase in the newer ED categories (Hay et al., 2017). The transition from DSM-IV to DSM-V broadened the diagnostic criteria for AN and BN and introduced binge eating disorder (BED),[14] avoidant restrictive food intake disorder (ARFID),[15] and the ill-defined category of other specified feeding or eating disorders (OSFED)[16] (Jenkins et al., 2021). In global terms, BED and OSFED now account for the majority of the ED cases in disability adjusted life years (DALYs) (Santomauro et al., 2021). DALYs are an important measure because, compared with people without them, those with EDs are statically less likely to participate in gainful employment, have more time off work, earn less, accumulate higher healthcare and informal care costs, and die prematurely (Santomauro et al., 2021).

[12] Anorexia nervosa (AN) is a DSM defined mental disorder characterized by restriction of energy intake, relative to requirements, leading to significantly low body weight. Individuals with anorexia also display a fear of gaining weight or becoming fat, or persistent behavior that interferes with weight gain as well of specific disturbances in relation to perception or experience of their own body, weight, and shape (see APA, 2013, pp. 338–345).

[13] BN or Bulimia Nervosa is a DSM defined mental disorder characterized by frequent episodes of binge eating followed by inappropriate behaviors such as self-induced vomiting to avoid weight gain (see APA, 2013, pp. 345–350).

[14] BED or Binge Eating Disorder is a DSM defined mental disorder characterized by recurrent episodes of binge eating in the absence of regular compensatory behavior such as vomiting or laxative abuse (see APA, 2013, pp. 350–353).

[15] ARFID or • Avoidant/Restrictive Food Intake Disorder is a DSM defined eating or feeding disturbance, whose most significant diagnostic feature is avoidance or restriction of food intake manifested by clinically significant failure to meet requirements for nutrition, and insufficient energy intake through oral intake of food (see APA, 2013, pp. 334–338). The criteria for ARFID have altered in DSM-V-TR (APA, 2022), with the following statement eliminated from the text: "as manifested by persistent failure to meet appropriate nutritional and/or energy needs."

[16] OSFED or Other Specified Feeding or Eating Disorder is a DSM category which applies to presentations in which symptoms characteristic of a feeding and eating disorder that cause clinically significant distress or impairment in social, occupational, or other important areas of functioning dominate, but which do not meet the full criteria for any of the disorders in the feeding and eating disorders diagnostic class (see APA, 2013, pp. 353).

Thirty to fifty percent of those with a diagnosis of BED will also be diagnosed as obese (McCuen-Wurst et al., 2018), creating an obvious link between overweight and mental disorder.[17] Since a high portion of those with low socioeconomic status (SES) and from minority ethnic groups will also be diagnosed with BED, it amounts to the pathologizing of social inequality. Yet studies suggest that when people of lower SES do seek out ED services, they may face longer waiting times and receive lower levels of care and attention from providers (Huryk et al., 2021). This serves to further stigmatize those in economically and socially disadvantaged communities.

At least some of the growth in numbers of reported eating disorders can be attributed to an increased emphasis on early detection and better knowledge of EDs among health professionals and others working in the community (BEAT, 2024a; Schaumberg et al., 2017). One fall out from this is that in the last decade, the number of children and young adults diagnosed with an eating disorder (ED) has greatly outstripped hospital capacity (Milliren et al., 2023). In the UK, child and adolescent referrals to the UK NHS eating disorder services increased by 46 percent in 2020 alone (Jayanetti, 2021). Many of the professionals operating in the UK public healthcare sector are left to carry out their difficult work within an underfunded, patchwork ED service (Galmiche et al., 2019). The situation has worsened since the Covid pandemic, with more referrals and longer waiting lists for ED treatment (Ayton et al., 2022; Cook et al., 2022). UK Liberal Democrat peer Kate Parminter pointed out how, despite these trends, the present government was failing to address the "woeful shortages of beds" and was instead sending very sick patients hundreds of miles across the border from England to Scotland for treatment at great expense (Marsh, 2023). According to the Royal College of Psychiatrists (2022), EDs among young people in the UK rose by 90 percent between 2016 and 2021. Additionally, there has been a notable shift in the gender and ethnic distribution of eating disorders in the UK and US, with males in these countries now representing 20–40 percent of cases (BEAT, 2024a, b; NEDA, 2024). Recent NHS figures show an

[17] In a large-scale study of community surveys by Kessler et al. (2013), most respondents with lifetime binge eating disorder also met the criteria for one or more DSM disorder.

increase in hospital admissions between 2017 and 2020 of 53 percent for those from ethnic minorities compared to 31 percent from white communities (BEAT, 2024a, b). There are also known disparities in eating disorder diagnosis and treatment according to weight status, race/ethnicity, socioeconomic background, and gender (Sonneville & Lipson, 2018).

Those who find themselves hospitalized face the difficulties and consequences of in-patient treatment, voluntary or otherwise. Receiving the initial diagnosis may be a relief, but once in the mental health system, it can be difficult not only to access care but later to exit it. In these times of subjectivity and social comparison, this has consequences for individuals who find themselves labelled. In spite of all the efforts of public awareness campaigns, having a mental health diagnosis can still be highly stigmatizing (Hazell et al., 2022). In a society in which medical and social care systems are overloaded, those diagnosed with a serious ED may find themselves treated in a similar manner to a criminal, in that they may be detained involuntarily, force-fed, and their every movement monitored. The association between mental illness and criminality means that those living in social disadvantage, and also with an ED, are more likely to end up in jail (Treatment Advocacy Center, 2016). Women detained in prisons are also more likely to have been diagnosed with an ED than the general population (The Sentencing Project, 2022). This makes eating disorders as much a matter of social justice as one of biomarkers and genetics, yet increasingly the latter are the areas in which research is being targeted and funded.

Approach of the Book

This book attempts to rebalance this field of study by challenging the dominance of psychiatric terminology and arguing for a broader recognition of the socially constructed nature of disordered eating. The central argument of the book is that disordered eating is never an individual concern, the discussions and practices shaping what it means to be a "disordered eater" are constructed by an expanding range of groups who claim investment, experience, and expertise in their diagnosis and management—and sometimes their continuation. The world of disordered eating has evolved through the efforts of biomedical, psychiatric, legal, pharmaceutical, media, marketing, and consumer interest groups, frequently in competition and conflict with one another. It is a messy history, involving fierce physical and psychological battles over the control of bodies and eating regimes. There are risks to reputation at stake in these battles, as well as huge economic consequences. Wrestling for control are the industries and sectors who stand accused of complicity in the eating disorder epidemic through their encouragement of "unhealthy" eating choices, but the sectors who treat and profit from the social and medical problems associated with disordered eating. As we shall see, even seemingly neutral agencies, such as charities and public education bodies, are not without vested interests. As a result of these forces, the diagnostic process itself has been undergoing change, from being a top-down process to one that involving with many more players and stakeholders, from different sectors and walks of life, all encouraged to engage in the detection and labeling of mental disorders.

Terminology

Regarding the terminology used in this book, there are various ways of denoting aberrant/abnormal eating behaviors which can confuse those studying or reading about them. For the sake of clarity, I (largely) employ the term "disordered eating" when discussing these phenomena in their more general sense and as often allied with a physiological condition. Conversely, I use "eating disorder" or its abbreviation, ED, when referencing diagnosis as outlined in *The Diagnostic and Statistical Manual of Mental Disorders* (DSM) and *International Classification of Diseases* (ICD), encompassing atypical food habits, weight concerns, and shape control beliefs and actions falling within psychiatric classifications. It should also be noted that other published manuals of psychiatry exist,[18] and most, but not all, comments made in the book concerning psychiatry's taxonomy apply to these manuals. I have tended to use the full title of an ED, such as "anorexia nervosa," when referring to the condition in

[18] Other manuals of psychiatry include the Chinese Classification of Mental Disorders (CCDM).

broad, cultural, and historical terms, and its abbreviation AN when specifically referring to the DSM/ICD classification. In practical terms there are frequent overlaps between the way disordered eating and eating disorders are addressed and managed. The term "disordered eating" is not employed to pass judgment on individuals' dietary choices but rather to illustrate how certain forms of eating deemed unnatural are socially, morally, and medically constructed within society. All forms of disordered eating have at some time been framed as imposing social and financial burdens on governments and broader society, with the considerable costs to the global economy of poor dietary decisions emphasized in recent epistemological literature (Santomauro et al., 2021). While our main concern is not with numbers, statistics are cited in the book where relevant to an argument.

Theoretical Position

While a few writers have adopted a social constructionist approach to eating disorders (Duran et al., 2000; Hepworth, 1999), this volume is the first known to present original work and critical discussion on a range of topics related to the social, political, and industrial construction of eating disorders and disordered eating. Its singularity lies not solely in focusing on psychiatry and health, cultural representations, or the politics of eating disorders and disordered eating but in bringing these topics together in a single volume.

The contents of the book venture into the realms of social constructionism, poststructuralism, deconstructionism,[19] and symbolic interactionism[20] to unravel the complex, multifaceted nature of disordered

[19] A theoretical approach connected with French philosopher Jacques Derrida (1930–2004) to indicate that the meaning of work is unstable and could have multiple meanings. Postcolonial studies use the term deconstructionism to attest to the way that, throughout history, reality has been defined in ways which ensure domination over others, for example, people of color. New terms are therefore needed to overcome this legacy.

[20] Symbolic interactionism is a social theory primarily linked to George Herbert Mead (1863–1931) and Max Weber (1864–1920). This perspective broadly views society as constructed through shared symbols, such as language. Individuals assign meanings to things based on their interpretations of verbal and non-verbal interactions with others.

eating and eating disorders as they manifest at different levels and in different contexts. For those unfamiliar with social constructionism, broadly this approach regards social reality as constructed and shaped by human discourse and interests. In other words, what we take as fact or knowledge is both grounded in and mediated by the world views (i.e., the implicit basic values, assumptions, and beliefs) of specific sociocultural groups at certain times and places. Would EDs as we know them exist in a world beyond that which has been socially created? History suggests they might not. The social constructionist/interpretive approach offers a range of theoretical and practical tools[21] for exploring disordered eating and eating disorders, and a number of these are elucidated in the following chapters. Social constructionism explains how behind diagnoses and social labels exists a kaleidoscope of human experience which constitute variations of normality and deviance, familiarity, and strangeness (Pikäinen, 2015). As an approach it helps to explain why in contemporary society certain restrictive eating behaviors such as dieting can be considered as normal and even desirable, while others such as intentional purging for weight loss are pathologized or regarded as deviant (Becker, 1963; Taub & McLorg, 2011). It also explains why at different times groups evolve, who attempt to change prevailing attitudes and conditions in society, for example, how user-led movements such as *Recovery in the Bin*[22] seek to change the research and policy agendas around mental health and to align them with the lived experiences of "survivors."

[21] Social constructionism covers many different disciplines and standpoints. Gergen (1992) describes social constructionism as not a reflection or a map of the world but as an artefact of communal exchange. Burr (2015) describes it as a flexible amalgamation of various perspectives, such as deconstructionism, critical theory, poststructuralism, discourse analysis, and discursive psychology. Some regard as its starting point the ethnographic work of sociologist Garfinkel's on everyday activities (Weinberg, 2009). Others regard Berger and Luckmann's phenomenological work, *The Social Construction of Reality* (1967), as the real origin of social constructionism. The authors assume a middle path to reality in their book, proposing that society exists as both an objective and a subjective reality, with our social world a dialectical process of externalization, objectification, and internalization, i.e., "society is a human product. Society is an objective reality. Man is a social product" (p. 61).

[22] *Recovery in the bin* is a "user-led critical theorist group" who challenge the dominant narratives and technologies of recovery. https://recoveryinthebin.org/neorecovery-a-survivor-led-conceptualisation-and-critique-mhrn2019/

To understand the discourses and practices around the diagnosis and treatment of disordered eating, I have looked to poststructuralism and the work of Michel Foucault (1978, 1982, 1985, 2001) concerning power and discourse relating to the disciplining of "docile" and "unruly" bodies in society. At its core, poststructuralism urges us to question the stability of meaning and the constructed nature of reality. It posits that our understanding of eating disorders is entangled in a web of shifting discourses, power structures, and linguistic constructs that shape our perceptions. Foucault has been critiqued for his obsession with power (Marx, 2019),[23] yet his work was seminal in recognizing discourse as extending far beyond language to actively shape all social practices. Discursive power for Foucault is everywhere but is arguably most evident in those "big narratives" that devolve from institutions to popular speech such as the "mental health epidemic" or the "war on fat." These discourses are very powerful because they are communicated not just through words but statistics, images, and the policies and practices arising from them. Much of the book is devoted to exploring how these relatively familiar discourses around eating disorders (EDs) and disordered eating are constructed.

Foucault was interested in discourse in connection to how society deals with those who live outside of societal norms, such as people considered as criminal and/or insane (Foucault et al., 2013). His concept of disciplinary power emphasizes how institutions, such as the medical establishment, contribute to the surveillance and regulation of bodies (Ransom, 1997). However, Foucault rejects the notion of a top-down model of knowledge and power in contemporary society, instead proposing the concept of "bio-power" (Foucault et al., 2008), which involves the regulation and control of populations through various institutions. Biopower has, with the diminution of the sovereign state, become the prevailing form of power over bodies, which brings "life and its mechanisms into the realm of explicit calculations" (Foucault, 1978, p. 187). We witness and experience this aspect of biopower in the ongoing collection of

[23] In his book on surveillance G.T. Marx (2019) critiques Foucault for insisting that the sole purpose of surveillance is power, ignoring other reasons such as verification, discovery, documentation, profit, organizational, government, administration, etc.

population-level health statistics via censuses, "big data" collection, and surveillance cameras, which have now become an accepted part of our lives.

Foucault's analysis of the medicalization of society highlights how medical knowledge shapes our understanding of health and illness. In the case of eating disorders, medical expertise remains largely responsible for the classification and treatment of these conditions. The medical discourse surrounding eating disorders can both empower and disempower individuals, depending on how it is deployed. Foucault's theory of biopower also sheds light on the ways in which responsibility for health and welfare has, under neoliberalism, shifted away from the state to the individual subject. What Foucault calls "care of the self" is not simply a personal ethic or practice, it is the basis on which institutions and individuals measure normality, success, and market viability. Neoliberal governance has been highly preoccupied with developing a specific form of personhood that is amenable to techniques and technical interventions aimed at shaping the modern citizen and making them fit for work (Cohen, 2016; Rose, 1990, 1998, 2019). However, counter discourses and resistance have increasingly taken on self-care as their own projects, no more so than in the realm of body shape and eating. In the so-called post-truth age, characterized by the proliferation of information and the blurring of lines between fact and opinion, alternative health narratives, often challenging mainstream medical perspectives, have gained much traction. The implications of this for those experiencing mental distress in relation to aberrant eating are explored in various chapters of this book, including that on the proposed "healthy eating" disorder, orthorexia nervosa.

Central Arguments

This book is not simply a textbook; it is a call to action for those who read it to become conscious participants in looking behind the veil that conceals certain discourses which shape and command what and how we should consume. Central to the book is a critique of the current focus on individual solutions and the dominance of psychiatry in the field. Instead, I explain how colonialism, capitalism, western medical ideology, food conglomerates, food poverty, and media have all been involved in the construction of disordered eating and EDs. Socioeconomic disadvantage is now recognized as a fundamental determinant of mental health outcomes (WHO, 2024b), yet emphasis on individual diagnosis has led to a blurring out of the structural conditions and institutions of power which create and reproduce intergenerational inequalities. Psychiatry acknowledges that people exposed to more unfavorable social circumstances are more vulnerable to poor mental health over their life course[24]; however, its diagnostic focus has increasing been that of bringing more people into the psychiatric and therapeutic fold.

From a governance perspective, the continued expansion of psychiatric categories has implications for how society defines and manages deviance. Above and beyond the protestations of critics and mental health service "survivors" that we must all ascribe to some perfect state of mind or body, are the pressures to identify those who are unable to feel, behave, or eat in a normative way. As persons in non-medical spheres of life are asked to be on lookout for any signs of psychological or emotional distress that might resemble a mental health disorder, it creates an expectation of hidden irregularities in our own and others' mental states. The result is a diagnostic culture in which being given a psychiatric label is not just acceptable but commonplace, overlooking the issue that a label itself requires the person to reconfigure their identity and possibly rethink their future. There is also the potential disappointment or distress when a specific label is denied, or a drug or treatment program fails to deliver the required effect. When it used largely to combat social or moral deviance,[25] psychiatric labeling not only undermines individual autonomy but stifles the potential for social change, medically enforcing conformity rather than allowing for the questioning or challenging of convention.

Worse still are those situations where psychiatric diagnoses are used to oppress or punish. Western medical imperialism resulted in exporting the

[24] To quote psychiatrists Kirkbride et al. (2024), "there is now compelling evidence that the risk of developing any mental health condition is inextricably linked to our life circumstances, meaning that a higher burden of population psychiatric morbidity is disproportionately experienced by those closer to the margins of our societies" (p. 58).

[25] An example of this was the classification of homosexuality as a mental disorder in DSM-I in 1952.

ideologies and practices of western psychiatry across the globe[26] and continues to be applied in places reeling from the legacy of western colonialism. Current investigations of political regimes attest that the absolute power of psychiatry continues to be misused to incarcerate those with different views or practices in large numbers, including persecuted ethnic or political minorities (Lyons & O'Malley, 2002; van Voren, 2016). In countries such as the UK, these types of practices are frowned upon. Nevertheless, there are notable inequalities in the delivery of serious and legally enforceable psychiatric diagnoses. Those from black communities remain far more likely to be "sectioned" (detained involuntarily) under the UK Mental Health Act than their white counterparts. A recent press release by the Royal College of Psychiatrists (2024) pointed out the ongoing inequalities within mental health, with many black people in the UK feeling abandoned within a system rife with structural, institutional, and interpersonal racism.

While the conceptualization of eating disorders (ED) as psychiatric categories is largely a medical concern, disordered eating is a societal matter, which must be approached from a variety of angles. Changing food landscapes, globalization and colonial legacies, overemphasis on subjectivity and self-cultivation, idealistic and stereotypical representations of bodies in the media, socioeconomic inequalities and food poverty, the expansion of fast-food industries, the "war on fat" and fat stigma, healthism and body extremism, and the algorithms of social media—along with various processes by which bodies are defined as normal or deviant in their appearance or eating practices—have all been instrumental in the construction of disordered eating. Yet, most health policies seeking to making changes to disordered eating practices focus on shifting individual patterns of thinking and behavior, with the inability to understand or follow official advice put down to some personal defect, requiring some type of pharmaceutical, cognitive, or biotechnical solution—resulting in thriving markets in all these areas.

[26] The history of racism in psychiatry must remain the subject of other books. One famous historical example is "drapetomania," a diagnosis invented in the 1850s for a "mental illness" in which the slave takes it into the head to flee a plantation. This failed to enter the DSM.

Not everyone will agree with these arguments or the approach to EDs and disordered eating taken in this book. Social constructionism's apparent opposition to biological determinism and foundational claims about the nature of mental illness (Fixsen, in print; Horwitz, 2012) can be problematic when considering these topics from a neuroscientific, biomedical, or therapeutic perspective. The book's lack of practical guidance for persons and policymakers may also be seen as a flaw. Sociologist Ian Hacking (1999) has argued that it is all too easy to declare the eating disorder, anorexia nervosa, a "social construct," but this seems of little practical use to the patient or parent faced with the day-by-day stresses of disordered eating and statistics suggesting the consequences of severe food restriction to be potentially fatal (Van Eeden et al., 2021). The arguments put forward in this work are neither straightforward or unambiguous. The reader of this book is going to see "rough edges" and unresolved issues, with some sections throwing up more questions than answers. Highlighting the problematic nature of medicalization does not deny the importance of human experience. Professionals and others—including those who generously gave up their time to be interviewed for studies—perform incredible work, frequently within underfunded and piecemeal healthcare systems. Similarly, many researchers in more science-based fields continue to seek better solutions to the complex and distressing issues around eating disorders.

Yet in our search for therapeutic solutions, we must not forget about the politics around bodies and the dangers of psychiatric hegemony. My conversations with those working in the ED field suggest that arguments concerning the social and political factors potentially undermining people's health and well-being are largely missing from educational curricula, in favor of understanding medical terminology and learning treatment strategies such as cognitive behavioral therapy (CBT) and other types of cognitive and emotional re-conditioning. This is not to deny the importance of these treatment approaches; however, focusing on diagnosis and treatment alone is like chipping away at the tip of the iceberg. Receiving an ED diagnosis might increase the chances of gaining access to therapy; however, it also holds the potential to encroach further on a person's right to make decisions about their own life and even death. Without addressing the inherent flaws and inequities of neoliberal capitalism and the legacies of colonialism, we risk witnessing a continual rise in the number of individuals receiving official or unofficial diagnoses of eating disorders, typically alongside that of one or more other mental disorder. Many will face the prospect of limited access to timely, cost-free treatment. At the same time, the cultural, social, and economic conditions fostering these behaviors and disorders often escape meaningful scrutiny and, like eating disorders themselves, remain highly resistant to change.

Disordered eating and eating disorders are now topics of widespread interest, due to their far-ranging and complex nature, their links to mental health, and their association with chronic morbidity and premature mortality. These problems accompany the reshaping and potential destruction of our food landscapes, at least as we recognize them today. My hope is that this book proves a valuable resource for researchers, students, and professionals who wish to gain a better appreciation of eating disorders and disordered eating as they are perceived today, and the markets which influence and profit from them. Its novel approach to topical and controversial issues is aimed to appeal to the critical, enquiring reader, and indeed anyone interested in understanding the social and industrial construction of eating disorders in the twenty-first century.

Further Chapters

A broad range of issues are covered in the book, including those related to the history of disordered eating and its past and current diagnoses and treatments, global and public health, medical ethics, cultural representations, gender issues, health and eating disorder markets, digitalization and disordered eating, and the many matters relating to human and social justice. All chapters feature empirical studies (several by the author) of persons operating in sectors which have been associated with disordered eating such as modeling, fitness training, and bodybuilding, and those involved in the treatment of eating disorders such as medical doctors and nurses, clinical psychologists, dieticians, and more recently fitness instructors. The book also investigates true-life and fictional portrayals of eating disorders on screen and digital platforms, descriptions and discussions of eating disorders on social media, the development of new disorders based on health anxieties and obsessions, and biotechnological and AI (artificial intelligence) developments in the ED field.

Chapter 2, "Bodies Beyond Conformity" probes into the sociology of non-conforming bodies, and more specifically those to whom the idiom of an "eating disorder" is attached. It explains how, across different historical and geographical contexts, bodies come to be perceived as divergent in their atypical and "unhealthy" eating practices and behaviors, and how society endeavors to regulate these rebellious bodies. Drawing extensively from sociological literature on bodies, with a focus on feminist studies, the chapter considers historical and contemporary perspectives on how we shape our own bodies and how societal influences impact them. Topics explored include the concept of embodiment in relation to the disordered body, the body as a project for identity development, the body under medical scrutiny, and the commodification of the bodies in the context of neoliberalism and post-feminism. The chapter concludes with a brief consideration of the impacts of artificial intelligence (AI) and other forms of technologies which can be used for surveillance on the construction and perception of bodies, both by corporate entities and the broader public.

Chapter 3, "Anorexia Nervosa: The Making of the First Eating Disorder," looks at the historical context of anorexia nervosa (AN) and the interlinking of religious, social, and medical perspectives on the fasting body. Sociological studies of anorexia nervosa highlight the multifaceted nature of the disorder and the importance of considering social, cultural, and structural factors in both understanding its causes and developing effective prevention and intervention strategies. The chapter considers the evolution of AN as a medical phenomenon, from the early professional battles over its naming and interpretation through to its categorization as a psychiatric condition by the American Psychiatric Association. Current diagnostic categories and treatments for AN are then explored, and the risks and ethics of involuntary treatment considered. The clinical features of AN have been thoroughly investigated, but AN must also be understood in relation to the neoliberal "tyranny of the body." The chapter concludes with accounts from those with lived experience of anorexia, providing us with unique insights into the realities of undergoing treatment, and what "being" and "doing" anorexia mean beyond its clinical description. The chapter concludes with arguments supporting the assertion that anorexia as a phenomenon is deeply embedded in the capitalist economy. Through examining the ways that meanings, identities, and behaviors are shaped by social interactions and cultural contexts, anorexia nervosa emerges, not as an individual pathology but as a product of broader historical, medical, and cultural constructions.

Chapter 4, "ED Diagnosis and Therapeutic Frameworks," takes a critical approach to the present diagnostic system, focusing on the power structures inherent in these processes and then highlighting gaps in funding, communication, and long-term support within the current UK mental health system. In the case of disordered eating, understanding the multidimensional nature of the diagnostic process is crucial due to its potential to propel the individual on a journey which may involve distressing procedures, loss of personal liberty, and a host of unintended consequences. The chapter explores some of the controversies around psychiatric labeling, including the exploitative potential of diagnosis and the stigma attached to mental illness. The rising numbers of people now diagnosed with an eating disorder have yet to be matched by available treatment, and while digital technology has allowed an expansion of online treatments for EDs, long-term support for those with EDs remains inadequate. The chapter includes qualitative research into the perceptions and experiences of ED professionals with an examination of its key themes, including the stresses of working in an underfunded service, patient resistance, and the relational problems associated with diagnostic labels. Diagnostic categories fulfil medical and social functions, yet inevitably lead to a one-size-fits-all approach in treatment which, for patients, can result in disappointment and competition over labels, denial of treatment, or loss of autonomy.

Chapter 5, "Disordered Eating, Food Landscapes, and Public Health," explores the complex and often contentious relationship between food landscapes, food policy, and disordered eating. The chapter also focuses on various epistemological and sociological discourses concerning the changing patterns of eating disorders (EDs). The evolving food landscape, marked by globalization and socioeconomic inequalities, has challenged traditional dietary practices and exacerbated health disparities.

Modern technology has revolutionized the promotion of health behaviors with key public health initiatives targeting normative and disordered eating and disseminating "biopedagogic" messages which shape public understanding of fitness and health according to neoliberal public health principles. However, the effectiveness of these health messages remains inconsistent, particularly across different socioeconomic and cultural groups. Policies often hinge on the idea that individuals are solely responsible for their health, perpetuating stereotypes and inequalities. The politicization of food, influenced by the "post-truth" society and media dynamics, further complicates the landscape of dietary advice and health behaviors. The chapter then delves into the ambiguous and complex role of digital technology in regulating our eating behaviors.

Chapter 6, "Biopolitics of Weight and Disordered Eating," looks at the emerging narratives and technologies which have led to the forms of governmentality which constitute what Michel Foucault calls biopower, in relation to weight and disordered eating. It examines ideas around the operations of biopower with examples such as the "normative" biological standard set by body mass index (BMI). Three seemingly polarized narratives are examined. The "War on Fat," as widely advocated by western governments, supports the capitalist notion of the overweight individual as a social and moral failure. Fatness is seen as a matter of self-control and a burden to the rest of society. The obesogenic environmental theory, on the other hand, contests the idea of weight as solely a matter of individual control, laying emphasis instead on structural inequalities, ethnicity, place of residence, and lack of access to institutional care or self-care opportunities. "Fat talk" and its role in marking out certain groups is then discussed in relation to the perpetuation of weight stigma and discrimination in the workplace and wider society. While feminists argue that women have been marked out for fat talk, men's experiences of weight discrimination and ridicule should not be dismissed. The tactics used by weight-loss and health foods industries are also examined, and their financial links with medical and nutritional experts. Finally, the chapter turns to the trend in body positivity, questioning whether it continues to be a counterforce to capitalism or has been turned into another form of "brand possibility."

Chapter 7, "Disordered Eating and the Media Industry," takes a critical look at the relationship between mass media and disordered eating. The chapter examines the considerable part that the media plays in both the representation and commodification of bodies, and in the construction of public narratives around EDs and disordered eating. It explores how media representations intersect with medicine, psychology, the influence of various forms of feminism, and the emergence of "commodity feminism." Several mechanisms come into play when considering the impact of media on ED diagnosis, the development of new categories and treatment programs. Documentaries often medicalize disordered eating, portraying it as a mental disorder rooted in a specific psychological profile. The identification effect occurs as individuals, influenced by the experiences of actors and celebrities with eating disorders, may self-diagnose or seek diagnosis and treatment. Entertainment value is also found in emotionally charged or humorous storylines about characters grappling with the indignities of an eating disorder, while graphic depictions of behaviors such as binging and purging are largely deemed acceptable. Examples of portrayals of bodies and individuals with eating disorders in drama, comedy, and documentary are also scrutinized. Finally, the chapter considers the implications of the media industry's eagerness to feature a greater range of body sizes and to use plus-size actors, and the potential for the latter becoming targets of media exploitation.

Chapter 8, "Disordered Eating in the Virtual World," explains how, for scholars and researchers, Internet platforms and the forums, videos, blogs, podcasts hosted by them have created an archive of information concerning the lived experiences of disordered eating from the perspective of the online generation. Social media platforms also provide a particularly fertile ground from which to gather "digital footprints" to analyze and predict, not just activities, but user location, age, gender, level of education, health status, political preferences, and so on. This chapter focuses on four key aspects of disordered eating discourse in the virtual world. First, it touches on the topic of digital surveillance and data gathering on the Internet. Second, and in relation to the more covert spaces on social media, it delves into the dynamics of discourses surrounding eating disorders and mental health within the context of what have been loosely named pro-eating disorders (pro-ED) forums. The third point concerns the impact of the "selfie society" on the shaping of discourses about disordered eating online, and the use of adapted psychiatric and psychological terminology to describe personal experiences. Finally, it explains how the illness narratives elucidated in recent online videos have taken a decidedly entrepreneurial turn, with the authors of these videos gaining followings on their subscription channels and diversifying, for example, from beauty product promotion to their "my anorexia story."

Chapter 9, "Orthorexia Nervosa: Eating Disorder for a Pro-Health Era," examines the making of a new putative eating disorder characterized by an extreme focus on healthy eating—orthorexia nervosa (ON)—in the light of the social and medical ambiguities and disagreements around "right" food consumption and definitions of health. Beginning with the origins and recognition of ON, the chapter examines the uncertain clinical parameters and overlaps with other EDs and mental disorders. Also discussed are philosophical and sociological explanations for society's seeming obsession with food provenance, including radical changes to food ecologies and institutional structures, neoliberal capitalism's emphasis on self-cultivation, and the promotion of healthism as a means of diverting attention from social and economic ills. A secondary analysis of several distinct perspectives on health-conscious eating is then described and discussed featuring the following: individuals self-identifying as deeply engrossed in healthy eating practices, body builders, professionals specializing in eating disorders, fitness instructors, and posts on eating disorder forums. By juxtaposing the narratives of those adopting varying stances regarding the intersection of health and dietary habits, insights can be gained into the sociopolitical and psychological tensions surrounding the medical labeling of health-conscious persons as troubled and misguided. Deeply rooted in sociocultural factors, ON, arguably more than any other form of "disordered eating," reflects broader societal, political, and economic shifts and struggles.

Chapter 10, "Cultural and Technological Transformations," integrates the central themes of this book, bringing together insights from sociology, cultural studies, and other disciplines. While the contemporary body is often viewed as a flexible project for individuals to shape, it remains largely influenced by external forces within the political economy. Examples are given of this in medicine, culture, fashion, sports, fitness and entertainment, and biotechnological and genetic industries, and their implications for the construction of disordered eating are discussed. The illusion of dietary freedom is discussed, emphasizing the costs for those living and working in the countries where these goods are produced. Disparities in food quality between high- and low-income neighborhoods create a paradox where malnutrition and obesity coexist, even within the same communities. The chapter goes on to explain how the reach of diagnostic culture can give the impression that psychiatry has been democratized, but in practice it remains a largely uncontested system of power. With state sponsorship, psychiatry has gained cultural legitimacy, institutional authority, and political influence, providing governments with ethical justification and practical tools to manage their most challenging citizens. While involuntary treatments, such as tube feeding, may be deemed necessary to save lives, these measures can result in a loss of autonomy, erosion of trust, and subsequent stigma and social isolation. The chapter then shifts its focus to the ongoing crisis in mental health services, pointing out how ethnic and intersectional disparities, intergenerational racial trauma, and microaggressions have undermined trust in psychiatry. Finally, advancements in biomedicine, genetic engineering, and other advanced technologies are considered. These and other technological innovations are prompting us to question the nature of our own bodies and minds in ways previously only imagined in fiction.

References

Albert, M. (1993). *Capitalism vs. capitalism: How America's obsession with individual achievement and short-term profit has led it to the brink of collapse.* Basic Books.

American Psychiatric Association (APA). (2013). *Diagnostic and statistical manual of mental disorders: DSM-V* (5th ed.). American Psychiatric Association Publishing.

American Psychiatric Association Publishing. (2022, August 6). *DSM5-TR-diagnostic statistical manual of mental disorders.* https://www.appi.org/products/dsm

Anekwe, C. (2020, July 8). *Managing weight gain from psychiatric medications.* Harvard Health Publishing. Retrieved August 22, 2024, from https://www.health.harvard.edu/blog/managing-weight-gain-from-psychiatric-medications-202207182781

Angell, M. (2009). Drug companies & doctors: A story of corruption. *The New York Review of Books, 56*(1), 8–12.

Ayton, A., Viljoen, D., Ryan, S., Ibrahim, A., & Ford, D. (2022). Risk, demand, capacity and outcomes in adult specialist eating disorder services in South-East of England before and since COVID-19. *BJPsych Bulletin, 46*(2), 89–95.

BEAT. (2023, March 4). *Semaglutide weight loss medication "very dangerous" for those with eating disorders.* Retrieved August 22, 2024, from https://www.beateatingdisorders.org.uk/news/semaglutide-weight-loss-medication-very-dangerous-for-those-with-eating-disorders/

BEAT. (2024a, April 8). *How many people have an eating disorder in the UK?* Retrieved August 22, 2024, from https://www.beateatingdisorders.org.uk/get-information-and-support/about-eating-disorders/how-many-people-eating-disorder-uk/

BEAT. (2024b, April 8). *Statistics for journalists. How many people in the UK have an eating disorder?* Retrieved August 22, 2024, from https://www.beateatingdisorders.org.uk/media-centre/eating-disorder-statistics/

Becker, H. (1963). *Outsiders: Studies in the psychology of deviance.* Free Press.

Berger, P. L., & Luckmann, T. (1967). *The social construction of reality: A treatise on the sociology of knowledge.* Penguin.

Boltanski, L., & Chiapello, E. (2005). The new spirit of capitalism. *International Journal of Politics, Culture, and Society, 18*, 161–188.

Bredström, A. (2019). Culture and context in mental health diagnosing: Scrutinizing the DSM-V revision. *Journal of Medical Humanities, 40*(3), 347–363.

Brinkmann, S. (2016). *Diagnostic cultures: A cultural approach to the pathologization of modern life.* Routledge.

Bruch, H. (1978). *The golden cage: The enigma of anorexia nervosa.* Harvard University Press.

Bruch, H. (1982). Anorexia nervosa: Therapy and theory. *American Journal of Psychiatry*, 139, 1531.

Burr, V. (2015). *Social constructionism.* Routledge.

Claudino, A. M., Pike, K. M., Hay, P., Keeley, J. W., Evans, S. C., Rebello, T. J., et al. (2019). The classification of feeding and eating disorders in the ICD-11 results of a field study comparing proposed ICD-11 guidelines with existing ICD-10 guidelines. *BMC Medicine, 17*, 1–17.

Cohen, B. M. Z. (2016). *Psychiatric hegemony: A Marxist theory on mental illness.* Palgrave Macmillan.

Cook, B., Mascolo, M., Bass, G., Duffy, M. E., Zehring, B., & Beasley, T. (2022). Has COVID-19 complicated eating disorder treatment? An examination of comorbidities and treatment response before and during the COVID-19 pandemic. *The Primary Care Companion for CNS Disorders, 24*(1), 39313.

Cosgrove, L., & Wheeler, E. E. (2013). Industry's colonization of psychiatry: Ethical and practical implications of financial conflicts of interest in the DSM-V. *Feminism & Psychology, 23*(1), 93–106.

Coveney, J. (2006). *Food, morals and meaning: The pleasure and anxiety of eating.* Routledge.

Das, S., & Ungoed-Thomas, J. (2023, March 12). *Orchestrated PR campaign: How skinny jab drug firm sought to shape obesity.* The Guardian. Retrieved August 22, 2024, from https://www.theguardian.com/society/2023/mar/12/orchestrated-pr-campaign-how-skinny-jab-drug-firm-sought-to-shape-obesity-debate

Duran, T. L., Cashion, L. B., Gerber, T. A., & Mendez-Ybanez, G. J. (2000). Social constructionism and eating disorders: Relinquishing labels and embracing personal stories. *Journal of Systemic Therapies, 19*(2), 23–42.

Eriksson, G., & Machin, D. (2020). Discourses of 'Good Food': The commercialization of healthy and ethical eating. *Discourse, Context & Media, 33*, 100365.

Erskine, H. E., Whiteford, H. A., & Pike, K. M. (2016). The global burden of eating disorders. *Current Opinion in Psychiatry, 29*(6), 346–353.

Fixsen, A. (in press). *The social construction of mental illness* (Wiley-Blackwell encyclopedia of health, illness, behavior, and society) (2nd ed.).

Fixsen, A., Barrett, D. S., & Shimonovich, M. (2022). Supporting vulnerable populations during the pandemic: Stakeholders' experiences and perceptions of social prescribing in Scotland during Covid 19. *Qualitative Health Research, 32*(4), 670–682.

Food and Agriculture Organization of the United Nations (FAO). (2024, August 21). *The state of food security and nutrition in the world,* 2024. Retrieved August 22, 2024, from https://openknowledge.fao.org/items/4bdbfa10-dae9-465e-b197-b7023f44aca5

Foucault, M. (1978). *The history of sexuality. Volume 1, The will to knowledge.* Penguin Books.

Foucault, M. (1982). The subject and power. *Critical Inquiry, 8*(4), 777.

Foucault, M. (1985). *The history of sexuality. Volume 2, The use of pleasure.* Random House.

Foucault, M. (2001). *Interviews with Michel Foucault: Power, The essential works of Foucault, 1954–1984* (Vol. 3).

Foucault, M., Davidson, A. I., & Burchell, G. (2008). *The birth of biopolitics: Lectures at the Collège de France, 1978–1979.* Springer.

Foucault, M., Murphy, J., & Khalfa, J. (2013). *History of madness.* Routledge.

Frances, A. (2013). Saving normal: An insider's revolt against out-of-control psychiatric diagnosis DSM-V, big pharma and the medicalization of ordinary life. *Psychotherapy in Australia, 19*(3), 14–18.

Freeborn, A. (2022). *Review of: Horwitz, Allan V.: DSM: A History of Psychiatry's Bible.* Johns Hopkins University Press 2021. *The FASEB Journal,* 1–4.

Galmiche, M., Déchelotte, P., Lambert, G., & Tavolacci, M. P. (2019). Prevalence of eating disorders over the 2000–2018 period: A systematic literature review. *The American Journal of Clinical Nutrition, 109*(5), 1402–1413.

Gergen, K. J. (1992). The social constructionist movement in modern psychology. In R. B. Miller (Ed.), *The restoration of dialogue: Readings in the philosophy of clinical psychology* (pp. 556–569). American Psychological Association.

GOV.UK. (2024, April 8). *Accessing Wegovy for weight loss.* Department of Health and Social Care Centre. Retrieved August 22, 2024, from https://healthmedia.blog.gov.uk/2023/09/04/accessing-wegovy-for-weight-loss-everything-you-need-to-know/

Graham, L., Friedman, J., & Vega, X. (2022). Forbidding your cake and eating it too: Health performance strategies in U.S. middle class families. *Social Theory of Health, 20,* 237–259.

Hacking, I. (1999). *The social construction of what?* Harvard University Press.

Hay, P., Mitchison, D., Collado, A. E. L., González-Chica, D. A., Stocks, N., & Touyz, S. (2017). Burden and health-related quality of life of eating disorders, including Avoidant/Restrictive Food Intake Disorder (ARFID), in the Australian population. *Journal of Eating Disorders, 5,* 1–10.

Hazell, C. M., Fixsen, A., & Berry, C. (2022). Is it time to change the approach of mental health stigma campaigns? An experimental investigation of the effect of campaign wording on stigma and help-seeking intentions. *PLoS ONE, 17*(8), e0273254.

Hepworth, J. (1999). *The social construction of Anorexia Nervosa.* Sage.

Horwitz, A. (2012). Social constructions of mental illness. In *Oxford Handbook of Philosophy of the Social Sciences* (pp. 1–23).

Horwitz, A. V. (2021). *DSM. A history of psychiatry's bible.* JHU Press.

Horwitz, A. V., & Grob, G. N. (2016). The troubled history of psychiatry's quest for specificity. *Journal of Health Politics, Policy and Law, 41*(4), 521–539.

Huryk, K. M., Drury, C. R., & Loeb, K. L. (2021). Diseases of affluence? A systematic review of the literature on socioeconomic diversity in eating disorders. *Eating Behaviors, 43*, 101548.

Jackson, C., & Rizq, R. (2019). *The industrialisation of care: Counselling, psychotherapy and the impact of IAPT*. PCCS Books.

Jayanetti, C. (2021, February 20). *NHS sees surge in referrals for eating disorders among under-18s during Covid.* The Guardian. Retrieved August 22, 2024, from https://www.theguardian.com/society/2021/feb/20/covid-eating-disorder-referrals-rise-under-18s

Kessler, R. C., Berglund, P. A., Chiu, W. T., Deitz, A. C., Hudson, J. I., Shahly, V., et al. (2013). The prevalence and correlates of binge eating disorder in the World Health Organization World Mental Health Surveys. *Biological Psychiatry, 73*(9), 904–914.

Kirkbride, J. B., Anglin, D. M., Colman, I., Dykxhoorn, J., Jones, P. B., Patalay, P., Pitman, A., Soneson, E., Steare, T., Wright, T., & Griffiths, S. L. (2024). The social determinants of mental health and disorder: Evidence, prevention and recommendations. *World Psychiatry, 23*(1).

Kutchins, H., & Kirk, S. A. (2003). *Making us crazy*. Simon and Schuster.

Lyons, D., & O'Malley, A. (2002). The labelling of dissent–politics and psychiatry behind the Great Wall. *Psychiatric Bulletin, 26*(12), 443–444.

Marsh, S. (2023, September 12). *Some English patients with eating disorders sent to Scotland for treatment*. The Guardian. Retrieved August 22, 2024, from https://www.theguardian.com/society/2023/sep/12/england-patients-with-eating-disorders-sent-hundreds-of-miles-for-treatment

Marx, G. T. (2019). *Windows into the soul: Surveillance and society in an age of high technology*. University of Chicago Press.

McCuen-Wurst, C., Ruggieri, M., & Allison, K. C. (2018). Disordered eating and obesity: Associations between binge-eating disorder night-eating syndrome, and weight-related comorbidities. *Annals of the New York Academy of Sciences, 1411*(1), 96–105.

Melamed, O. C., Selby, P., & Taylor, V. H. (2022). Mental health and obesity during the COVID-19 pandemic. *Current Obesity Reports, 11*(1), 23–31.

Mezzich, J. E. (2002). *Culture and psychiatric diagnosis: A DSM-IV® perspective*. American Psychiatric Pub.

Milliren, C. E., Richmond, T. K., & Hudgins, J. D. (2023). Emergency department visits and hospitalizations for eating disorders during the COVID-19 pandemic. *Pediatrics, 151*(1), e2022058198.

National Eating Disorders Association (NEDA). (2024). *Men and eating disorders.* Retrieved August 22, 2024, from https://www.nationaleatingdisorders.org/men-eating-disorders.

Pikäinen, P. (2015). *Madness: A history*. Routledge.

Puhl, R., & Suh, Y. (2015). Stigma and eating and weight disorders. *Current Psychiatry Reports, 17*(10).

Ransom, J. S. (1997). *Foucault's discipline. The politics of subjectivity.* Duke University Press.

Rose, N. (1990). *Governing the soul: The shaping of the private self.* Taylor & Frances/Routledge.

Rose, N. (1998). *Inventing ourselves: Psychology, power, and personhood.* Cambridge University Press.

Rose, N. (2019). Forward. In C. Jackson & R. Rizq (Eds.), *The industrialisation of care: Counselling, psychotherapy and the impact of IAPT* (pp. v–x). PCCS Books.

Ross Arguedas, A. A. (2020). "Can naughty be healthy?": Healthism and its discontents in news coverage of orthorexia nervosa. *Social Science & Medicine, 246*, 112784.

Royal College of Psychiatrists. (2022, May 18). *Hospital admissions for eating disorders increased by 84% in the last five years.* Retrieved August 22, 2024, from https://www.rcpsych.ac.uk/news-and-features/latest-news/detail/2022/05/18/hospital-admissions-for-eating-disorders-increased-by-84-in-the-last-five-years

Santomauro, D. F., Melen, S., Mitchison, D., Vos, T., Whiteford, H., & Ferrari, A. J. (2021). The hidden burden of eating disorders: An extension of estimates from the Global Burden of Disease Study 2019. *The Lancet Psychiatry, 8*(4), 320–328.

Schaumberg, K., Welch, E., Breithaupt, L., Hübel, C., Baker, J. H., Munn-Chernoff, M. A., et al. (2017). The science behind the academy for eating disorders' nine truths about eating disorders. *European Eating Disorders Review, 25*(6), 432–450.

Scull, A. (2022). *Desperate remedies: Psychiatry and the mysteries of mental illness*. Penguin.

Shanouda, F., & Orsini, M. (2023, August 20). *Ozempic. The miracle drug and the harmful idea of a future without fat.* The Conversation. Retrieved August

22, 2024, from https://theconversation.com/ozempic-the-miracle-drug-and-the-harmful-idea-of-a-future-without-fat-211661

Sonneville, K. R., & Lipson, S. K. (2018). Disparities in eating disorder diagnosis and treatment according to weight status, race/ethnicity, socioeconomic background, and sex among college students. *International Journal of Eating Disorders, 51*(6), 518–526.

Steel, C. (2021). *How food can save the world.* issuu. Retrieved August 22, 2024, from https://issuu.com/landscape-institute/docs/12421_landscape_issue_1-2021_v8a_issuu/s/11604694.

Sweet, P. L., & Decoteau, C. L. (2018). Contesting normal: The DSM-V and psychiatric subjectivation. *BioSocieties, 13*, 103–122.

Taub, D. E., & McLorg, P. A. (2011). Eating disorders as deviance. In C. R. Bryant (Ed.), *The Routledge handbook deviant behaviour*. Routledge.

The Economist. (2023, November 23). *The obesity pay gap is worse than previously thought.* Retrieved August 22, 2024, from https://www.economist.com/finance-and-economics/2023/11/23/the-obesity-pay-gap-is-worse-than-previously-thought

The Sentencing Project. (2022). *Incarcerated women and young girls.* Retrieved August 22, 2024, from https://www.sentencingproject.org/publications/incarcerated-women-and-girls

Treatment Advocacy Center. (2016). *Serious Mental Illness (SMI) prevalence in jails and prisons.* Office of Research and Public Affairs.

van Eeden, A. E., van Hoeken, D., & Hoek, H. W. (2021). Incidence, prevalence and mortality of anorexia nervosa and bulimia nervosa. *Current Opinion in Psychiatry, 34*(6), 515.

van Voren, R. (2016). Ending political abuse of psychiatry: Where we are at and what needs to be done. *BJPsych bulletin, 40*(1), 30–33.

Weinberg, D. (2009). Social constructionism. *The new Blackwell companion to social theory*, 281–299.

Welch, S., Kalssen, C., Borsova, O., & Clotheir, H. (2013). The DSM- 5 controversies: How should psychologists respond? *Canadian Psychology, 54*(3), 166–175.

Whitaker, R., & Cosgrove, L. (2015). *Psychiatry under the influence: Institutional corruption, social injury, and prescriptions for reform.* Palgrave Macmillan.

Williams, C. (2014, November 20). *Obesity rivals smoking and war among self-inflicted health risk.* Los Angeles Times. Retrieved August 22, 2024, from https://www.latimes.com/world/europe/la-fg-global-obesitycosts-20141120-story.html

Wilson, M. (1993). DSM-III and the transformation of American psychiatry: A history. *American Journal of Psychiatry, 150*, 399–399.

World Health Organization. (2019). *International Classification of Diseases 10th revision: Ch. 5 Mental and behavioural disorders.* Retrieved August 22, 2024, from https://icd.who.int/browse10/2019/en#/F50.0

World Health Organization. (2022, June 16). *World mental health report: Transforming mental health for all.* Retrieved August 22, 2024, from https://www.who.int/publications/i/item/9789240049338

World Health Organization. (2024a, March 1). *Obesity and overweight.* Retrieved August 22, 2024, from https://www.who.int/news-room/fact-sheets/detail/obesity-and-overweight

World Health Organization. (2024b, August 5). *Social determinants of health.* Retrieved August 22, 2024, from https://www.who.int/health-topics/social-determinants-of-health#tab=tab_1

Children's Commissioner. (2024). Major conditions strategy consultation response. Retrieved August 24, 2024, from https://assets.childrenscommissioner.gov.uk/wpuploads/2023/07/Major-Conditions-Strategy-response_final.pdf

Royal College of Psychiatrists. (2024). It's time to tackle the trap of inequality and mental illness. Retrieved August24, from https://www.rcpsych.ac.uk/news-and-features/latest-news/detail/2024/01/25/it-s-time-to-tackle-the-trap-ofinequality-and-mental-illness

Young, G. (2013). Breaking bad: DSM-5 description, criticisms, and recommendations. *Psychological Injury and Law, 6*, 345–348.

2

Bodies Beyond Conformity

The terrain of the human body is changing. Ancient Greeks and those in the Enlightenment era investigated the inner workings of the body, its health, and ailments, although this interest did not extend to viewing bodies as sites of medical power or gender oppression. The body has also long been a prominent theme in the arts,[1] natural sciences, and anthropology.[2] In sociology, it took what Turner (1992) calls the turn toward a "somatic society" for the body to be viewed as a critical subject of modernity and capitalism. In contemporary sociological discourse, the body now serves as a fundamental site of analysis, and as reflecting broader social, cultural, and political dynamics. Feminists have been critical of the way that women are encouraged to "wage war" on their bodies, through the machinations of the cosmetic, fashion, food, diet, anti-aging, surgical, wellness, pharmaceutical, and fitness industries (Orbach, 2019). Critics of colonialism have drawn attention to bodies upon which the legacies of oppression and imperialism have inflicted profound and

[1] In the arts, for example, the dominant political concerns and anxieties of society have often been portrayed through disrupted, disjointed, and disturbed images of the body (as in the "ravages" of famine, plague, or death) (Turner, 2012).

[2] Anthropologist Marcel Mauss' essay on "body techniques" is seen as an important contribution to the study of bodies in society.

A. Fixsen, *The Construction of Eating Disorders*, The Politics of Mental Health and Illness, https://doi.org/10.1007/978-3-031-70318-8_2

enduring wounds and violence (Fanon, 1952), and those that continue to be persecuted because of their color, gender, or appearance. Recent developments—such as body positivity, #MeToo movement, artificial intelligence, gender realignment, epigenetics, and the selfie culture—all demand new ways of thinking about and studying bodies (Orbach, 2019).

This chapter proposes a sociology of bodies beyond conformity and more specifically those to whom the idiom of an "eating disorder" is attached. The aim of such a study is to illuminate how, across different historical and geographical contexts, certain bodies are perceived as divergent in their atypical and "unhealthy" eating practices and behaviors, and the ways in which society endeavors to regulate these rebellious, nonnormative bodies. Ultimately, the study of the disordered or transgressive body reveals such bodies as existing, not just at the margins but as the locus of social and political critique concerning the construction, regulation, and control of difference and nonconformity. Given the breadth of this subject, the following is a summary of significant sociological and feminist concepts related to bodies that merit deeper exploration. Adopting Foucault's genealogical approach (1973, 1977, 1978), the inquiry begins by considering some important historical, phenomenological, and feminist interpretations of the body, with the latter illustrated up by a recent empirical study of models in the fashion industry. The chapter concludes with a brief consideration of the impacts of artificial intelligence (AI) and other forms of surveillance technologies on the construction and perception of bodies, both by corporate entities and the broader public.

Materialism and Embodiment

In the twenty-first century, the human body occupies a pivotal role in the utilization of disease and disorder as productive elements in the emerging economy (Turner, 2012). It is the central subject of many modern industries including biotechnologies, pharmaceuticals, media, and mental and physical therapies. Utilizing a particular concept of the body to support a broader institutional or philosophical structure goes far back in history. Ancient Eastern metaphysical paradigms for the human body include the chakras in Hinduism and the Chinese philosophical theory of meridians. Many of an alternative persuasion still hold by these more esoteric interpretations of the workings of the human body. In western cultures, professional tensions between metaphysical and emerging scientific theories about the body became pronounced during the Western Renaissance when scientists were captivated by the intricacies of bodily mechanisms. Rene Descartes (1596–1650) is often referenced for likening the body to a composition of mechanical components, a viewpoint that influenced western science's establishment of the idea of mutual exclusivity between the mind and body, as well as the body and soul. This conceptualization has persisted and led to criticisms of western medicine for adhering to "Cartesian dualism" (Iwakuma, 2006). Nevertheless, others have felt compelled to reconsider bodies in less mechanistic and more philosophical and even metaphysical terms.

An early example was Immanuel Kant (1724–1804), who saw the body as necessary for the recollection and connection of representations outside of the mind, although he regarded these as of a different and inferior substance to the soul (Carpenter, 1998). Mathematician and philosopher Edmund Husserl (1859–1939) later proposed a distinct method for depicting human existence in the world called "transcendental phenomenology," which turned directly to the evidence derived from lived experiences (Husserl, 1989). Martin Heidegger (1879–1976), a former student of Husserl, developed his own phenomenological perspective, an "ontology of being," grounded in the belief that human life is not solely, or primarily, rooted in conscious thought. He introduced the term "Dasein," or "being in-the-world," to describe a person's intimate engagement with everyday activities within their surroundings (Overgaard, 2004). It should be noted that Heidegger used his concepts to promote Nazi ideology and discredit Jewish academics including Husserl (Farías, 1987), indicating how susceptible philosophical ideas about bodies are to both economic and political manipulation.

Another way of observing and analyzing the relationship between the human body and its physical and social surroundings has been through the lens of embodiment. Embodiment has proved a difficult concept to define but is often characterized as a non-conceptual, somatic form of knowledge distinct from rationalism and rigid facts (Longo et al., 2008).

The term "embodiment" is largely attributed to twentieth-century phenomenologist philosopher Maurice Merleau-Ponty (1908–1961), who emphasized the pivotal role that perception plays in human experience of the world. Drawing from the ideas of phenomenology and Existentialism,[3] Merleau-Ponty (1945/2013) argued that neither rationalism nor empiricism could fully elucidate phenomena such as why a woman might exhibit physical symptoms of a false pregnancy when strongly desiring or believing in conception (Merleau-Ponty, cited in Iwakuma, 2006, p. 77). Embodiment theory claims to enable researchers to anchor enquiry into the body by shifting the vantage point from an externally driven orientation to the subjective experience of the "body-subject" that is experientially aware and connected to feelings and sensations of the corporeal body (Merleau-Ponty, 1945/2013).

The notion of embodiment has continued to captivate contemporary audiences seeking less mechanistic explanations for the experiences of being in a body. In particular, the experience of embodiment is frequently emphasized in studies related to illness and its treatment. Leder (1990) made a distinction between the "incorporation of the body"—representing the seamless operation of the body as a mostly unnoticed state of physical existence—and the "dys-appearing body," where bodily parts and sensations attract a person's attention during moments of dysfunction, pain, and discomfort. The "dys-appearing body" is the one that individuals are most aware of, often in an unpleasant manner. Interestingly, the notion of the smoothly functioning body finds widespread application in Eastern and alternative medicine, suggesting an unobstructed flow of energy within the body. Embodiment, when used as a tool, implies for the therapist a focus beyond the biology of disease, with attention to personhood and "the broader landscape that underlies human suffering" (Mount, 2003, p. 42). For example, due to their closer relations to patients and families, nurses cultivate "embodied knowledge" and "relational knowledge," which more distant figures such as consultants lack. In contrast, too much emphasis on technological progress and

[3] Existentialism is a term used by philosophers who consider the nature of human existence as a key philosophical problem and share the view that this problem is best addressed through ontology. It was particularly popular in the nineteenth and twentieth centuries (Guignon, 2024).

target setting over human contact threatens the quality of care and diminishes human values such as "empathic attunement" (Wright & Brajtman, 2009, 2011). Technology turns the body to object and away from subject.

Nancy Krieger (2005) outlines three main points underlying embodiment: bodies cannot be studied when divorced from the conditions of our existence; bodies tell stories which do not always align with people's stated accounts; and the body conveys stories that people may be unable or unwilling to reveal to others. These three aspects suggest that "body-knowledge" is externalized, readable by those trained to detect it, and open to being acted upon by others, as well as by the self. A therapist, for instance, will not only physically examine and question the patient but scrutinize their demeanor and gestures when making their assessments, often giving more weight to these observations than their verbal responses. Following this line, eating disorders can be viewed as "embodied acts" used to cope with internal and external demands perceived as overwhelming, which need to be treated accordingly (Pellegrini et al., 2021). Many studies have linked the development of disordered eating behaviors, in terms of their prevalence, presentations, and severity, with physical and sexual trauma and/or physical neglect at an early age, noting its subsequent effects on attachment, emotional regulation, and identity development (Chen et al., 2010; Pellegrin, et al., 2021; Vanderlinden & Palmisano, 2018). One theory is that violation of the body may lead the person (usually depicted as a woman) to seek to reclaim a sense of self or to release herself from her body or to experience herself as disembodied (Lester, 1997).

It is therefore unfortunate that the objectification of the female body on the part of clinicians and researchers may mirror the pathological legacy of abuse, with lack of empathy and insensitive treatment potentially resulting in further damage rather than to healing of body and mind (Malecki et al., 2018). This effect was borne out in one study of survivors' accounts of their medical treatment for an ED following childhood trauma, which mirrored the patient's own experiences of disordered eating, rather than acting as a vehicle for expressing and coping with unspeakable trauma (Gur, 2018). For victims of sexual abuse, disordered eating may be enacted as a form of self-harming, often coexisting with other harms like cutting and substance misuse. In Hodge and Baker's interview study (2021), fasting and purging offered a perception of cleanliness and renewal which was attractive to participants who experienced overwhelming shame, enabling them to transfer their emotional pain to a place where it became visible and tangible. The authors conclude that it is crucial that understandings and treatment of EDs move beyond the abstract model of psychiatric illness and pathology, and account for the material and corporal components of disordered eating.

Despite their popularity to contemporary audiences, medicalized concepts of embodiment can be problematic from the constructivist perspective, in that they rest on assumptions concerning the need for experts to interpret the sufferings of others through a specific therapeutic model and its language. Some have argued that our reliance on therapy has changed the way we view, not just our troubled bodies but our ways out of the suffering. The "therapy culture" has resulted in a radical redefinition of selfhood, wherein personal well-being is portrayed as constantly at risk of being harmed or damaged (Furedi, 2004). Cultivation of "true" embodiment becomes a never finished project, which requires an expensive mixture of professionally administered treatments and purchased self-care practices. This individualistic approach to treatment supports an elitist, largely privatized health model resting on one's ability to pay. For Eckermann (2009), the term embodiment itself creates divisions between people whose bodies are deemed to be "ideal" and those considered wanting or flawed. In a society founded on competition, those more able to access the resources required to participate in embodiment exercises and activities also gain prestige and social approval for doing so. Embodiment theories face other challenges when applied to realms of human exploitation and oppression. When considering the buying and selling of body parts, Lesley Sharp (2000) contends that the commodification of bodies in biomedicine, reproductive technologies, organ transplants, cosmetic and transsexual surgeries expose the limitations of embodiment theory, as these processes prioritize the objectification of the body over the subjective experience of a person's intact and integral body. In the twenty-first century, we can add AI chemistry and synthetic biology to this list (Orbach, 2019). This suggests that different approaches to the study of embodiment and dis-embodiment are required, which account for diverse and novel modes of human transformation.

A further critique of embodiment as a theory is that it neglects the influence of social and political processes on its formation. In this respect, Pierre Bourdieu's (1984) work on habitus and lifestyle played a major role in placing the work on Merleau-Ponty and sociologist-anthropologist Marcel Mauss (1872–1950) on "techniques of the body" firmly in a socioeconomic context. According to Mauss (1979), techniques of the body encompass a range of bodily behaviors, practices, and dispositions acquired by individuals as part of their enculturation as fully fledged members of society. The concept of habitus indicates that although these techniques may seem natural, they ultimately result from social rather than individual processes, meaning that they are linked with such things as class, income, and education. More recently, the concept of embodiment has been used to draw attention to political and social inequality issues linked with western imperialism. Approaching embodiment from a post-colonialist perspective, Shaw (2006) writes about the "embodiment of disobedience," focusing on what she calls fat, black, women's unruly political bodies. Shaw argues that western society has acquired the ideological erasure of both blackness and fatness to attain western acceptability. She cites the examples of black female icons such as Aretha Franklin whose magnetism and sexual energy on stage defiantly transgressed the white western body norms of thinness. Nevertheless, as Coffey (2021) points out, even in the wake of the body positivity movement, social media and diet culture continue to exert a strong influence on the way that young girls think about food and eating and their bodies.

A final ontological concern arising from the idea of experiencing "embodiment" is its implication of a "self" distinct from anything shaped through social discourse—an idea explicitly rejected by most constructionists, including Foucault (Foucault, 1982).[4] While these arguments may seem a matter of philosophy or religion, the concept of a self with an identity which needs to be tended and cultivated is integral to capitalist profit-making, which requires the raising of consumer expectations and desires. Whatever one's views concerning the utility of the term embodiment, as a concept it clearly has implications for the ways in

[4] Foucault (1997) regarded the self as a social act, and something to be created and invented, as in "technologies of the self."

which those with eating disorders are perceived and treated in contemporary settings.

The Sociological Body

Sociologists have always concerned themselves with people's movements and positionalities within a society. While Emile Durkheim (1858–1917) never fully engaged in a sociology of the body, he drew attention to the diminishing quality of life in urban capitalist society, which necessarily impacted on people's bodies as well as their minds (Durkheim, 1897, 1912). Although most of his writings were of a more strictly political nature, philosopher Karl Marx (1818–1883) expressed concern about the condition of bodies under capitalism, asserting that a person's economic class influenced their bodily experiences. In terms of bodies and governmentality, Foucault's work on "docile bodies" explains how the contemporary body is now predominantly shaped, not through brutal punitive regimes but through an ideological process, by which subjects actively seek to pacify their own bodies. According to Foucault (1978), authority over bodies now takes place largely through biopower, a force intimately tied in with population regulation, economic power, knowledge production, and "*alèthurgy*," that are the various truth manifestations recognized and validated in society, which serve the authorities that legitimize them (1978, p. 20). Biopower is, as Foucault states bluntly, "the power to let live or let die" (Foucault, 2003, p. 240). It is enacted through innumerable practices that may be assumed to fall outside the scope of power.[5] Certain modes of operation over bodies *en masse* (e.g., population censuses, medical and

[5] In *Society Must be Defended*, Foucault (2003) explains the link between discipline and biopower in this way: "Discipline tries to rule a multiplicity of men, to the extent that their multiplicity can, and must be dissolved into individual bodies that can be kept under surveillance, trained, used, and needs to be punished. And that new technology that is being established is addressed to a multiplicity of men, not to the extent that they are nothing more than individual bodies, but to the extent that they form, on the contrary, a global mass that is affected by overall processes, characteristic of birth, death, production, illness, and so on. After a first seizure of power over the body in an individualistic mode, we have a second seizure of power that is not individualising … What does this new technology of power, this biopolitics, this biopower, that is beginning to establish itself involve? … a set of processes, such as the ratio of births and deaths, the rate of reproduction, opportunity of a population, and so on" (pp. 242–243).

legal records) are not concerned with directly exerting power over individuals but in keeping a statistical watch over sectors of the population—examples being the number of people under 16 who have been diagnosed with a mental health disorder or an eating disorder. Since Foucault's lifetime, new techniques and technologies have been brought in to record and maintain control over populations, many of which align with the neoliberal goals of bolstering and creating markets (Fixsen et al., 2017).

One of the most popular ways of thinking about the social body in contemporary sociology is to view it as an ongoing, individualized project. Anthony Giddens, a key theorist in this area, writes of how in late modernity[6] the body has become a reflexive project to be worked on by everyone, resulting in a reconfiguration of identity around the body. People now use their bodies to consciously construct an image of what they want to present to others through a process Giddens (1991) calls "reflexive mobilization." Since modernity tends to be self-referring rather than looking to tradition, its trajectory is one of reflexivity on the self, through observation of bodies and body awareness. Here Giddens distinguishes between the kind of body awareness associated with Eastern spiritual practices aimed at dissolution of ego, and awareness predicated on the differentiation of self. Self-reflexivity under late modernity is aimed at finding oneself through an *active* process of self-construction. Being on a diet, Giddens writes, "In the narrow meaning of the phrase is only a particular version of a much more general phenomena—the cultivation of bodily regimes as a means of reflexivity influencing the project of the self" (1991, p. 105). Anorexia and its opposite, compulsive eating, should, according to Giddens, be understood as part of the need and responsibility of the individual to attain a distinctive self-identity, though he also points out how in most pre-modern societies the thin female shape was not regarded as at all desirable (Giddens, 2009). However, Giddens finally conceives anorexia to be a striving for security in the world of plural, but ambiguous options; "the tightly controlled body is an emblem of a safe existence in an open social environment" (1991, p. 107).

[6] Modernity has been variously defined, but in simple terms means a condition of social existence which is significantly different from all past forms of existence or tradition. The age of modernity is thought by some to begin in the seventeenth century with the writings of Hobbs.

This compulsive mastery is quite different from authentic reflexive monitoring, as the anorectic person may feel herself taken over by the very regime to which she submits her body. The individual only feels worthy based on a regime of self-regulation, such that the slightest lapse becomes threatening.

Giddens' theory of the body as a self-chosen project has been subject to criticism for its neoliberal orientation. For example, Shilling and Mellor (1996) critique Giddens' analysis of bodies for privileging the reflexive mind and offering a view of the social actor as disembodied. Giddens has been accused of accepting and even celebrating the turn to the individual within a narrow collective agency, which is best kept within the limits of neoliberal accumulation (Boyle, 2013). While he points out some of the problems of "late modernity," Giddens essentially normalizes the idea of the individual as the freely chosen agent within contemporary society. He barely addresses the specificity of the relationship between the body and gender (Budgeon, 2003). Felski (1995) fiercely challenges the male-centered theories of modernity of Giddens and others, pointing out how modernity itself has been built on myths around feminine aesthetics and sexuality and arguing that any text or ideas about bodies and modernity must be re-examined through a feminist lens.

Bryan Turner presents a more politicized discussion of the body in contemporary society regarding it as more *operated on* than freely operating in the changing society. The body is not the free subjective agent suggested by Giddens; it is a product and one that is pivotal to the success of the new technological economy (Turner, 2006, 2012). Bodies in society, Turner argues, should be studied from the angle of reproduction, regulation, constraint, and representation (Turner, 2008). The human body is central to economic growth in various biotechnology industries, with developments including genetic engineering and cloning affording it a more plastic, mutable status than mere "flesh and blood." The contemporary body is subjected to intense commercial, digital and medical scrutiny (Boero & Mason, 2021; Shilling, 2012). The disordered body has long been the object of the "medical gaze" (Foucault, 1973; Hatty & Hatty, 1999), but in contemporary societies it is the consumer themselves who—spurred on by medical marketing hype—stores pharmaceuticals in their cupboards as magic bullets for every physical, psychological, and domestic issue (Fox & Ward, 2008). The push to medicalize the body involves the erasure of the patient's individual differences and personal history, replacing it with a clinical examination focused on anatomical and biological features. For individuals with eating disorders, this has led to increasing emphasis on specific diagnostic categories, BMI measurements, blood and urine tests, and potential genetic screening.

Those from the symbolic interactionist tradition have also turned their attention to the ways in which actors perform their roles under the medical gaze. Even when ill, the way we conduct our bodies is shaped by social norms and expectations around such things as compliance with medical advice on dietary and medication regimes. Goffman's systematic examination of the social codes governing our encounters with others helps to explain why individuals, even when extremely unwell, feel compelled to comply with social expectations (1961, 1967). Within in-patient settings, contacts with the outside world are limited, and the rules around bodily and verbal behavior are very rigid; hence, the patient is more likely to act out the official view of self (as in playing the part of the psychiatric patient, an "anorexic," and so on). In a study of pro-anorexia sites online and in the clinic, Lavis (2011) noted how anorexia is acted out by patients and staff very differently within in-patient settings. For the AN patient, both daily life and in-patient treatment assumes and conflates "anorexia" with bodily thinness, such that the "more-thin" body equates to being "more anorexic." Patients learn what being an anorexic means to others and how to behave as an anorexic in recovery or resisting it.

O'Connell (2020), in her autobiography on "being" and "doing" anorexia nervosa, also explains how, in treatment settings, individuals develop a diagnostically informed anorexic identity to grapple with their diagnosis and its implications for self-understanding and identity. By following anorexic "scripts" and learning a diagnostically informed anorexic identity in treatment contexts, the author O'Connell and others in her situation performed the various phases of their illness. Nursing staff in ED patient units in one of our own studies (Fixsen et al., 2023b) were conscious of this effect of institutionalization. Some expressed concerns that in-patient treatments and physical surveillance, such as force-feeding or staff standing guard outside toilets, led to an atmosphere of distrust and even competition among patients to be sicker. Clearly, there is a rationale to safeguarding practices in hospital settings. However, staff also thought that the desire to achieve the status label of anorexia nervosa was due in part to an emphasis on low BMI when screening patients for treatment. Paradoxically, the "deviant/disordered" body from the taxological and medical standpoint may equate to the "good" anorexic in the performative sense.

The Female Body

Women have long been aware of the extent to which their lives are informed by the appearance of their bodies, which in recent times has been in accordance with cultural messages and images whose content is "suffused with the dominance of gendered, racial, class, and other cultural iconography" (Bordo, 1993, p. 250). The female body is precariously positioned between idealization and romanticism and sexual and economic exploitation; hence, women have continued to find themselves at the sharp end of social judgment concerning the look, shape, and size of their bodies. Misogynistic ideologies conveniently justify women's subordinate social positions by confining them within bodies portrayed as fragile, imperfect, unruly, unreliable, and susceptible to various mental intrusions beyond conscious control (Bordo, 1994, 1996; Grosz, 1994). The inequalities in economic, social, and cultural status between men and women reproduce the conditions conducive for women to experience low self-esteem and low levels of control over individual circumstances. While division of labor within the domestic household has shifted, the instructing of women on how to achieve desirable bodily attributes through the purchase of advertised commodities remains the central theme of women's magazines and much of media specifically directed at women.

Tyler and Wilkinson (2007) consider "corporate anorexia" a metaphor for our age which captures the oppressive societal emphasis on slenderness. The woman who does not eat much is the woman beyond hunger—often portrayed exquisite, flawless, and innocent. Yet, in the slimmed down workplace, women are expected to put aside their appetites and to occupy minimum space. Eating disorders, according to this argument, result from internalizing these social and marketing pressures, leading women to experience an alienated sense of self and to engage in dieting, as they are driven into a largely ascetic form of competition with one another (Bordo, 1994; Tyler & Wilkinson, 2007). Similarly, compulsive eating and weight gain are seen as responses to social oppression and the relentless focus on women's weight (Orbach, 1978). On a more general level, the intentional framing of women as the "weaker sex" for hundreds or thousands of years continues to impact the way that women are treated in contemporary society and described in institutional discourses, such as in the "beautiful rape victim" (Brownmiller, 1975). Some stereotypes change, yet a look at the fictional and real crime literature shows how women are still portrayed as guilty victims on account of "over-sexualizing" their own bodies.

Western beauty standards are such that "not one part of a woman's body is left untouched, unaltered. No feature or extremity is spared the art, or pain, of improvement" (Dworkin, 1974, p. 112). Almost from babyhood, girls are schooled on how the desirable female body should look, through the images around them, and the representations of female forms with which they are encouraged to play. For over half a century, the ultra-slender female body has been fondled and handled in the countless reproductions of one of the world's most profitable toys, the Barbie doll. Barbie has been called a "truly global citizen" because, in addition to being the figurehead of the US company *Mattel Inc*, her body parts are manufactured from materials originating from several continents (Giddens, 2009, p. 135; Tempest, 1996).[7] In the interest of diversity and to create new market opportunities, Barbie now comes in different colors and sizes including a "curvy" Barbie (Dockterman, 2023). This family friendly stereotype was given something of a girl-power makeover in the Hollywood blockbuster, *Barbie*. The movie attracted big audiences but left the critics unsure whether to applaud its audacity or regard it as another piece of neoliberal fashion and beauty marketing (McIntosh, 2024). *Barbie* the film presents the twenty-first-century woman as an

[7] Along with other well-loved toys sold in the west, Barbie dolls are manufactured under exploitative and sometimes hazardous working conditions, with staff earning less than one dollar per hour (Chamberlain, 2016).

active agent who can choose to present herself in a seemingly objectified manner when it suits their liberated interests to do so. The movie follows in the wake of celebrities like *Beyoncé* and the *Kardashians* who have been celebrating and profiting from displaying their curvaceous bodies for decades, while also speaking out about female power, reinforcing an association between the "manufactured" body shape and increased social and economic status. The iconic feminist magazine *Ms* made no apologies for naming *Beyonce* as one of their Top 2022 Feminists, praising the pop icon for "connecting women of all genders, races, sexualities and communities through her music art" (Ms, 2023). The message is that if women want it, women should get it, regardless of what it costs in terms of the money and the effort required to create a look (this new imagining of the female body is also toned and flawless). These arguments about appearance are compounded by other demands for changes to the way that women are viewed and treated in society.

Attempts by women to take more ownership of their bodies are not new, as those who have studied the history of feminism can attest.[8] The suffragette movement of the early twentieth century was not merely about ideology; members of the movement employed their bodies in shocking and sometimes violent ways, including staging prolonged hunger strikes, to draw maximum attention to the political rights of other women (Miller, 2016). However, while traditional forms of feminism were largely politically motivated and sought to liberate their sex from the shackles of patriarchy (Greer, 1970; Farrell, 1998), a different kind of feminism emerged from the 1980s which welcomed the paradoxes and contradictions in representations of women. This so-called third wave or post-feminism recast gender equality, not as an anti-capitalist movement but as an "entrepreneurial project that can be inculcated by the self" (Gill, 2017; Gill & Orgad, 2015, p. 334). Post-feminists such as Naomi Wolf (1994) dismissed the antiquated ideas of "second wave" feminism with its victimization mentality and its failure to inspire modern women, who were looking to the mainstream media discourses for role models. Best-selling books such as *Lean in* (Sandberg, 2013) urged women who

[8] For an in-depth account of the development of feminism, including its historical phases, Nancy Fraser's book *Fortunes of Feminism* (2013) is a good source.

complain about gender inequalities to address their personal confidence issues and find their inner power, with variations of this archetype modified to fit with new guidance on equality, diversity, and inclusivity (EDI).

The ferocity of debate among feminist writers concerning representations of female bodies indicates just how complex and problematic these issues have become, especially where one group of women are claiming to be spokespersons for women across the world. These issues are no less challenging in relation to feminist accounts of disordered eating. There is no doubt that the classical feminist literature on eating disorders has greatly contributed to our understanding of the shaping of women's bodies under capitalism (Day & Keys, 2008). However, a limitation of much of the traditional feminist discourse concerning disordered eating has been its reliance on psychoanalytic theory. Those studying Freud may be tempted to depict girls and women with eating disorders as deluded and their mothers as needy (Bruch, 1978), even if they acknowledge the influence of sociocultural factors in creating this situation. Another common theory, as suggested by Orbach (1986), is that some young girls and women choose to starve their bodies as a form of protest. According to Orbach, the woman who overrides her hunger and systematically refuses to eat is effectively on hunger strike and does so (consciously or unconsciously) to draw attention to the illegitimacy of the jailer, the moral righteousness of their cause, or the necessity for action. Eckermann (1997) points out the contradictions in depicting women and girls who practice self-starvation as both defiant rebels (as in defying the dictates of the medical and health professions and the needs of their own bodies) and "super-compliant" (as in wanting to be the best at school, complying to the demands of the thin ideal). Our own empirical studies suggest that, at least from the perspective of clinicians, both features are seen as characterizing eating disorder patients, resulting in tensions and contradictory emotions within practitioners concerning the seeming willfulness and extreme vulnerability of their eating disorder patients (Fixsen et al., 2023a, b).

A further criticism of traditional feminist studies of eating disorders has concerned their ethnic and gender specificity. Until recently, virtually all qualitative studies of eating disorders featured white, westernized girls and young women, thereby limiting their relevance to a wider audience.

One of the foundational theories of feminism argues that media imagery and popular culture degrades and objectifies women; however, the promotion of idealized representations of people's bodies has never been wholly confined to those who are born as female. The expansion of eating disorder diagnoses among male and transgender populations, including in the traditionally masculinized field of weight training (Håman et al., 2017), fits awkwardly with some of the accepted feminist theories around female subjection and eating disorders. Although women have typically been the catchment audience for weight-loss programs, fitness regimes, Botox injections, lip and breast enlargements, and buttock implants, since neoliberalism appears to be more concerned with profit than with the politics of gender, people of all genders are subjected to the pressures of fashion and marketing concerning the beautifying or modifying of their bodies.

The freedom and permission given to individuals to choose their own identities can be seen as a positive turn in contemporary society. Some gender activists might say it has been *the* great achievement of the twenty-first century and a step toward greater social justice. There is no denying the lure of these arguments; however, they fail to justify the extent to which the media and its marketing strategies infiltrate people's lives. Numerous studies have linked the viewing of idealized and hyper sexualized body images with such things as body shame, negative attitudes toward the obese, and the development of disordered eating behaviors in young persons of all genders (e.g., Hargreaves & Tiggemann, 2004; Monro & Huon, 2005; Van den Berg et al., 2007). From the labeling perspective a desire to modify one's body through gender realignment may still result in a diagnosis of gender dysphoria in DSM-V (APA, 2013)—renamed as gender incongruence in ICD-11 (World Health Organisation, 2023), but still carrying the stigma of a psychiatric disorder. The everyday body ideal is also markedly shifting from "wafer-thin" toward a stronger, muscular body type, not only creating new marketing opportunities for promoting diets and food supplements but also opening the door to more people being diagnosed with muscle dysmorphia. Judging by the different ways that idealized body shapes change, and the role played by diet in this process, the future diagnostic categories of eating disorders may look very different from those of today.

The Selling of Skinny: Qualitative Study

Although body positivity and third- and fourth-wave ("cyber") feminists have challenged the idea of an idealized body, the slender look has never really fallen out of fashion. Post-feminism does not appear to have greatly eased societal pressures on women's bodies, especially in professions such as modeling, where slimness is prized. The industry's fixation on youthful, slim figures has long raised concerns about its role in promoting eating disorders. After decades of superficial or non-existent interest in the well-being of young female subjects in fashion and media, the collective outcry from feminists and model activists has prompted some action. In 2011, amidst growing concerns about the surge in eating disorders, the UK government engaged in discussions with magazine editors, women, and feminist Susie Orbach to establish a code of practice discouraging the use of size 0 models in fashion and beauty images. While the value of such initiatives is widely acknowledged, the editors and journals themselves have been prone to overlooking these codes. Within months, glossy magazines were once again featuring images of models with skeletal legs (McRobbie, 2011). Since a model's physique and appearance are their "tools of the trade," the relationship between work, body, and identity in models is likely to be fraught (Holla, 2016). Hence, the perceived connection between modeling and disordered eating is an old one, with some suggesting a predisposition to EDs among those attracted to the industry (Zancu & Enea, 2017).

Methods and Findings

To understand the lived experiences of models themselves, a qualitative study was conducted on this topic, as outlined below (Fixsen et al., 2023a, b). An interpretative phenomenological approach (IPA) was chosen for the study's conceptual framework and to guide its methodology (Smith et al., 2021). Our research utilized a multi-vocal analysis approach to ensure that all voices and experiences were represented, leading us to view the work in an idiographic yet integrated manner (Montague et al., 2020). The study, which received University Research Ethics approval, included female participants who were 24 years or older and had at least 5 years of professional experience as fashion models. We excluded non-English speakers and those currently undergoing treatment for an eating disorder. The final sample comprised nine female models of diverse nationalities (Poland, the UK, Russia, Ukraine, Australia, and Denmark), consistent with the homogeneity and sample size recommendations by Smith et al. (2021).

Our data provided vivid and insightful accounts of participants' experiences in the modeling world, detailing their journey from novice to experienced model. Narratives told of how, from an early age, models' lives and bodies were "shaped" to adhere to the industry's stringent body standards, regardless of the physiological and psychological repercussions. It was universally recognized that to attract the attention of modeling agencies and, most importantly, to become a "runway model,"[9] one had to be super skinny. Most of the participants had been recruited to the industry in their early teens and soon found themselves subjected to judgments about their vital measurements, as illustrated in the following quote:

> I was being treated as a professional working model at the age of 13. And you know you're expected to be able to work, able to communicate with adults at such a young age and, you've got that whole thing of … your value being judged on how you look like and I think … as a young woman that can be very tough.

One model spoke of how she was scouted as a 14-year-old girl when she was "a stick" and the agency had not liked it when she had got "curvier" as she went through puberty; "It's not fair because you were scouted as a child," she declared. In some cases, penalties had been imposed on teenage models who had gained or failed to lose weight, such as removal of pocket money. Idioms such as "feeling like a piece of meat" and "being a hanger of clothes" were used by participants to convey their deep sense of degradation and objectification. Rules about maintaining a low body weight through dieting instilled at a formative age continued to influence

---

[9] A professional who models clothes while walking down the length of a T-shaped stage.

their self-image and eating patterns, indicating an industrial role in the construction of eating disorders.

Simultaneously, a model's body shape was expected to adapt to the specific demands of each show or season. This added to the feelings of frustration and rejection whenever the body standards shifted: "I was told I was too big at first, and then too skinny. It was a constant struggle. They just sent me home without offering any guidance, saying, 'You're too skinny, you're in; you're too big, you're out.'" While becoming a professional model might have seemed like a dream come true to new recruits, their later stories reveal a professional journey marked by a loss of personal autonomy concerning body size and appearance, coupled with minimal guidance from managers on maintaining a healthy diet. Although there were some exceptions, most agents were perceived as money focused and ruthless to the young women in their care, to the extent of stranding them in foreign places. The selection process left participants feeling reduced to a set of body statistics or worse—"feeling like a piece of meat"—sentiments that resonate with Sharp's (2000) observations concerning the objectification of body parts for commercial gain in contemporary society.

From the health perspective, our study underscores the industry's potentially negative impact on the well-being of those recruited to the modeling world at an early age and the exploitative nature of the industry.

Disordered eating may be seen as a way of life in the industry, while infantilization, sexism, and other unethical elements can become normalized in poorly regulated industries like fashion, leading to enduring consequences for the health and well-being of employees (Fixsen et al., 2023a, b. Similar and more distressing conclusions concerning the toxic side to this glamorous industry have emerged from other investigations into the international modeling world. Described as "brutal," the competition in the fashion world compels models to take extreme measures to secure casting opportunities (Lewak & Ridley, 2017; Rodgers et al., 2021). Beyond the glamor of catwalks, real-life stories of models reveal the darker aspects of the industry, encompassing sexual harassment, self-starvation, drug addiction, and suicidal feelings (Clarke, 2022; Dauxerre & Peronnet, 2017; Helmore, 2017). In the US and France, legislation has been enacted to include private changing areas and medical certificates to shield models from pressures to maintain an extremely thin physique. However, recent surveys suggest these interventions have not fully achieved their intended goals (Rodgers et al., 2021). Meanwhile, the concept of "heroin chic," glamorizing low weight, stringy hair, and a pallid complexion, remains prevalent. Initially popularized in the 1990s by models like Gia Carangi and Kate Moss, the waiflike-rich-kid-look persists. Diaz (2022) notes even the "bootydelicious" Kardashians have appeared increasingly slender lately. In these media portrayals, possessing a sexy body is presented as a woman's key to success.

The Modified Body

Digital technology has allowed anyone with a little technical know-how to be able to manipulate and enhance images of their own bodies and others and to disseminate them privately or to a potentially unlimited public. While it is too early to predict the effects of AI technology on how people will come to perceive their physical selves, studies suggest that these digital representations are instrumental in the drive toward what is regarded by contemporary standards as bodily perfection (Fischer & Klazar, 2020). The exploitation of deep fake images[10] has already made considerable waves in official and unofficial circles. Beyond the everyday creation and sharing of videos and images, there are the malign and sometimes criminal activities (such as blackmailing and extortion) that digital editing allows, including the posting of deep fake AI pornography to be viewed by millions across social media, as in a recent Taylor Swift deep fake controversy (Beaumont-Thomas, 2024). However, the repercussions of viewing largely fake images of oneself and others in terms of both social engineering and eating behaviors are less clear (Ioannidis & Chamberlain, 2021). In one study investigating their effects, young female participants who watched deep fake "self-celebrity" videos reported feeling better about themselves after viewing these videos. The authors suggest that these types of technologies could play a future role in enhancing body esteem in those with poor body image (Wu et al., 2021).

[10] Extremely manipulated digital images.

Antognini and Woods (2023), on the other hand, argue that AI technology can lead to harms such as body dysmorphia and pressure to sexualize images. Policymakers and scholars are rightly concerned with deep fakery; however, the problems of deception on social media are, the authors argue, more subtle and more endemic than a few actors disseminating malicious content. These platforms are awash with fakery, but many of these images are superficial tweaking of self-presentations using filters and presenting bogus or enhanced versions of images. Whether harmful or not, the business model of today's biggest social media platforms depends on bringing users to their platforms to monetize their attention to advertisements. The popularity of *Instagram* filters set off an arms race for digital beautification. *Snapchat* has introduced video filters which aggressively alter the appearance of one's face, while *TikTok* may apply filtered images, even when the user had selected "no filter."

Another result of the constant viewing of fake bodies is a reduced social tolerance to bodily "imperfection" both online and in real life. Body shaming, where people repeatedly express unsolicited, negative opinions and comments about a target's body (Schlüter et al., 2021), has been widely linked to low self-esteem, especially where it happens in the formative years of childhood and adolescence (Gilbert & Thompson, 2014; Troop & Redshaw, 2012). Body shaming online is harder to avoid than other forms of bullying and body teasing (Day et al., 2022) (due to the ease with which messages and images can be sent to the target, day and night. Furthermore, digital technology means that it is extremely easy to manipulate images to suit the intentions of the sender. Another concern for those involved in the study of eating disorders is the apparent popularity of social media sites which use enhanced images and messages to promote disordered eating. "Pro-eating disorder" forums have been around since the advent of the Internet; however, the greater sophistication of algorithms means that within the space of a few clicks, any child or young person can be directed to this moral universe, where ideas about "good" and "bad" foods are reversed and the ultra-thin body is celebrated (Christodoulou, 2012; Tragantzopoulou et al., 2024). How these platforms operate and what they mean for users and the wider public is explored at length in Chap. 8: "Disordered Eating in the Virtual World."

The consequences for a life largely played out in virtual spaces are many. On a physical level, being constantly on a screen means that the body is no longer an active agent of production but is reduced to a mere commodity and a byproduct of production. On a surveillance level, the advent of biometrics and artificial intelligence (AI) has significantly amplified the capacity to track and monitor people's behaviors for political, economic, and medical purposes. Facial recognition is frequently highlighted as a cutting-edge surveillance tool, while biometric measurements can identify numerous aspects of bodies. Nonetheless, not all individuals are subjected to the same levels of surveillance; those categorized as belonging to an outlier group face heightened monitoring, ostensibly for public safety or for their own well-being (as in psychiatric cases). Many surveillance and predictive tools exhibit racial bias, thereby perpetuating a historic network of discrimination, power, and control (Minocher & Randall, 2020). On an everyday level, as our bodies serve more as tools of technology than independent entities, a rapid erosion of human autonomy and democratic sovereignty (Zuboff, 2023) is taking place. Yet with vast profits to be made through automation, the world's most powerful corporations are thoroughly invested in harvesting, analyzing, and selling data about people who use their products (Venkatesh, 2021). Big data harvesting now includes not just gathering information on people's online shopping and browsing preferences but extracting and selling on data on every possible aspect and dimension of their bodies that could be known or predicted. For Zuboff (2023) this is akin to robbing people of their human rights. Whether or not Elon Musk's prediction that AI will lead to a society where no one needs to work holds true, the potential impact on human bodies of further advanced technological developments must be enormous. In the meantime, most of us will continue to participate in this transformative process, willingly or reluctantly playing the part of the "entrepreneur of the biological self."

The following chapter, "Chapter 3: Anorexia Nervosa: The Making of the First Eating Disorder," takes a critical look at the processes by which the phenomenon of self-starvation came to be conceived not as a miraculous or religious matter but as a mental and moral affliction of women, to be interpreted and presided over by (predominantly male) medical "experts." The chapter begins with its history up to its inclusion in

DSM-I, then goes on to examine feminist and contemporary definitions and treatments for AN. Finally, first-hand sociological accounts of anorexia are explored, providing with unique insights into the lived experience beyond clinical description.

References

American Psychiatric Association. (2013). *Diagnostic and statistical manual of mental disorders: DSM-V* (5th ed.). American Psychiatric Association Publishing.

Antognini, A., & Woods, A. K. (2023). Shallow fakes. *Penn State Law Review, 128*, 69.

Beaumont-Thomas, B. (2024, January 24). *Taylor Swift fake pornography Sparks renewed calls for US legislation.* The Guardian. Retrieved August 22, 2024, from https://www.theguardian.com/music/2024/jan/26/taylor-swift-deepfake-pornography-sparks-renewed-calls-for-us-legislation

Boero, N., & Mason, K. (2021). In N. Boero & K. Mason (Eds.), *The Oxford handbook of the sociology of body and embodiment.* Oxford University Press.

Bordo, S. (1993). *Unbearable weight: Feminism western culture and the body.* University of California Press.

Bordo, S. (1994). Feminism, Foucault and the politics of the body. In *Reconstructing Foucault* (pp. 219–243). Brill.

Bordo, S. (1996). Hunger is ideology. In C. Luke (Ed.), *Feminisms and pedagogies of everyday life.* SUNY Press.

Bourdieu, P. (1984). *Distinction: A social critique of the judgement of taste.* Routledge.

Boyle, B. O. (2013). Reproducing the social structure: A Marxist critique of Anthony Gidden's structuration methodology. *Cambridge Journal of Economics. [Online], 37*(5), 1019–1033.

Brownmiller, S. (1975). *Against our will: Men, women, and rape.* Fawcett Books.

Bruch, H. (1978). *The golden cage: The enigma of anorexia nervosa.* Harvard University Press.

Budgeon, S. (2003). Identity as an embodied event. *Body and Society, 9*(1), 35–55.

Carpenter, A. N. (1998). Kant, the body, and knowledge. In *The Paideia archive: Twentieth world congress of philosophy* (Vol. 45, pp. 47–53).

Chamberlain, G. (2016). *The grim truth of Chinese factories, producing the Westside Christmas toys*. The Observer. Retrieved August 18, from https://www.theguardian.com/business/2016/dec/04/the-grim-truth-of-chinese-factories-producing-the-wests-christmas-toys

Chen, L. P., Murad, M. H., Paras, M. L., Colbenson, K. M., Sattler, A. L., Goranson, E. N., et al. (2010). Sexual abuse and lifetime diagnosis of psychiatric disorders: Systematic review and meta-analysis. In *Mayo Clinic proceedings* (Vol. 85, No. 7, pp. 618–629). Elsevier.

Christodoulou, M. (2012). Pro-anorexia websites pose public health challenge. *The Lancet, 379*(9811), 110.

Clarke, R. (2022*). Former Victoria's Secret model Bridget Malcolm lifts the veil on toxic modelling industry.* Grazia. Retrieved August 22, 2024, from https://graziamagazine.com/articles/bridget-malcom-toxicmodelling-industry

Coffey, J. (2021). *Everyday embodiment: Rethinking youth body image*. Palgrave Macmillan.

Dauxerre, V., & P'eronnet, V. (2017). *Size zero: My life as a disappearing model*. William Collins.

Day, K., & Keys, T. (2008). Starving in cyberspace: A discourse analysis of pro-eating-disorder websites. *Journal of Gender Studies, 17*(1), 1–15.

Day, S., Bussey, K., Trompeter, N., & Mitchison, D. (2022). The impact of teasing and bullying victimization on disordered eating and body image disturbance among adolescents: a systematic review. *Trauma, Violence, & Abuse, 23*(3), 985–1006.

Diaz, A. (2022, November 2). *Bye-bye booty: Heroin chic is back*. New York Post Lifestyle. Retrieved August 22, 2024, from https://nypost.com/2022/11/02/heroin-chic-is-back-and-curvy-bodies-big-butts-are-out/

Dockterman, E. (2023). Barbies got a New Body. *Time*. https://time.com/barbie-new-body-cover-story/

Durkheim, E. (1897) [1951]. *Suicide: A study in sociology*. The Free Press.

Durkheim, E. (1912) [2021]. *The elementary forms of the religious life*. Translated from the French by Joseph Ward Swain, MA.

Dworkin, A. (1974) *Woman-Hating*. Dutton.

Eckermann, L. (1997). Foucault, embodiment, and gendered subjectivities: The case of voluntary self-starvation. In A. Peterson & R. Bunton (Eds.), *Foucault, health, and medicine*. Routledge.

Eckermann, L. (2009). Theorising self-starvation: Beyond risk, governmentality and the normalizing gaze. In H. Malson & M. Burns (Eds.), *Critical feminist approaches to eating dis/orders* (pp. 9–21). Routledge.

Fanon, F. (1952). *Black skin, White masks*. Penguin Classics.
Farías, V. (1987). *Heidegger and Nazism*. Temple University Press.
Farrell, A. E. (1998). *Yours in sisterhood: Ms. magazine and the promise of popular feminism*. The University of North Carolina Press.
Felski, R. (1995). *The gender of modernity*. Harvard University Press.
Fischer, R., & Klazar, E. (2020). Facts, truth, and post-truth. *The International Journal of Information, Diversity, & Inclusion, 4*(3/4), 5–19.
Fixsen, A., Cranfield, S., & Ridge, D. (2017). Self-care and entrepreneurism: An ethnography of soft Skills development for Higher Education staff. *Studies in Continuing Education, 40*(2), 181–197.
Fixsen, A., Kossewska, M., & Bardey, A. (2023a). I'm skinny, I'm worth more: Fashion models' experiences of aesthetic labor and its impact on body image and eating behaviors. *Qualitative Health Research, 33*(1–2), 81–91.
Fixsen, A., Ridge, D., Ponsford, O., Holder, M., & Saran, G. (2023b). Battles over 'unruly bodies': Practitioners' interpretations of eating disorders and the utility of psychiatric labelling. *Sociology of Health & Illness, 45*(3), 560–579.
Foucault, M. (1973). *The birth of the clinic. An archaeology of medical perception*. Routledge.
Foucault, M. (1977). *Discipline & punish: The birth of the prison*. Vintage Books.
Foucault, M. (1978). *The history of sexuality. Volume 1, The will to knowledge* [Book]. Penguin Books.
Foucault, M. (1982). The subject and power. *Critical Inquiry, 8*(4), 777.
Foucault, M. (1997). *The ethics of the concern of the Self as a practice of freedom. Ethics: Subjectivity and truth* (pp. 281–302). Ed. Paul Rabinow. Trans. R. Hurley. New.
Foucault, M. (2003). *Society must be defended*. Lectures at the College de France 1975–76. Picador.
Fox, N. J., & Ward, K. J. (2008). Pharma in the bedroom … and the kitchen … The pharmaceuticalisation of daily life. *Sociology of Health & Illness. [Online], 30*(6), 856–868.
Furedi, F. (2004). *Therapy culture: Cultivating vulnerability in an uncertain age*. Routledge.
Giddens, A. (1991). *Modernity and self-identity: Self and society in the late modern age*. Polity.
Giddens, A. (2009). *Sociology* (6th ed.). Polity.
Gilbert, S. C., & Thompson, J. K. (2014). Body shame in childhood and adolescence: Relations to general psychological functioning and eating disorders. *Body shame*, 55–74.

Gill, R. (2017). The affective, cultural and psychic life of postfeminism: A post-feminist sensibility 10 years on. *European Journal of Cultural Studies, 20*(6), 606–626.
Gill, R., & Orgad, S. (2015). The confidence cult(ure*). Australian Feminist Studies, 30*(86), 324–344.
Goffman, E. (1961). *Asylums: Essays on the social situation of mental patients and other inmates*. Aldine Transaction.
Goffman, E. (1967). *Interaction ritual.* Penguin Books.
Greer, G. (1970). *The female eunuch*. MacGibbon & Kee.
Grosz, E. (1994). *Volatile bodies*. Routledge.
Guignon, C.B. (2024, August 18). Existentialism. *Routledge encyclopedia of philosophy*. https://www.rep.routledge.com/articles/thematic/existentialism.
Gur, A. (2018). *Foreign bodies: Eating disorders, childhood sexual abuse, and trauma-informed treatment*. Routledge.
Håman, L., Lindgren, E. C., & Prell, H. (2017). "If it's not Iron it's Iron f*cking biggest Ironman": Personal trainers's views on health norms, orthorexia and deviant behaviours. *International Journal of Qualitative Studies on Health and Well-Being, 12*(sup2), 1364602.
Hargreaves, D. A., & Tiggemann, M. (2004). Idealized media images and adolescent body image. Comparing boys and girls. *Body Image, 1*(4), 351–361.
Hatty, S. E., & Hatty, J. (1999). *Disordered Body, The: Epidemic disease and cultural transformation*. State University of New York Press.
Helmore, E. (2017, October 19). *Model Cameron Russell calls out the fashion industry on sexual harassment*. The Guardian. Retrieved August 22, 2024, from http://www. theguardian.com/fashion/2017/oct/19/modelcameron-russell-fashion-sexual-harassment
Hodge, L., & Baker, A. (2021). Purification, punishment, and control: Eating disorders, self-harm, and child sexual abuse. *Qualitative Health Research, 31*(11), 1963–1975.
Holla, S. (2016). Justifying aesthetic labor: How fashion models enact coherent selves. *Journal of Contemporary Ethnography, 45*(4), 474–500.
Husserl E. (1989). *Ideas pertaining to a pure phenomenology and to a phenomenological philosophy, second book. Studies in the phenomenology of constitution.* In Collected works of Edmund Husserl (Vol. 3). Trans. R. Rojcewicz, & A. Schuwer. Springer.
Ioannidis, K., & Chamberlain, S. R. (2021). Digital hazards for feeding and eating: What we know and what we don't. *Current Psychiatry Reports, 23*, 1–8.

Iwakuma, M. (2006). The body as embodiment: An investigation of the body by Merleau-Ponty. In M. Corker & T. Shakespeare (Eds.), *Embodying disability theory*. Continuum books.

Krieger, N. (2005). Embodiment: A conceptual glossary for epidemiology. *Journal of Epidemiology & Community Health, 59*(5), 350–355.

Lavis A (2011) *The boundaries of a Good Anorexic: Exploring pro-anorexia on the internet and in the clinic.* Doctoral thesis. Goldsmiths, University of London.

Leder, D. (1990). *The Absent body*. University of Chicago Press.

Lester, R. J. (1997). The (dis)embodied self in anorexia nervosa. *Social Science & Medicine (1982), 44*(4), 479–489.

Lewak, D., & Ridley, J. (2017, February 8). *Inside the terrifying tactics models use to stay thin.* The New York Post. Retrieved August 22, 2024, from https://nypost.com/2017/02/08/models-tell-all-before-newyork-fashion-week/

Longo, M. R., Schüür, F., Kammers, M. P., Tsakiris, M., & Haggard, P. (2008). What is embodiment? A psychometric approach. *Cognition, 107*(3), 978–998.

Malecki, J., Rhodes, P., & Ussher, J. (2018). Childhood trauma and anorexia nervosa: From body image to embodiment. *Health Care for Women International, 39*(8), 936–951.

Mauss, M. (1979). Body techniques. In *Sociology and Psychology* (Essays) (pp. 95–123). Routledge.

McIntosh, S. (2024, January 24). *Oscar nominations: Barbies snubs and more five talking points*. BBC News. Retrieved August 22, 2024, from https://www.bbc.co.uk/news/entertainment-arts-68067403

McRobbie, A. (2011). Beyond post-feminism. *Public Policy Research, 18*(3), 179–184.

Merleau-Ponty, M. (2013). *Phenomenology of perception.* Routledge & Kegan Paul. (Original work published 1945).

Miller, I. (2016). *A history of force feeding: Hunger strikes, prisons and medical ethics, 1909–1974* (p. 267). Springer Nature.

Minocher, X., & Randall, C. (2020). Predictable policing: New technology, old bias, and future resistance in big data surveillance. *Convergence, 26*(5–6), 1108–1124.

Monro, F., & Huon, G. (2005). Media-portrayed idealized images, body shame, and appearance anxiety. *International Journal of Eating Disorders, 38*(1), 85–90.

Montague, J., Phillips, E., Holland, F., & Archer, S. (2020). Expanding hermeneutic horizons: Working as multiple researchers and with multiple participants. *Research Methods in Medicine & Health Sciences, 1*(1), 25–30.

Mount, B. M. (2003). Existential suffering and the determinants of healing. *European Journal of Palliative Care, 10*, 40–42.

Ms Magazine. (2023, December 26). *The Ms Top feminists of 2022.* Retrieved August 22, 2024, from https://msmagazine.com/2022/12/26/the-ms-top-feminists-of-2022/

O'Connell, L. (2020). *Being and doing anorexia nervosa: An exploration of diagnosis identity, work and performance of illness.* Ph.D. thesis, University of Essex. Retrieved August 22, 2024, from https://repository.essex.ac.uk/28205/1/Thesis_OConnell_July2020.pdf

Orbach, S. (1978). *Fat is a feminist issue: The anti-diet guide to permanent weight loss*. Paddington Press.

Orbach, S. (1986). *Hunger strike: The anorectic's struggle as a metaphor for our age.* Faber & Faber.

Orbach, S. (2019). *Bodies*. Profile books.

Overgaard, S. (2004). Heidegger on embodiment. *Journal of the British Society for Phenomenology, 35*(2), 116–113.

Pellegrini, R. A., Finzi, S., Veglia, F., & Di Fini, G. (2021). Narrative and bodily identity in eating disorders: Toward an integrated theoretical-clinical approach. *Frontiers in Psychology, 12*, 785004.

Rodgers, R. F., Ziff, S., Lowy, A. S., & Austin, S. B. (2021). Disordered eating behaviors and sexual objectification during New York fashion week: Implementation of industry policies and legislation. *International Journal of Eating Disorders, 54*(3), 433–437.

Sandberg, S. (2013). *Lean in: Women, work and the will to lead.* Alfred A Kopf.

Schlüter, C., Kraag, G., & Schmidt, J. (2021). Body shaming: An exploratory study on its definition and classification. *International Journal of Bullying Prevention*, 1–12.

Sharp, L. A. (2000). The commodification of the body and its parts. *Annual Review of Anthropology, 29*, 287–328.

Shaw, A. S. (2006). *The embodiment of disobedience: Fat black women's unruly political bodies*. Lexington Books.

Shilling, C. (2012). *The body and social theory*. Sage.

Shilling, C., & Mellor, P. (1996). Embodiment, structuration theory and Modernity: Mind/body dualism and the repression of sensuality. *Body & Society, 2*(4), 1–15.

Smith, J. A., Flowers, P., & Larkin, M. (2021). *Interpretative phenomenological analysis: Theory, method and research*. Sage.

Tempest, R. (1996, September 22). *Barbie and the world economy. Los Angeles Times.* Retrieved August 25, 2024, from https://www.latimes.com/archives/la-xpm-1996-09-22-mn-46610-story.html

Tragantzopoulou, P., Fixsen, A., Ridge, D., & Cheshire, A. (2024). 'You are not alone, we've got you': Power plays, devotion, and punishment on Healthy Eating and Pro-Eating disorder websites. *Qualitative Health Research.* https://doi.org/10.1177/10497323241238628

Troop, N. A., & Redshaw, C. (2012). General shame and bodily shame in eating disorders: A 2.5-year longitudinal study. *European Eating Disorders Review, 20*(5), 373–378.

Turner, B. S. (1992). *Regulating bodies: Essays in medical sociology*. Routledge.

Turner, B. S. (2006). Body. *Theory, Culture & Society, 23*(2–3), 223–229.

Turner, B. S. (2008). *The body and society* (3rd ed.). Blackwell.

Turner, B. S. (2012). Introduction: The turn of the body. In *Routledge handbook of body studies* (pp. 16–32). Routledge.

Tyler, M., & Wilkinson, A. (2007). The tyranny of corporate slenderness: 'corporate anorexia' as a metaphor for our age. *Work, Employment and Society, 21*(3), 537–549.

Van den Berg, P., Paxton, S. J., Keery, H., Wall, M., Guo, J., & Neumark-Sztainer, D. (2007). Body dissatisfaction and body comparison with media images in males and females. *Body image, 4*(3), 257–268.

Vanderlinden, J., & Palmisano, G. L. (2018). *Trauma and eating disorders: The state of the art* (pp. 15–32). Springer Publishing Company.

Venkatesh, N. (2021). Surveillance Capitalism: A Marx-inspired account. *Philosophy, 96*(3), 359–385.

Wolf, N. (1994). *Fire with Fire: The new female power and how to use it.* Fawcett Columbine.

World Health Organisation. (2023). *Gender in congruence and transgender health in the ICD.* Retrieved August 22, 2024, from https://www.who.int/standards/classifications/frequently-asked-questions/gender-incongruence-and-transgender-health-in-the-icd#:~:text=ICD%2D11%20has%20redefined%20gender,incongruence%20of%20childhood%E2%80%9D%2C%20respectively

Wright, D., & Brajtman, S. V. (2009). Human relationships at the end of life: An ethical ontology for practice. *Palliative Nursing, 11*, 219–227.

Wright, D., & Brajtman, S. (2011). Relational and embodied knowing: Nursing ethics within the interprofessional team. *Nursing Ethics, 18*(1), 20–30.

Wu, F., Ma, Y., & Zhang, Z. (2021). "I Found a More Attractive Deepfaked Self": The self-enhancement effect in deepfake video exposure. *Cyberpsychology, Behavior, and Social Networking, 24*(3), 173–181.

Zancu, S. A., & Enea, V. (2017). Eating disorders among fashion models: A systematic review of the literature. *Eating and Weight Disorders-Studies on Anorexia, Bulimia and Obesity, 22*, 395–405.

Zuboff, S. (2023). The age of surveillance capitalism. In *Social theory re-wired* (pp. 203–213). Routledge.

3

Anorexia Nervosa: The Making of the First Eating Disorder

Over the years, many efforts have been made to understand the nature and causes of anorexia nervosa (AN), although few have approached this from a social constructionist lens. For over a century, the discourse around AN centered around girls and young women, as in the cases published by Hilde Bruch (1979, 1988), who is credited for bringing this condition to public attention (Lucas et al, 1991). Even after AN was observable in non-western populations, with some symptom variations (Lee et al., 1993), the western model continued to dominate the medical narrative. Those in biomedicine, cognitive psychology, and genetic screening have also formulated their own opinions and solutions to this complex and potentially fatal disorder. Feminists also have had much to say about the role of chauvinistic society in laying the foundations for anorexia, while autobiographical literature has highlighted a gap between the meanings that anorexia holds for those affected and the perceptions held by medical professionals and wider society. From a social labeling[1] perspective, AN has been interpreted as a "deviant identity" (Taub, 2011), wherein the

[1] Here I adopt Durkheim's (1897) conception of labeling as one of identifying and creating social deviance so that society can protect itself from deviance. Suicide for Durkheim was an example of social deviance.

A. Fixsen, *The Construction of Eating Disorders*, The Politics of Mental Health and Illness, https://doi.org/10.1007/978-3-031-70318-8_3

individual's deviance manifests in their refusal to maintain a minimum weight for their age and height and their strong resistance to treatment. The paradox here is that, rather than intending to defy social norms, anorexic individuals often emerge in studies as high achievers who set excessively high standards for themselves (Halmi et al., 2000; Wonderlich et al., 2005).[2] In this context, AN might be viewed as an inverted form of deviance, where the individual over-conforms to specific social and cultural norms regarding body shape and dietary discipline.

This chapter explores anorexia nervosa (AN) beyond its individual symptoms, examining how social, cultural, and institutional factors contribute to its construction. While psychiatry and medicine focus on diagnosis and treatment, historians and sociologists highlight the role of powerful institutions, cultural contexts, and social interactions in shaping the disorder. The chapter begins with a review of the historical roots of AN, its early treatments, and the influence of feminism on contemporary definitions and treatments, before presenting sociological perspectives that offer deeper insights into the lived experience of AN. Current diagnostic categories and treatments for AN are then explored, and the risks and ethics of involuntary treatment considered. The chapter concludes with arguments supporting the assertion that anorexia as a phenomenon is deeply embedded in the capitalist economy.

Historical Precedents

For many years, anorexia nervosa was considered a "culture-bound syndrome," meaning it was thought to exist only in western cultures or those influenced by them (Swartz, 1985). This idea was supported by the DSM-IV-TR (2000), which defined a culture-bound syndrome as a disorder that only occurs in a specific cultural context, with diagnosis and treatment based on that culture's beliefs. Some scholars, however, have argued that anorexia can also be found in non-western societies, describing it as a "culturally reactive syndrome" (DiNicola, 1990) or a

[2] It is also acknowledged that there are many variations in personality type and that emotional instability is probably the most prevailing characteristic.

"metaphor for our time" (Orbach, 1986). Yet, historical evidence indicates that self-restricted eating has occurred in various places and times, throughout recorded history. It is believed that a variety of health and humanitarian approaches have advocated periods of abstinence, such as fasting or avoiding specific foods, as methods of physical, mental, and spiritual purification (Dell'Osso et al., 2016; Gordon, 2015). These practices were often endorsed by religious or medical institutions. As the age of science moved on, so eating became more medicalized and medicine more institutionalized. Consequently, specific interpretations of eating as pathological became focused on their causes and treatment. For individuals engaging in self-harm through restricted eating, a host of explanations and treatments were proposed. While some of these approaches have been discarded in favor of more culturally appropriate and humane medical management, others like forced feeding persist, regardless of ongoing debates surrounding the best interests of individuals and potential human rights infringements (Umezulike, 2020).

From a western historical perspective, extreme fasting has been framed as largely women's business. According to Bemporad (1997), the intensification of fasting behaviors in European culture can be traced back to the incorporation of Eastern beliefs regarding spiritual purification through physical abstinence from bodily pleasures. Forcen (2013) notes that while not strictly approved by the Catholic church, self-starvation was a relatively common practice in mediaeval Europe. However, this explanation does not account for the gender disparity observed in the adoption of *anorexia mirabilis* or "holy anorexia" (Dell'Osso et al., 2016).[3] Apart from a few male exceptions, such as St. Symeon the Stylite, these instances were part of a set of practices observed by women, aimed at emulating the life of Christ. Bemporad (1997) describes the phenomenon of holy anorexia emerging as "a rash of cases of willful female starvation, particularly in southern Europe" (p. 405). Historian Rudolph M. Bell (1985) documented 181 such cases of self-imposed starvation between the 1200s and 1600s, a figure which is probably an underestimation given the broad

[3] Abstinence from food is also a feature of non-western cultures, notably Hindu ascetic practices in India. As part of the *bhakti* tradition, fasting is practiced mostly among male devotees, but also women.

distribution of population and gaps in communication during the period.[4]

Various theories have been put forward for the fasting of women in the name of religion. In a patriarchal society where the church wielded considerable power, wealth, and corruption at the highest levels, extreme religiosity provided one of the few avenues through which women could leave a lasting impact. Regardless of the Catholic church's criticism of self-starvation, some fasting women—as living embodiments of flesh renunciation—gained local celebrity status, and a select few were canonized as saints. The allure of accounts featuring fasting women persisted, perhaps due to their sensational nature, as seen in stories and depictions of figures like Catherine of Siena engaging in self-starvation, flagellation, and performing miraculous feats such as drinking the purulent matter from a female breast cancer victim and multiplying food (Bynum, 1985). These narratives of fasting women held a peculiar fascination, extending into the present day.[5] Stories of female saints like St. Catherine underscored their commitment to sexual abstinence and unwavering dedication to aiding the sick and suffering in their communities. It is important to note that during periods of scarcity, particularly in times of war, plague, and famine during the medieval era, women, especially mothers, often sacrificed their own sustenance to protect others. Regardless of the true motivations behind these women's actions, they were upheld as moral exemplars of humility and chastity, highlighting the importance of voluntary caregiving to the sick and poor. This narrative of willing service and self-denial stands in contrast to the experiences of young women coerced into unwanted marriages or convents, exposing other dimensions of gender politics in medieval Europe (Walker, 2003).

It is tempting in our age of popular psychology to interpret the feelings and behaviors of these mediaeval women through modern eyes, but

[4] According to Dell'Osso et al. (2016), in the Middle Ages deprivation of food (except for the ritual of Eucharist) was an element of spirituality along with reclusion, self-flagellation, humble dressing, and other practices.

[5] The number of published articles on so-called "pro-Ana" websites (sites which advocate extreme slimness and offer advice on ways to lose significant amounts of weight) is far too numerous to list. This topic appears to be of particular interest to master's and PhD students, who may well be of a similar generation to those posting comments on sites. This can be a source of worry for University Research Ethics Committees.

seeking parallels between these practices and modern day anorexia is problematic. Bell (1985) and Bynum (1985) agree that both mediaeval fasting and contemporary anorexia take place within a paternalistic society. However, while Bell considers both to represent a quest for liberation, Bynum argues that fasting for mediaeval women was but one aspect of a complex of experiences concerned with piety and spirituality. Brumberg (1987, 1997) suggests that although Saint Catherine's slender appearance and restricted food consumption may resonate with contemporary issues, drawing parallels between medieval saints and female anorexics overlooks the sociocultural meanings embedded in fasting. In Brumberg's studies on young American girls, the body itself becomes their primary project, contrasting with medieval women who fasted for spiritual and pious reasons. "The modern anorectic strives for perfection in terms of society's ideal of physical, rather than spiritual, beauty" (Brumberg, 1987, p. 46). Bordo (1993) challenges this differentiation, asserting that "it does not follow that the contemporary slender obsession is without deep spiritual dimensions and that these cannot share important – that is, illuminating – affinities with ascetic ambitions of medieval saints" (p. 68).

During medieval Europe, particularly in the era of witch hunts, women were often targeted with accusations of possessing mysterious powers or engaging in activities considered unnatural or heretical. The intersection of religious intolerance, wars, and plagues created an environment where women's actions, such as self-starvation, were interpreted through a lens of demonic possession (Hepworth, 1999). The "Black Fast," said to be practiced by a woman in sixteenth-century Lancashire, exemplifies how certain behaviors were perceived as evidence of involvement with the devil (Jones & Zell, 2005). Reports of fasting women persisted, albeit in smaller numbers, from the end of the Renaissance to the Victorian era (Bemporad, 1997). The ability to survive through abstinence from food was viewed as a sign of spiritual nourishment compensating for the physical effects of fasting. The explanations for such abilities were often a blend of spiritual and material beliefs, although a shift toward medical explanations was gaining prominence in the eighteenth century. The testing of fasting women, as in the case of Moore of Tutbury in 1808, illustrates a growing skepticism and the attempt to debunk non-scientific assertions (Henderson, 1813).

Reflecting on the long-standing relationship between self-starvation and religious ideals, Banks (1992) argued that this aspect of restricted eating in girls and young women still needed to be considered in a modern context. Recent studies of "pro-Ana" platforms appear to support this idea, with their incorporation of devotional elements such as creeds, psalms, commandments, penitence, bodily purity, and invocations to their god, Ana (Day & Keys, 2008; Stapleton et al., 2019; Tragantzopoulou et al., 2024). However, unlike the fasting girls of the past, the self-inflicted acts of "mortification" described on these sites are now considered symptoms of a mental disorder, arousing concern rather than admiration from the broader public gaze. Moreover, it is debatable whether ascetic and religious influences can be entirely separated from other concerns, which nowadays include body image or dieting. What the historical context does shed light upon is the entanglement of religious, social, and medical perspectives and the need for psychological and emotional expression during times of significant cultural and intellectual shifts.

Anorexia as a Medical Discourse

The classification of anorexia nervosa as a medical condition unfolded during a period marked by intense debates over the identification and naming of newly recognized phenomena. A growing skepticism toward self-starvation practices gained traction, particularly within scientific circles, as empiricism and rationalism supplanted occultism and folklore in the realm of medicine. Baptist van Helmont (1580–1644), a theologian, physician, and chemist, attributed alimentary diseases like anorexia nervosa to disruptions in the fermentation process, leading to the production of so-called "bad acids" in the stomach. The first truly medical description of AN is often credited to Dr Richard Morton who, in 1689, reported on two clinical cases of a 16-year-old boy and an 18-year-old girl (Mitchell, 1980). Morton described his patients as having a nervous consumption (phthisis nervosa), characterized by low mood and anxiety along with shortness of breath, lack of appetite, and emaciation

(Silverman, 1985, 1989). Around a century later, Dr Robert Willan documented a case of a man who, after isolating himself from work and friends and abstaining from solid food for 78 days, ultimately starved to death (Silverman, 1987, 1992). In 1694, Morton—convinced that he had identified a nonspecific form of tuberculosis—described a young woman who did not exhibit the typical symptoms of shortness of breath and fever but rather suffered from loss of appetite, disrupted menstruation, and cachexia. This case is regarded as a potentially early "medical" depiction of anorexia (Moncrieff-Boyd, 2016).

In the nineteenth century, more reports began to emerge concerning cases of disordered eating. Initial descriptions dealt with cases of vomiting and starvation attributed to the patients' subjective belief that they were unable to swallow or to eat due to stomach pains. Mostly these cases were interpreted as manifestations of hysteria, which was considered a neurasthenic condition almost peculiar to women. In 1840, French alienist Luis Marcé published a work entitled *Traité théorique et pratique des maladies des femmes.* In his book, Marcé distinguishes between gastrointestinal anorexia (anorexie gastrique) and anorexia nervosa (anorexie nerveuse) and confirmed that most of these cases were in women (Silverman, 1989). The origins of the latter come from the Greek "nervous loss of appetite," where the adjective "nervosa" indicates the functional and non-organic nature of the disorder and marks it out from simple loss of appetite. This was also the age of biological classification and taxonomy, and Marcé was probably the first to describe the nosology of what came to be known as anorexia nervosa and to distinguish it from other forms of cachexia or wasting (Dell'Osso et al., 2016).

The term *anorexia nervosa* is also used in a medical paper by Sir William Withey Gull in 1874, who claimed the discovery as his own (Gull, 1874). Simultaneous to Gull's discovery was that of his French rival Dr Laseque, who regarded the cause of anorexia to be some disturbance in a woman's marital sexual or emotional life.[6] The rivalry between the English and French doctor prevented Gull from being able to claim anorexia nervosa

[6] The intense rivalries between Sir William Gull and Charles Lasègue are well documented, including the latter's furious response to Gull's reading of his seminal report on anorexia nervosa to the Clinical Society of London (Silverman, 1992).

to be an exclusively British medical discovery. He did however win the argument concerning the naming of the condition as "anorexia nervosa," rather than "hysterical anorexia" (Hepworth, 1999). From the onset, anorexia was introduced in the medical literature as a female condition, with recorded cases in males being extremely rare. It was considered a nervous disease observed to affect "high born" girls from wealthy families (Brumberg, 1997; Gooldin, 2003), which distinguishes it in this sense from the early recorded cases of self-starvation and is probably more an indication of the physician's client base.

Disagreements arose about the typical profile of the patient with anorexia nervosa, with Laseque observing abnormal quietude in female patients and Gull emphasizing severe agitation, the latter aligning with Victorian notions of women as prone to hysteria. Quietness and separation from family and friends therefore became the first line of treatment in anorexia nervosa. In the late nineteenth century, the French neurologist Jean-Martin Charcot drew from his theory of female hysteria to stress the importance of an unstable psychology and the family environment in the development of anorexia. Others continued to search for the biological origins of food aversion. German physician and pathologist Morris Simmonds, whose name is associated with Simmonds disease (Escamilla & Lisser, 1938), linked anorexia to hypothyroidism or pituitary gland necrosis, shifting the focus from psychological factors. Subsequent research discounted Simmonds' perspective, indicating that pituitary damage in his patients was likely a consequence rather than a cause of the disease. Attention then moved more toward psychological factors.[7] Through the means of its "discovery" by men of science, the term "anorexia nervosa" transformed the experiences of women who refuse food in their position as subjects to objects of the medical gaze (Hepworth, 1999). As we will see in the following sections, this definition secured the continued management of such individuals within the medical system and the development and reproduction of clinical and legal practices that exist in eating disorder treatment units today.

[7] Similar conclusions could be reached about the morphological brain changes noted in patients with severe anorexia (e.g., Seitz et al., 2016) which is likely to be a consequence of self-starvation rather than a cause.

Early Treatments of Anorexia

To understand how the medicalization of anorexia came to be, it needs to be studied within the context of institutionalization. Foucault's (1973) concept of the "medicine of social spaces" provides insights into this process. At some point in history, individuals deemed threats, including those classified as sick or insane, were segregated and removed from the general population, finding themselves confined within clinics, asylums, and sometimes prisons. The more complex the social space in which a "disease" is situated, the greater the likelihood that it is "denatured"[8] by this separation, and the individual becomes an object of disease. The emergence of the clinic in the eighteen century was clearly a step in this direction, with its separate functions from the hospital and a more specialist type of training required for its medical personnel. Within the clinic, a new alliance was forged between "words and things, enabling one to 'see and say'" (Foucault, 1973, xii). Medical treatment methods nevertheless remained very crude. Andrew Scull (2022) notes the extraordinary vulnerability of the mentally ill to the "scientific" enthusiasms of the time. The pressures on medical men to *do something* about conditions which they poorly understood were accompanied by a corresponding lack of restraints on the zeal for therapeutic experimentation.[9] The result was the emergence of a "host of dubious interventions aimed at these recalcitrant disorders" (Scull, 2022, p. xiv).

As women sought greater emancipation in the late nineteenth and early twentieth centuries, those who transgressed societal norms were liable to be labeled as deviant. At least some of these became subjects of medical experimentation, particularly for conditions perceived as moral, nervous, or psychiatric in origin. Since anorexia nervosa was framed as a medical condition, it necessitated specialized treatment from trained professionals. Those from wealthier classes were likely to have access to clinics. What followed however amounted to the careful controlling of the

[8] Foucault (1973) explains how the original or "true" nature of the disease is effectively removed in medical spaces such as hospitals and clinics.

[9] Gull himself admitted the absence of any relationship between the medical preparations prescribed and the patient's subsequent recovery from anorexia, stating that "the medical treatment probably needs not to be considered as contributing much to the recovery" (Gull, 1874, p. 24).

afflicted woman within the physician-patient relationship. The female patient was not consulted, and effective communication was neither established nor deemed desirable (Hepworth, 1999). While the patient was seen as not to be trusted, so too were her family and friends sent away or kept at a distance. In this scenario, the physician and his attendants assumed complete moral and medical authority, overseeing the treatment and recovery of the anorexic patient. The exclusion of women from the medical profession made them more vulnerable as medical subjects, as men could exert full control over bodies and behaviors which they were not able to fully understand.[10]

Hepworth (1999) points out how, once the conversation had moved away from organic causations, a moral or psychoanalytic explanation for anorexia nervosa became imperative. The ideological hegemony of psychoanalysis in American psychiatry was especially important to the framing of early anorexia nervosa treatments. One of Freud's theories was that repulsion toward food in adolescent girls was a manifestation of aversion to sexuality (Lawrence, 2008), an idea that persisted in psychotherapy (Beech, 1959). *In Conversations with Anorexics* (1988), psychotherapist Hilda Bruch wrote of how, for the anorexic, denial of the body is both an attitude and painful daily practice, which makes them feel stronger, more in control, and less vulnerable. In one case study she scolds an anorexic patient for her childish thinking and resistance, when this young person expresses her anxiety about her developing female body. Bruch was convinced that all the efforts and striving for affection and excessive thinness of the anorexic were directed toward "hiding the fatal flaw of her fundamental inadequacy" (Bruch, 1988, p. 6). The role of the therapist is to "find the person within the patient" (1988), to encourage them to look at their own development in more realistic terms, and to actively explore what is going on within.

Like Bruch (1979), psychiatrist Arthur Crisp (1980) regarded anorexia as resulting from faulty development and contended that the presence of parents and other family members hindered rather than helped the anorectic's process of inner change. Superficially, congenial relationships to

---

[10] Hesse-Biber et al. (2004) point out how the medical "colonisation" of women and their bodies took place at a time when imperial colonialism was at its height.

parents could be maintained but only through excessive conformity on the part of the child. After the illness has existed for some time, the hostility toward parents comes into the open, making it necessary to modify the family interaction. Nowadays, this thinking has changed. The conversation has now moved away from "parentectomy" (enforced separation from both parents or a parent) or "parent-blaming" toward the idea of families and providers as "the best allies in treatment" (Schaumberg et al., 2017, p. 2). Even so, biological and genetic explanations for eating disorders retain the family pathology connection (Paolacci et al., 2020), while some therapists may harbor a conviction that faulty parental upbringing plays a major role in AN development.

In the second half of the twentieth century, Freudian techniques began to face competition from approaches with a quite different intellectual lineage. A large and increasing proportion of mental health outpatients were soon receiving psychotropic medication, often without the more expensive and time-consuming psychotherapy (Scull, 2022).[11] From 1970s, the technique of cognitive behavioral therapy (CBT) gained popularity, due in part to its short-term, structured treatment timeframe and its mounting evidence base. CBT could be supplied by psychologists, psychiatric social workers, and others, at far cheaper rates than those commanded by a medically trained psychiatrist, making it attractive to the modern proponents of managed care. It also aligns with the idea of certain parts of neuro cognitive processes as being largely responsible for faulty decision-making around food (Steinglass et al., 2019). CBT has subsequently become one the most popular treatments for eating disorders, including AN (Galsworthy-Francis & Allan, 2014; Hilbert et al., 2017), and continues to gain traction as a first-line therapy.

[11] For a detailed explanation of the psychoanalytic perspective on anorexia nervosa, see Brenner (2022).

Criteria and Comorbidity

When DSM-1 was first published in 1952, it categorized anorexia nervosa (AN) as a "psychophysiologic gastrointestinal dysfunction." Since then, there have been significant revisions to its definition, to diagnostic criteria, and to the understanding of its variability. According to DSM-V (APA, 2013), individuals with anorexia nervosa or AN exhibit a damaging relationship with food, eating, exercise, and possess a distorted self-image, often accompanied by obsessive behaviors related to weight gain. The manual delineates three primary diagnostic criteria for AN (2013, pp. 338–339). The first criterion involves restricting energy intake leading to significantly low body weight considering various factors. The second criterion encompasses an intense fear of weight gain or becoming fat, along with persistent behaviors hindering weight gain despite being underweight. The third criterion involves a disturbance in body weight or shape perception, its impact on self-evaluation, and/or a persistent lack of recognition of the seriousness of low body weight. The minimum severity level, based on body mass index (BMI) percentile, is set at less than 17. Two recognized subtypes of AN exist: the restricting type, involving minimal caloric intake, fasting, and exercise for weight loss; and the binge-eating/purging type. Additionally, the ICD-10 and DSM-V-TR include *atypical anorexia.*[12] The DSM (along with other clinical literature) emphasizes the comorbidity of AN with other mental health disorders including major depressive disorder, substance use disorder, social anxiety disorder, obsessive compulsive disorder, and suicidality (APA, 2013; Thornton et al., 2016; Wade et al., 2000).

Statistics suggest that while anorexia nervosa remains relatively rare,[13] an increase in cases among individuals aged 15 or younger has occurred (Smink et al., 2016; van Eden et al., 2021). Previously considered as confined to middle-class, western women (Bruch, 1979; Darmon, 2009), associations between AN prevalence and specific sociocultural norms have been challenged, with many suggesting a complex interplay between

[12] There remains some controversy over whether fear of weight gain needs to be present in AN. Subtypes and atypical categories allow for this variation.

[13] Lifetime prevalence for AN is estimated to be about 0.6 percent.

genetics and environment (Paolacci et al., 2020; Schaumberg et al., 2017). The high diagnosis rates in females can also be partly attributed to gender differences in detection rates (Holland et al., 2016), while studies are divided on whether the incidence of AN reported in females correlates with a greater likelihood of mortality from this disorder (Edakubo & Fushimi, 2020; Gueguen et al., 2012; Keshaviah et al., 2014). Overall, AN is credited as having the highest mortality among mental illnesses, from both natural causes and suicide (Arcelus et al., 2011). Premature mortality in older adults appears to be related to lack of treatment, while social support is regarded a mitigating factor (Keshaviah et al., 2014). Determining the cause of death in AN patients can be difficult, with common medical complications linked to heart abnormalities and irregularities induced by psychotropic medications (Mehler & Anderson, 2022).

Current Treatment Guidelines

Despite developments in its clinical diagnosis, preventing and treating anorexia nervosa remains highly challenging (Schaumberg et al., 2017). According to DeJong et al. (2011), dropout rates from anorexia nervosa treatments are high, even where individuals are made aware of the impact and consequences of untreated anorexia, such as infertility, brittle bones, deterioration of organs, and an early death range. Standard treatment comprises weight restoration and normalization of eating behavior followed by relapse prevention, which needs to include convincing patients to overcome their drive to lose weight (Guarda et al., 2007). The UK National Institute of Clinical Excellence (NICE)[14] guide (2021) sets out how acute medical care should be provided for people who have an eating disorder with severe electrolyte imbalance, severe malnutrition, severe dehydration, or signs of incumbent organ failure. Although psychological therapy may be utilized in the involuntary treatment of the anorectic, medical hospitalization is primarily aimed at stabilizing the patient

[14] The National Institute for Health and Care Excellence (UK) provides evidence-based recommendations for the health and social care sector, developed by independent committees, which include professionals and lay members and consulted on by stakeholders.

through weight restoration and nutritional supplementation, with longer-term psychological treatments more likely to take place at home or in outpatient settings (Kells et al., 2017). The use of artificial feeding in the treatment of severely compromised anorexia nervosa patients remains a problematic issue. The risk of refeeding syndrome[15] is inherent in this procedure, and the utilization of a nasogastric feeding tube may inflict pain and trauma.

Current UK treatment guidelines also emphasize addressing the emotional, educational, employment, and social needs of individuals with AN, and the requirement to abide by the rules of confidentiality, privacy, and dignity (NICE, 2021). Alongside vitamin and mineral supplements and nutritional rehabilitation, psychological therapy is considered the cornerstone of AN treatment for adult anorexic patients. Recommended treatments for AN in adults include cognitive behavioral therapy (CBT) and Maudsley Anorexia Nervosa Treatment, with specialist supportive clinical management also being mentioned. Health professionals are cautioned to be alert for signs of bullying, teasing abuse, and neglect. Psychotropic medications such as olanzapine have been used on- and off-prescription as adjunctive therapy to weight restoration but with inconsistent results. ICD-10 (WHO, 2019) states that antidepressant medication may be prescribed for anxiety and depression in AN and to reduce "ruminations" that sufferers describe. Garner et al. (2016) found antidepressants to be widely prescribed to adults and adolescents with AN, regardless of recommendations to the contrary in treatment guidelines. Family based therapy is now a common treatment modality for patients referred with AN. This pathway is based on the premise that the patient has lost control over his or her ability to self-feed and requires the assistance of parents or other family members to monitor and enforce meal times until decision-making capabilities have been restored (Kells et al., 2017).

The notion that the anorexic body requires involuntary detention for the treatment of their eating disorder remains a debated topic in many

[15] Refeeding syndrome can be defined as the potentially fatal shifts in fluids and electrolytes that may occur in malnourished patients receiving artificial refeeding, whether through gastric means or intravenously (Mehanna et al., 2008).

countries. International approaches to this span a wide range of clinical ethical and legal positions which in places like the US may vary from one part of the country to another. The UK medical and legal position is that AN falls into the category of serious mental illness resulting in diminished autonomy (NICE, 2021). Unconsented clinical interventions lie within the rights of medical practitioners and do not constitute a violation of the person's rights. Studies suggest that involuntary treatment of AN occurs in around 13–44 percent of admissions (Clausen, 2020). While the context in which involuntary detention takes place are varied, it is generally associated with psychiatric symptoms, comorbidity, long illness duration, and previous submissions (Clausen & Jones, 2014; Clausen, 2020). When considering the imposition of involuntary treatment on patients with severe anorexia, it needs to be asked for whom and by whom is it justified—by the family, the medical profession, or society at large? (Yager, 2020). Over and above the idea of sustaining life irrespective of its quality, there are the emotional and psychological effects of involuntary treatment to consider. Involuntarily treated individuals typically feel a loss of autonomy, dignity, and respect, accompanied by feelings of disempowerment (Saya et al., 2019; Umezulike, 2020). While interventions like nasogastric tube feeding may find justification under the Mental Health Act due to diminished responsibility, Umezulike (2020) underscores how such treatments might sever the connection with the subjective significance associated with self-starvation.

The author also emphasizes the overarching power and paternalism of medical intervention and its potential encroachment on the human right to make decisions about one's life and death.

Studies examining anorectic patients' experiences of assessment and detention under mental health legislation suggest it to be frightening and distressing, and to include physical force and restraint (Akther et al., 2019). Among the recommendations made by Akther et al. (2019) are providing a voice and more collaboration with patients and designing physical and social environments which are more conducive to recovery. While most patients acknowledge involuntary treatment interventions as necessary and lifesaving, they also view it as a form of punishment, which should be either short-lived or prohibited (Clausen, 2020). People's experiences can be influenced by the degree of actual or perceived person-centered care, and a therapeutic bond with clinicians was seen as a key factor in positive experiences of in-patient detention in Seed et al.'s (2016) study. In line with this, several studies suggest focusing on quality of life for patient, rather than their eating disorder symptoms (Kaplan & Miles, 2016; Miles, 2020; Yager, 2020).

For those who live with anorexia, the journey toward recovery can be prolonged and arduous. However, an encouraging glimpse into the life prospects of individuals developing AN during their younger years emerged from one of the limited outcome studies. This longitudinal study, conducted in Sweden, followed individuals born in 1970 and screened for AN in 1985 over a span of 30 years. Despite 23 percent of patients not receiving psychiatric treatment, the study reported no mortalities within the sample, and only one in five went on to develop a chronic eating disorder. The authors suggest that in the long-term perspective, most individuals with AN can fare well. This positive outcome may be attributed in part to the quality of healthcare in Sweden, renowned for having one of the world's best public health systems. More than half of the individuals in the study received some form of treatment, and the majority lived in communities with accessible treatment facilities (Dobrescu et al., 2020). This suggests that improving accessibility to treatment must remain a priority for eating disorders services.

Feminism and Anorexia Nervosa

Over the years, feminist scholars have provided alternative and sometimes radical explanations for self-starvation, often linking it to the cultural emphasis on the thin female body or its sexualized objectification, along with evolving social and cultural expectations on women since the latter half of the twentieth century. Feminist psychoanalyst Susie Orbach presents a compelling critique of paternalistic interpretations regarding both weight gain and weight loss. In her work, *Hunger Strike: A Metaphor for Our Age* (1986), Orbach describes anorexia nervosa as a dramatic outcome of society's cultural obsession with regulating body size and fostering body insecurities in women. She compares AN to the diagnosis of hysteria in late nineteenth-century Europe, with both expressing the internal compromise faced by western women navigating their passions and desires amidst extraordinary confusion. Starvation amid abundance, denial juxtaposed with desire, and the dichotomy of striving for invisibility versus the wish to be seen are identified by Orbach as key features of AN, portraying it as a "metaphor for our age" (1986, p. 4). Orbach (1986) points out the uncomfortable parallels between such things as force-feeding and enforced bedrest and general cultural attitudes toward women which allow for their intrusion in brutal and invasive ways. Anorexia represents a bid to "negotiate conflicted desire" which takes place using body and food as a metaphor (Orbach, 1986, xiv).

Orbach's "hunger strike" analogy is powerful but has also been seen as exaggerating the political nature of anorexic behaviors. Brumberg (1987, 1997) contends that if refusal to eat is a political act it is a limited, infantile form primarily directed at parents and oneself, lacking allegiance to broader connectivity. While acknowledging biological and psychological roles in anorexic development, Brumberg, a social historian, delves into the changes in the cultural meaning of appetite in women's lives. Utilizing girls' diaries and archival material, she reveals that anorexia nervosa predates the widespread cultural imperative for the thin female body. Bordo (1985, 1993, 1994, 2009), a feminist philosopher, focuses less on traditional causes of anorexia nervosa and more on articulating the complexities of cultural interpretations of individual weight loss. Drawing from Foucault's historical approach, she explores how women adopt disciplinary practices sanctioned in a patriarchal society, such as slimming and dieting. Bordo criticizes the pursuit of precise classifications, instead emphasizing cultural axes leading to anorexia, including the dualist axis (body-mind distinction), control axis (obsession with body control), and gender/power axis (distorted body images due to female misconceptions and external control from gender power relations). These psychopathologies, she argues, are expressions of the heterogeneous distress of our age.

Barkty (1988) also writes about the fragmentation and objectification of the female body under neoliberal capitalism and proposes two subjects involved in the process of objectification, the "objectifier" and the "objectified person." Employing Foucault's account of the deployment of power, Barkty recounts the various ways in which women are induced to systematically discipline their bodies through diet, exercise, restricted movement, make-up, skincare, and other forms of body grooming. Women are made to feel deficient and ashamed for trying but failing to measure up to unattainable ideals of feminine beauty. Naomi Wolf (1991) also examines the misogynistic nature of the philosophical underpinnings of western culture and its institutions, where women are taught that the male mind is to be valued while the female body is to be hated, and if possible, to be destroyed. A culture which fixates on female thinness is not an obsession about female beauty, Wolf argues, it is an obsession with female obedience. Anorectic women are not individually ill; rather, they are keen students of cultural expectations. Dieting serves as a potent political sedative, rendering a compliant population. Nevertheless, Wolf's work reflects the complexities within the feminist literature, concurrently serving as a critic and advocate of third-wave feminism.[16] In a later work, she criticizes what she perceives as outdated approaches and attempts to link feminist struggles with broader social inequality, asserting that second-wave feminist messages have failed to inspire women who now turn to mainstream media for role models: "Anti-capitalism, an insider-outsider mentality … once necessary and effective - are now getting in our way" (Wolf, 1994, p. 2).

Feminist theory has diverged from medical and psychiatric perspectives of anorexia nervosa (AN) by taking a broader view of women's lives and considering the cultural, familial, and political aspects. However, it is important to note that feminists do not adopt a uniform approach to eating disorders or broader issues of female inequality. While some feminist analyses aim to break away from the dominant medical viewpoint on AN and challenge its narrow definitions of women's experiences, many still utilize medical and psychiatric terminology, despite its patriarchal basis (Lester, 1997; Hepworth, 1999).[17] Anorexia nervosa has frequently been framed in both sociological and feminist literature as fundamentally bound up with western diet culture, with an underlying assumption that the condition largely exists due to the western fear of fatness. Yet, this

[16] A type of feminism which recasts gender equality not as an anti-capitalist movement but as an entrepreneurial project predicated on personal empowerment.

[17] An exception to this is Barbara Hepworth (1999), who has written extensively on the social construction of anorexia nervosa. Her thesis is both historically rooted and theoretically uncompromising in its insistence that this disorder is a medically constructed discourse.

culturally biased view of AN may obscure healthcare professionals' understanding of a patient's own cultural reasons for self-starvation and even hinder their recovery (Simpson, 2002). A further critique of earlier feminist studies is the relative absence of first-hand anorexic stories, voices, and experiences in this literature. A notable dichotomy exists between academic voice and subject, with one positioned as the enlightened feminist researcher and the other the politically unaware anorectic (Bordo, 1993).

The Anorectic Voice

While psychiatry and social scientists all seek to give their insights into what is going on in the mind of the person, the voice of anorectic subjects themselves may well be unheard, silenced, or misunderstood. Ultimately, only those who have lived with the condition can understand what it feels like to be diagnosed and treated with anorexia nervosa. In her autoethnographic account, Holmes (2016) considers her feelings and responses as an academic with AN to a feminist literature which constructs the anorectic experience as contingent on a diet of mass media fashion images and invites her to question her ability to extricate herself from this all-encompassing power. Poststructural readings of anorexia have been crucial in interrogating how the construction and treatment of anorexia is used to endorse and reject normal and abnormal ways of being a woman. However, in so doing this literature assumes a commonality of experience between all women, which discounts the uniqueness of experience in a similarly reductive way to medicalization. Moreover, the discrediting of the anorectic voice as deluded and disordered jarred with what Holmes (2016) regarded as her own academic insight and authority. Overall, Holmes questions what she calls the "metaphorical exploitation" of anorexia, which fails to do justice to "the complex subjectivities that anorexia may entail" (2016, p. 205). Holmes also critiques the absence of non-heterosexual women from the literature on AN, which presupposes that a woman's desire to be thin begins as a response to the sexual requirements of patriarchy.

Others have adopted a distinctly performative lens through which to interpret the experiences of the "being and doing" of anorexia nervosa. O'Connell (2023), for example, uses autoethnography and performative theory to explain how individuals (including herself) *learn* an anorexic identity in a diagnostically informed treatment context, which is subsequently partly embraced and partly rejected. Clinically based anorexic scripts shape how individuals perceive and manage their diagnosis, sometimes conforming to these scripts and evaluating their own illness performances against them. O'Connell's insights uncover the hidden consequences of being diagnosed and clinically treated, providing a depth of understanding that second-hand accounts cannot achieve. Darmon's (2008) study, albeit written from an outsider perspective, also employs interaction ritual theory to explore the adoption of an anorexic/anorectic identity and the internalization of institutional understandings of diagnosis during in-patient treatment. Through interviews with young anorexic girls and their teachers, the author notes the progress of the "anorectic career" unfolding in distinct phases—from committing to a diet to the repercussions of hospitalization and eventual recovery (Darmon, 2008). Taken together, these first-hand accounts of anorexia provide unique insights into the lived experience beyond clinical description, challenging the stereotypes and misconceptions that surround the disorder, and revealing the social, medical, and industrial pressures on subjects to conform to type.

Capitalism and Anorexia

If we consider the body as a political arena on which the hegemonic relationships of the outer world exist (Turner, 1992), then eating disorders must be conceived of as deeply embedded in the capitalist economy. Critical approaches to anorexia nervosa (AN) lay emphasis on how intertwined both term and condition are with the language of entrepreneurship, profit, and risk taking (Malson & Burns, 2009; Miles, 2020). Aside from historical instances of self-starvation, when viewed as a clinical disorder subject to extensive management and exploitation by markets, AN, along with other eating disorders, aligns with the "performative instrumental logic of capitalism" (Tyler & Wilkinson, 2007). Moreover, many of the circumstances around which eating disorders emerge are not ones that neoliberal clients can willingly buy themselves out of, like chronic stress or domestic abuse. Drawing on Ulrich Beck's (1999, 2009) distinctions between pre-modernity's "hazards" and modernity's calculable "risks," Miles (2020) notes how people in neoliberal society must simultaneously steer their way through the seductiveness of consumption and the perils of food production. The manufacturing of psychiatric illnesses requiring individual solutions then sets the scene for the moral judgment of citizens failing to conform to neoliberal and consumer norms. Within the consumer-led, neoliberal healthcare system, individual morality is measured against character and personality types who can manage and mitigate the risks of illness and disease (as in "resilience" or "inner strength"). The outcome of this is that we have morally glorified the slim client who exemplifies self-control and rationality (Gill & Arthurs, 2006), while at the same time separating those with an eating disorder into fighters and losers. Regarding the descriptive language used for anorexia, Wilson (2016) notes how the metaphors used in media and popular literature for EDs often employ militaristic language, addressing power, inner and outer conflict, rebellion, battles, and overcoming the illness, in a similar manner to cancer. For instance, if a woman succumbs to an eating disorder, as seen in cases like fashion models Ana Carolina Reston in 2006 and Isabelle Caro in 2010, the narrative often frames this as "losing the battle" against the condition. Yet, fashion continues to showcase images of ultra slim young models, including those who are well below what might be considered of normal weight in terms of body mass index (BMI).

Anorexia as a malady now exists within a framework that affects individuals across gender, age, and ethnicity (Fraad, 2009; Rodgers et al., 2018). Whereas once it seemed necessary to focus on the "cult of thinness" (Hesse-Biber, 2007) as devised by males for females, these gendered arguments can now distract from a study of neoliberal discourses of power which determine how all those in society must think, behave, and look. The western subject is supposed to know themselves inside out. They are expected to be truly embodied beings within a culture which changes its rules and expectations so rapidly that few subjects can keep up with it. These contradictions are evident in the self-care culture, which preaches the ideals of peace and harmony, while creating expectations around what such a lifestyle might look like and entail. Such expectations are not gender- or age-specific. Young males (Wooldridge & Lytle, 2012) and individuals within the lesbian, gay, bisexual, and transgender communities (Zamantakis & Lackey, 2022) all report body "image" concerns and weight anxieties, and now a need for muscular slimness, indicative of capitalism's "tyranny of the body."

Body politics highlights the way in which we try to control the body by creating boundaries and forcing performance by using the body, not just as a crucial locus of self-construction but as a means of protesting and expressing a range of emotions and struggles (Rodgers et al., 2018). Muldtofte (2018) rejects the notion that the anorectic mind is one out of control or mad. Her personal experience was that her shrinking body was applauded (she was approached by a modeling agency and admired in the gym), and she used her body in a calculated and political way. Instead of a refusal of the body, Muldtofte favors the idea of a series of interconnected practices concerned with mastering the disturbance of needs and signals of the body which seemed to her so claustrophobic. Not eating was a way of breaking with institutional rules, such as the 8 o'clock breakfast or 12 o'clock lunch. In this sense, the author concurs with Delouse and Guattari (1987) in seeing anorexia in terms of a flux of affects which produces micro-political effects contrary to power and control. Anorexia can be viewed as a political act against consumption but also as against being consumed by institutional structures. Essentially, however, this is local-level politics and a solution to an emptiness and a voicelessness; "I did micro-politics by performing the double act of the betrayal of systems that were threatening to constrain me," Muldtofte concludes (p. 18).

Marxist interpretations of anorexia nervosa are scarce, possibly due to the concept's development through an individualistic and family oriented lens. One exception is the work of Oxana Mikhaylova (2023), who draws from personal experiences to examine how macro-level discourses which blame mothers then manifest in micro-level examinations of those diagnosed with an eating disorder. She describes a long tradition of social institutions, which placed physical and emotional responsibility on mothers, backed up by early anorexic studies that linked women's ambitiousness and willingness to abandon family duties in favor of careers as equating with poor maternal parenting. "My mother-blaming behavior was mainly influenced by apparatuses of medicine, church, education, family, and culture," Mikhaylova (2023, p. 3) concludes.

As contact with other bodies becomes more distant and virtual, individuals find it increasingly challenging to discern what is expected of them to gain acceptance, both from themselves and others, in both the real and digital realms. Bombarded by incessant messages about their bodies, they often turn to sources with which they can readily relate—typically those with similar concerns and interests on social media platforms. These so-called "pro-ED" or "pro-Ana" forums have been expanding in scope and influence since the early 1990s (Fox et al., 2005) and, despite extensive criticism of them, appear to be gaining in traction (Tragantzopoulou et al., 2024). Many of the personal accounts online posted by current and former pro-Ana members endorse these mutually subversive behaviors, even while they must use the tools of capitalism which provide them with avenues and spaces for their discussions.

In summary, this chapter underlines the importance of examining AN, not simply in terms of its clinical characteristics, as a product of broader historical, medical, and cultural constructions. That such a condition exists, challenges society to rethink its ideals and question the messages it perpetuates about the connection between mind and body. By examining the ways that meanings, identities, and behaviors are shaped by social interactions and cultural contexts, anorexia nervosa emerges as borne out of broader historical, medical, and cultural constructions. Feminist literature and accounts from those with lived experience of anorexia also provide us with rare insights into the meaning of "being" and "doing" anorexia, as a process that lies far beyond its clinical description. In Chap. 4 we turn to the construction of EDs through classification, social labeling and stigma, medical and therapeutic interventions, and the experiences of patients concerning in-patient treatment and the perceptions of health professionals working in the ED field.

References

Akther, S. F., Molyneaux, E., Stuart, R., Johnson, S., Simpson, A., & Oram, S. (2019). Patients' experiences of assessment and detention under mental health legislation: Systematic review and qualitative meta-synthesis. *BJPsych Open, 5*(3), e37.

American Psychiatric Association (APA). (2013). *Diagnostic and statistical manual of mental disorders: DSM-V* (5th ed.). American Psychiatric Association Publishing.

Arcelus, J., Mitchell, A. J., Wales, J., & Nielsen, S. (2011). Mortality rates in patients with anorexia nervosa and other eating disorders: A meta-analysis of 36 studies. *Archives of General Psychiatry, 68*(7), 724–731.

Banks, C. G. (1992). 'Culture' in culture-bound syndromes: The case of anorexia nervosa. *Social Science & Medicine, 34*(8), 867–884.

Barkty, S. (1988). Foucault, femininity, and the modernization of patriarchal power. In I. Diamond & I. D. Quinby (Eds.), *Feminism and Foucault: Reflections on resistance* (pp. 63–64). Northeastern University Press.

Beck, U. (1999). *World Risk Society*. Polity Press.

Beck, U. (2009). World Risk Society and manufactured uncertainties. *European Journal of Philosophy and Public Debate, 1*, 291–299.

Beech, H. R. (1959). An experimental investigation of sexual symbolism in anorexia nervosa: Employing a subliminal stimulation technique: Preliminary report. *Psychosomatic Medicine, 21*(4), 277–280.

Bell, R. M. (1985). *Holy Anorexia*. University of Chicago Press.

Bemporad, J. R. (1997). Cultural and historical aspects of eating disorders. *Theoretical Medicine, 18*, 401–420.

Bordo, S. (1985). Anorexia nervosa: Psychopathology as the crystallization of culture. *Philosophical Forum, 17*(2), 73–103.

Bordo, S. (1993). *Unbearable weight: Feminism, western culture, and the body*. University of California Press.

Bordo, S. (1994). Feminism, Foucault, and the politics of the body. In *Reconstructing Foucault* (pp. 219–243). Brill.

Bordo, S. (2009). Not justa white girl's thing': The changing face of food and body image problems. In *Critical feminist approaches to eating dis/orders* (pp. 68–82). Routledge.

Brenner, N. (2022). P*sychoanalytic perspective on eating disorder treatment: A qualitative enquiry.* Capella University ProQuest Dissertations Publishing, Retrieved August 22, 2024, from https://www.proquest.com/openview/cce577ab1c91e6f958d6a095579ad311/1?cbl=18750&diss=y&pq-origsite=gscholar

Bruch, H. (1979). *The golden cage: The enigma of anorexia nervosa*. Vintage.
Bruch, H. (1988). *Conversations with anorexics*. Basic.
Brumberg, J. J. (1987). *Fasting Girls: The history of Anorexia Nervosa*. Plume.
Brumberg, J. J. (1997). *The body project. An intimate history of American girls*. Vintage Books.
Bynum, W. C. (1985). Fast, feast, and flesh: The religious significance of food to Medieval Women. *Representations, 11*, 1–25.
Clausen, L. (2020). Perspectives on involuntary treatment of anorexia nervosa. *Frontiers in Psychiatry, 11*, 533288.
Clausen, L., & Jones, A. (2014). A systematic review of the frequency, duration, type and effect of involuntary treatment for people with anorexia nervosa, and an analysis of patient characteristics. *Journal of Eating Disorders, 2*(1), 1–10.
Crisp, A. H. (1980). *Anorexia nervosa: Let me be*. Academic Press.
Darmon, M. (2008). *Devenire anorexique: Une approache sociologue. La Découverte*. Poche/Sciences humaines et sociales.
Darmon, M. (2009). The fifth element: Social class and the sociology of anorexia. *Sociology, 43*(4), 717–733.
Day, K., & Keys, T. (2008). Starving in cyberspace: A discourse analysis of pro-eating-disorder websites. *Journal of Gender Studies, 17*(1), 1–15.
DeJong, H., Broadbent, H., & Schmidt, U. (2011). A systematic review of dropout from treatment in outpatients with anorexia nervosa. *International Journal of Eating Disorders, 45*(5), 635–647.
Dell'Osso, L., Abelli, M., Carpita, B., Pini, S., Castellini, G., Carmassi, C., & Ricca, V. (2016). Historical evolution of the concept of anorexia nervosa and relationships with orthorexia nervosa, autism, and obsessive-compulsive spectrum. *Neuropsychiatric Disease and Treatment, 12*, 1651–1660.
Delouse, G., & Guattari, F. (1987). *A Thousand Plateaus: Capitalism and Schizophrenia*. University of Minnesota Press.
DiNicola, V. F. (1990). Anorexia Multiforme: Self-starvation in historical and cultural context: Part II: Anorexia Nervosa as a culture-reactive syndrome. *Transcultural Psychiatric Research Review, 27*(4), 245–286.
Dobrescu, S. R., Dinkler, L., Gillberg, C., Råstam, M., Gillberg, C., & Wentz, E. (2020). Anorexia nervosa: 30-year outcome. *The British Journal of Psychiatry, 216*(2), 97–104.
Durkheim, E. (1897) [1951]. *Suicide: A study in sociology*. The Free Press.
Edakubo, S., & Fushimi, K. (2020). Mortality and risk assessment for anorexia nervosa in acute-care hospitals: A nationwide administrative database analysis. *BMC Psychiatry, 20*(1).

Escamilla, R. F., & Lisser, H. (1938). Simmonds' Disease (Hypophyseal Cachexia): Clinical report of several cases with discussion of diagnosis and treatment. *Californian and Western Medicine, 48*(5), 343–348.

Forcen, F. E. (2013). Anorexia Mirabilis: The practice of fasting by Saint Catherine of Siena in the Late Middle Ages. *American Journal of Psychiatry, 17*(3), 370–371.

Foucault, M. (1973). *The birth of the clinic. An archaeology of medical perception.* Routledge.

Fox, N., Ward, K., & O'Rourke, A. (2005). Pro-anorexia, weight-loss drugs and the internet: An 'anti-recovery explanatory model of anorexia. *Sociology of Health and Illness, 27*(7), 944–971.

Fraad, H. (2009). Starving and hungry: Anorexia nervosa and the female body politic. *Class Struggle on the Home Front: Work, Conflict and Exploitation in the Household*, 116–136.

Galsworthy-Francis, L., & Allan, S. (2014). Cognitive behavioural therapy for anorexia nervosa: A systematic review. *Clinical Psychology Review, 34*(1), 54–72.

Garner, D. M., Anderson, M. L., Keiper, C. D., Whynott, R., & Parker L. (2016). Psychotropic medications in adult and adolescent eating disorders: Clinical practice versus evidence-based recommendations. *Eating and Weight Disorders, 21*(3), 395–402.

Gill, R., & Arthurs, J. (2006). Editors' introduction: New femininities? *Feminist Media Studies, 6*(4), 443–451.

Gooldin. (2003). Fasting women, living skeletons. *Body and Society, 9*(2), 27–50.

Gordon, R. (2015). The history of Bulimia Nervosa. In *The Wiley handbook of eating disorders* (pp. 25–38). Wiley.

Gueguen, J., Godart, N., Chambry, J., Brun-Eberentz, A., Foulon, C., Divac, S. M., et al. (2012). Severe anorexia nervosa in men: Comparison with severe AN in women and analysis of mortality. *International Journal of Eating Disorders, 45*(4), 537–545.

Guarda, A. S., Pinto, A. M., Coughlin, J. W., Hussain, S., Haug, N. A., & Heinberg, L. J. (2007). Perceived coercion and change in perceived need for admission in patients hospitalized for eating disorders. *American Journal of Psychiatry, 164*(1), 108–114.

Gull, W. W. (1874). Anorexia Nervosa, Apepsia Hysterica, Anorexia Hysterica. *Transactions of the Clinical Society, 7*, 22–27.

Halmi, K. A., et al. (2000). Perfectionism in Anorexia Nervosa: Variation by clinical subtype, obsessionality, and pathological eating behavior. *American Journal of Psychiatry, 157*(11), 1799–1805.

Henderson, A. (1813). *An examination of the imposture of Ann Moore called the Fasting Woman of Tutbury: Illustrated by remarks on other cases of real and pretended abstinence*. J. Moyes.

Hepworth, J. (1999). *The social construction of Anorexia Nervosa*. Sage.

Hesse-Biber, S. N. (2007). *The cult of thinness*. Oxford University Press.

Hesse-Biber, S. N., Howling, S. A., Leavy, P., & Lovejoy, M. (2004). Racial identity and the development of body image issues among African American adolescent girls. *The Qualitative Report, 9*(1), 49–79.

Hilbert, A., Hoek, H. W., & Schmidt, R. (2017). Evidence-based clinical guidelines for eating disorders: International comparison. *Current Opinion in Psychiatry, 30*(6), 423–437.

Holland, J., Hall, N., Yeates, D. G., & Goldacre, M. (2016). Trends in hospital admission rates for anorexia nervosa in Oxford (1968–2011) and England (1990–2011): Database studies. *Journal of the Royal Society of Medicine, 109*(2), 59–66.

Holmes, S. (2016). Between feminism and anorexia: An autoethnography. *International Journal of Cultural Studies, 19*(2), 193–207.

Jones, K., & Zell, M. (2005). The divels speciall instruments': Women and witchcraft before the 'great witch-hunt. *Social History, 30*(1), 45–63.

Kaplan, A. S., & Miles, A. (2016). The role of palliative care in severe and enduring anorexia nervosa. In *Managing severe and enduring anorexia nervosa* (pp. 223–230). Routledge.

Kells, M., Schubert-Bob, P., Nagle, K., Hitchko, L., O'Neil, K., Forbes, P., & McCabe, M. (2017). Meal supervision during medical hospitalization for eating disorders. *Clinical Nursing Research, 26*(4), 525–537.

Keshaviah, A., Edkins, K., Hastings, E. R., Krishna, M., Franko, D. L., Herzog, D. B., et al. (2014). Re-examining premature mortality in anorexia nervosa: A meta-analysis redux. *Comprehensive Psychiatry, 55*(8), 1773–1178.

Lawrence, M. (2008). *The anorexic mind*. Routledge.

Lee, S., Ho, T. P., & Hsu, L. G. (1993). Fat phobic and non-fat phobic anorexia nervosa: A comparative study of 70 Chinese patients in Hong Kong. *Psychological Medicine, 23*(4), 999–1017.

Lester, R. J. (1997). The (dis)embodied self in anorexia nervosa. *Social Science & Medicine (1982), 44*(4), 479–489.

Lucas, A. R., Beard, C. M., O'Fallon, W. M., & Kurland, L. T. (1991). 50-year trends in the incidence of anorexia nervosa in Rochester, Minn: A population-based study. *American Journal of Psychiatry, 148*(7), 917–922.

Malson, H., & Burns, M. (Eds.). (2009). *Critical feminist approaches to eating dis/orders*. Routledge.

Mantel, H. (2014). The heart fails without warning. In *The assassination of Margaret Thatcher and other stories*. Fourth Estate.

Mehanna, H. M., Moledina, J., & Travis, J. (2008). Refeeding syndrome: What it is, and how to prevent and treat it. *British Medical Journal, 336*(7659), 1495–1498.

Mehler, P. S., & Andersen, A. E. (Eds.). (2022). *Eating disorders: A comprehensive guide to medical care and complications*. JHU Press.

Mikhaylova, O. (2023). Mother blaming and anorexia: How ideological state apparatuses have informed my perception of my mother's role in the formation of my eating disorder. *Feminism & Psychology, 33*(1), 3–22.

Miles, K. (2020). Anorexia Nervosa: A late modern mind game. *Critical Reflections: A Student Journal on Contemporary Sociological Issues*. ojs.leedsbeckett.ac.uk

Mitchell, D. (1980). Anorexia nervosa. *The Arts in Psychotherapy, 7*, 53–60.

Moncrieff-Boyd, J. M. (2016). *"Vile bodies": Disgust, self-disgust, their measurement and prevalence in eating disorders*. Doctoral thesis, The University of Western Australia. https://research-repository.uwa.edu.au/en/publications/vile-bodies-disgust-self-disgust-their-measurement-and-prevalence

Muldtofte, L. (2018). The grace of my perfect skeleton: An autoethnographic analysis of the anorexic body. *Capacious: Journal for Emerging Affect Inquiry, 1*(3), 2–15.

National Institute for Clinical Excellence (NICE). (2021). *Eating disorders recognition and treatment*. Retrieved August 22, 2024, from https://www.nice.org.uk/guidance/ng69/chapter/Recommendation

O'Connell, L. (2023). Being and doing anorexia nervosa. An autoethnography of diagnostic identity and performance of illness. *Health (London, England: 1997), 27*(2), 263–278.

Orbach, S. (1986). *Hunger Strike: The Anorectic's struggle as a metaphor for our age*. Faber & Faber.

Paolacci, S., Kiani, A. K., Manara, E., Beccari, T., Ceccarini, M. R., Stuppia, L., et al. (2020). Genetic contributions to the etiology of anorexia nervosa: New perspectives in molecular diagnosis and treatment. *Molecular Genetics & Genomic Medicine, 8*(7), e1244.

Rodgers, R. F., Berry, R., & Franko, D. L. (2018). Eating disorders in ethnic minorities: An update. *Current Psychiatry Reports, 20*, 1–11.

Saya, A., Brugnoli, C., Piazzi, G., Liberato, D., Di Ciaccia, G., Niolu, C., & Siracusano, A. (2019). Criteria, procedures, and future prospects of involuntary treatment in psychiatry around the world: A narrative review. *Frontiers in Psychiatry, 10*, 271.

Schaumberg, K., Welch, E., Breithaupt, L., Hübel, C., Baker, J. H., Munn-Chernoff, M. A., et al. (2017). The science behind the academy for eating disorders' nine truths about eating disorders. *European Eating Disorders Review, 25*(6), 432–450.

Scull, A. (2022). *Desperate remedies. Psychiatry and the mystery of mental illness*. Penguin Books.

Seed, T., Fox, J. R., & Berry, K. (2016). The experience of involuntary detention in acute psychiatric care. A review and synthesis of qualitative studies. *International Journal of Nursing Studies, 61*, 82–94.

Seitz, J., Herpertz-Dahlmann, B., & B., & Konrad, K. (2016). Brain morphological changes in adolescent and adult patients with anorexia nervosa. *Journal of Neural Transmission, 123*(2016), 949–959.

Silverman, J. A. (1985). Richard Morton, 1637–2698, limner of anorexia nervosa: His life and times: A tercentenary essay. *Journal of Psychiatric Research, 19*(2–3), 83–88.

Silverman, J. A. (1987). An eighteenth-century account of self-starvation in a male. *International Journal of Eating Disorders, 6*(3), 431–433.

Silverman, J. A. (1989). Louis-Victor Marcé, 1828–1864: Anorexia nervosa's forgotten man. *Psychology of Medicine, 19*(4), 833–835.

Silverman, J. A. (1992). Lasègue's editorial riposte to Gull's contributions on anorexia nervosa. *Psychology of Medicine, 22*(2), 307–308.

Simpson, K. J. (2002). Anorexia nervosa and culture. *Journal of Psychiatric and Mental Health Nursing, 9*(1), 65–71.

Smink, F. R., van Hoeken, D., Donker, G. A., Susser, E. S., Oldehinkel, A. J., & Hoek, H. W. (2016). Three decades of eating disorders in Dutch primary care: Decreasing incidence of bulimia nervosa but not of anorexia nervosa. *Psychological Medicine, 46*(6), 1189–1196.

Stapleton, K., Evans, S. L., & Rhys, C. S. (2019). Ana as god: Religion, interdiscursivity and identity on pro-ana websites. *Discourse & Communication, 13*(3), 320–341.

Steinglass, J. E., Berner, L. A., & Attia, E. (2019). Cognitive neuroscience of eating disorders. *Psychiatric Clinics, 42*(1), 75–91.

Swartz, L. (1985). Anorexia nervosa as a culture-bound syndrome. *Social Science & Medicine, 20*(7), 725–730.

Taub, D. E. (2011). Eating disorders as deviance. In C. D. Bryant (Ed.), *Routledge handbook of deviant behavior* (pp. 298–305). Routledge.

Thornton, L. M., Welch, E., Munn-Chernoff, M. A., Lichtenstein, P., & Bulik, C. M. (2016). Anorexia Nervosa, Major Depression, and suicide attempts: Shared genetic factors. *Suicide & Life-threatening Behavior, 46*(5), 525–534.

Tragantzopoulou, P., Fixsen, A., Cheshire, A., & Ridge, D. (2024). 'You are not alone, we've got you': Powerplays, devotion and punishment on healthy eating and pro-eating disorder websites. *Qualitative Health Research*. https://doi.org/10.1177/10497323241238628

Turner, B. S. (1992). *Regulating bodies: Essays in medical sociology*. Routledge.

Tyler, M., & Wilkinson, A. (2007). The tyranny of corporate slenderness: Corporate anorexia as a metaphor for our age. *Work, Employment and Society, 21*(3), 537–549.

Umezulike, C. C. (2020). *The meaning-centred anorexic body: A human rights-based approach to involuntary treatment*. Doctoral thesis, Birkbeck, University of London.

van Eeden, A. E., van Hoeken, D., & Hoek, H. W. (2021). Incidence, prevalence and mortality of anorexia nervosa and bulimia nervosa. *Current Opinion in Psychiatry, 34*(6), 515–524.

Wade, T. D., Bulik, C. M., Neale, M., & Kendler, K. S. (2000). Anorexia nervosa and major depression: Shared genetic and environmental risk factors. *American Journal of Psychiatry, 157*(3), 469–471.

Walker, C. (2003). *Gender and politics in early modern Europe*. Palgrave Macmillan.

Wilson, S. (2016). Anorexia and its metaphors. *Exchanges: The Warwick Research Journal, 3*(2), 216–226. Retrieved September 22, 2023, from: http://exchanges.warwick.ac.uk/index.php/exchanges/article/view/84

Wolf, N. (1991). *The beauty myth: How images of beauty are used against women*. Morrow.

Wolf, N. (1994). *Fire with fire: The new female power and how to use it*. Fawcett Columbine.

Wonderlich, S. A., Lilenfeld, L. R., Riso, L. P., Engel, S., & Mitchell, J. E. (2005). Personality and anorexia nervosa. *International Journal of Eating Disorders, 37*(S1), S68–S71.

Wooldridge, T., & Lytle, P. (2012). An overview of anorexia nervosa in males. *Eating Disorders, 20*(5), 368–378.

World Health Organization. (2019). *International Classification of Diseases 10th revision: Ch. 5 Mental and behavioural disorders.* Retrieved August 22, 2024, from https://icd.who.int/browse10/2019/en#/F50.0

Yager, J. (2020). Managing patients with severe and enduring anorexia nervosa: When is enough, enough? *The Journal of Nervous and Mental Disease, 208*(4), 277–282.

Zamantakis, A., & Lackey, D. (2022). Dying to be (a) gendered: An exploratory content analysis of trans/nonbinary people's experiences with eating disorders. *Sociological Inquiry, 92*, 870–893.

4

ED Diagnosis and Therapeutic Frameworks

A medical diagnosis is a powerful thing. It can open the door to certain possibilities while simultaneously closing the door to others. Categories such as diagnoses are regarded as important to humans because they break up the continuum of nature into manageable parts. Diagnoses can provide an overarching structure to the experience of illness and punctuate the illness journey. As stated by Jutel (2011), diagnoses can create collective identities, removing the individual from the isolation of the suffering, and providing the person with new potential networks with support. Viewed through the lens of therapy, a diagnosis can enable a client to separate their "real self" from the "illness" (e.g., anorexia nervosa) blighting their own and their families' lives. Yet, beneath the surface of medical diagnosis lies the realm of human judgment, wherein certain beliefs and behaviors are categorized as deviant[1] or pathological. In the case of disordered eating, understanding the multidimensional nature of the diagnostic process is crucial due to its potential to propel the individual on a journey which may be involving distressing procedures, loss

[1] The term "deviance" may seem strange when used in the context of eating disorders. However, sociologists such as Becker (1963) used deviance to describe something not objectively real or tangible but created and recreated through human interaction.

A. Fixsen, *The Construction of Eating Disorders*, The Politics of Mental Health and Illness, https://doi.org/10.1007/978-3-031-70318-8_4

of personal liberty, and a host of unintended consequences. This chapter takes a critical approach to the present diagnostic system, focusing on the power structures inherent in its processes and then highlighting gaps in funding, communication, and long-term support within the current UK mental health system.[2] After presenting an overview of ED diagnosis and treatment, empirical work on perceptions of professionals working in the ED field is discussed. Findings from these studies indicate an ideological and practical divide concerning the use of diagnostic labels by those in the field. Diagnostic labels were seen as reductive but essential within the present system, while anecdotal evidence that labels like AN were sought after by patients deterred some practitioners from referring to these terms directly in patient consultations.

Diagnostic Labeling and Stigma

Sociologists of medicine have had to consider in the course of their work, whether to assume the role of accomplice or critic to health care professions and their medical processes (Conrad & Barker, 2010). In the area of medicine, the positivist view of mental illness as scientifically reducible to its constituent parts has generally prevailed. Social constructionists, on the other hand, argue that bio diagnoses are never morally or ethically neutral (Conrad & Barker, 2010), hence mental disorder categories themselves cannot entirely and faithfully mirror the objective realities they pertain to describe (Weinberg, 2021). In every day health practice, striking a balance between enhancing detection methods and avoiding over diagnosis and the stigmatization and discomfort accompanying certain psychiatric labels and allied treatments is fraught with ethical and human rights considerations. While some may welcome a diagnosis, the absence or presence of a particular diagnosis inevitably shapes how a person feels about themselves and is subsequently treated and looked at by professionals, relatives, and associates. The diagnosis itself creates an interpretive wall between a patient's lived experience of pain and discomfort and the

[2] In England, a 54 percent increase in referrals to public mental health services from 2016 to 2022 was accompanied by merely a 10.9 percent real-term increase in service funding.

physician's medically and technologically mediated picture of a "disease" (McGann et al., 2011). Moreover, after being given a professional diagnosis, the person is expected to fully engage in the "regimes of patienthood" (Jeske et al., 2024) and play the part of the "good patient" (Parsons, 1975), while also learning to adequately manage their own symptoms outside of institutional support and care. Following an ED diagnosis, patients may still attempt to hide their condition or resist prescribed treatments, resulting in friction and frustration on the part of the prescribing practitioner (Halmi, 2013). The diagnostic process is also deeply tied into resource allocation (Jeske et al., 2024) legitimizing and supporting those with certain conditions, while, through failure to acknowledge the existence of others, excluding them from medical care or financial backing. Those who fail to engage in treatment may be subject to disciplinary procedures, for example, a person diagnosed with schizophrenia who refuses to attend appointments or to take their medicine could find themselves forcibly detained. All these factors make giving a diagnosis much more than simply assigning a diagnostic name or "label" to a condition.

Labeling theory was brought to notice by Howard Becker (1963) who explained how social groups create deviance by making rules whose infringement creates deviance, then apply those rules to particular people, essentially labeling them as "outsiders." This theory has since been widely applied to mental illnesses[3] and has not lost its power. One of the issues associated with psychiatric "labels" is their propensity to perpetuate or create negative attitudes and stigma (Saguy & Gruys, 2010) toward and within those who are given a psychiatric diagnosis (Goffman, 1963; Hazell et al., 2022; Puhl & Suh, 2015). Corrigan and Watson (2002) noted how the stigma of mental illness carries the double misfortune of a lack of public understanding and a pervasive cultural stigma. In the last two decades much work has been done to reduce stigma though public education and mental health campaigns (Hazell et al., 2022). Yet arguably, it is only the more moderate forms of mental distress that have been destigmatized, while more serious disorders such as schizophrenia and

[3] Thomas Scheff (1966), an early proponent of labeling theory, directly linked the emergence of mental illness to societal reaction and its labeling. Others such as Link et al. (1989) proposed a modified labeling theory which suggests that labeling does have negative outcomes but does not directly produce a mental disorder.

psychosis are still widely viewed with fear and suspicion. Perversely, a belief in increased public awareness, along with an emphasis on positive thinking, has contributed to a pathologizing of self-stigma (Link et al., 2015). Those who feel negatively about themselves may therefore be portrayed as irrational or paranoid for seeing themselves as singled out and treated unfavorably by society and the medical profession. Similarly, since "insight" is seen as occurring when an afflicted person can *identify* themselves as mentally ill, a person may be shamed or stigmatized for failing to acknowledge or report personal mental health or eating issues. This is despite the fact that, in the present climate of reduced mental health funding, they may be unlikely to receive prompt or adequate treatment for their problems (BEAT, 2023).

Difference in societal terms appears to be sufficient reason for people to be ostracized and marginalized, on account of their weight, size, appearance, intelligence, or ability. Yet, while much research has documented the prevalence and negative health implications of stigma attached to having a mental health diagnosis, little has been written about stigma in relation to eating disorders. Obesity is known to be a significant source of social and self-directed stigma (Durso & Latner, 2008; Sikorski et al., 2011), and anti-fat attitudes to affect life chances and work opportunities (O'brien et al., 2008). Social attitudes to EDs in general appear more complex. One study found that individuals with eating disorders (EDs) were viewed as responsible for their disorder and were seen as more likely to be seeking attention than people with a disorder such as depression (Roehrig & McLean, 2010). However, attitudes were also found to be ambiguous, with some perceiving certain aspects of EDs such as weight loss as beneficial or even admirable. Yet the messages encouraging persons to come forward for diagnosis and treatment are far more dominant in contemporary western societies, with organisations such as BEAT (2023) in the UK urging people to seek medical help for disordered eating patterns. Many point out the benefits of having a psychiatric label in terms of validation (Wright et al., 2011), with studies suggesting that service users often expect or even demand a diagnostic label from practitioners, both for self-confirmation and to gain access to professional help (Kendell & Jablensky, 2003). This suggests that complex social and psychological factors need to be considered in relation to the medical labelling of an individual with an ED.

The "end goal" of ED diagnosis is another contested area. While it is recognized that ED "presentations" are complex, what is expected in terms of mode and length of treatment following an initial diagnosis will vary according to present policy guidelines, along with factors such as available financial and medical resources, and social support. Faced with these dilemmas, researchers and clinicians are constantly working on developing more accurate diagnostic scales along with more cost-effective treatment strategies. While the ideal end point may be set at full recovery, this may be neither realistic nor something which is wholly sought after by the patient themselves. Both clinical and personal memoire ED literature present a spectrum of experiences (Bullitt-Jonas, 2000), including scenarios in which individuals may not return to "normal" eating but lear to manage the chronic cycle of disordered eating (D'Abundo & Chally, 2004). Given the different meanings that people can attribute to treatment experiences, sociological studies have focused more on the treatment "journey," including how the person under study goes about performing their role as the "anorexic" to navigate their way through tortuous social and institutional settings (Darmon, 2008; O'Connell, 2023).

Diagnostic Institutions

So far in the book, it has been emphasized that eating disorders, at least as we conceive of them, are constructed by powerful institutions. Traditional psychiatry has taken a unitary approach to mental disorders and a Cartesian[4] view of human life: one of separating the mind from the body and body parts from one another. Diagnosis is regarded as the very backbone of medical practice, with diagnostic accuracy at the heart of medical research. While aspects of medical institutions such as their modern architecture, greater diversification and specialization of roles, and widespread use of technologies are relatively recent developments, other institutional features remain. The political demand for "patient-centeredness" has not diminished the ultimate authority of the medical profession over a person's body or their medical status. Psychiatric

[4] Relating to the ideas of Rene Descartes and metaphysical dualism (mind and body as distinct).

categorization, as laid out in the DSM by an "expert" committee (APA, 2013), continues to largely determine the way that EDs are detected, assessed, discussed, and managed in medical institutions. Psychiatric discourse, through a social diffusion process, also largely shapes the ways that EDs are discussed in health education, and (as illustrated in chapters 7 & 8) are portrayed in media, film, literature and the arts. Medical sociology is a possible exception to this largely consensual discourse,[5] as debates within it have been decidedly polemic over the issue of diagnosis (Weinberg, 2021). Some sociologists continue to adopt the language of psychiatry; however, others have strongly contested the idea of diagnoses as neutral concepts, emphasizing instead their central role in the wider process of medicalization (Conrad & Barker, 2010; Conrad & Schneider, 1980) and the links between the various DSM committees and institutions and corporations wielding political, pharmaceutical, legal, and economic power (Cohen, 2016; Horwitz, 2012, 2021).[6] It is primarily due to these links that psychiatric categories and classifications have demonstrated remarkable success in recent decades, with much of this happening in relational and institutional spheres outside of the psychiatric profession (Dellwing & Harbusch, 2022). Psychiatric diagnoses today are not just the objects of psychiatry and other medical professions (Darmon, 2008), they are one of the principal ways in which members of society have come to "interpret, regulate and mediate various forms of self-understanding and activity" (Brinkmann, 2016, p. 2). The effects of diagnosis extend far beyond the initial patient/practitioner interaction. How a diagnosis is translated into treatment and is acted upon by employers, medical insurance companies, educational establishments, and criminal justice departments, has repercussions not just for individuals but everyone (as patients, workers and taxpayers). The contemporary diagnostic system plays a central role in shaping the economy, creating numerous opportunities for health, medical and therapeutic

[5] Although some of psychiatry's fiercest critics have also come from within its ranks, for example, Thomas Szasz (1960).

[6] While psychiatry may attest to having had a long-term fascination with the determinants of mental health across disorders (Kirkbride et al., 2024), its close association with institutions such as the pharmaceutical and biotechnological industries suggests that the psychiatry's focus remains that of observing, diagnosing, and medicating individuals.

markets. As Jutel (2011) points out, a diagnosis provides fodder for exploitation: medical, commercial, political, and personal. Exploitation is not restricted to the pharmaceutical industry; manufacturers of medical equipment, media, complementary therapies, nutritional supplements, food products, and biotechnologies all hope to gain from the expanding medical diagnoses.

While psychiatric diagnoses are institutional abstractions, the distresses they seek to describe are experienced by persons on an everyday level. As Sedgwick (1982) stated, debates regarding the existence or not of mental illness should not divert attention from the need for adequate health and welfare provision for all in society. Living with disordered eating can be devastating and disabling, and can have a profound effect on family, friends, and professional care givers. EDs are no longer seen as "diseases of affluence" (van Eeden et al., 2021) and have particularly adverse outcomes for those who cannot afford, or who are denied, access to treatment (Moreno et al., 2023). Persons with an ED have lower employment participation, greater absenteeism, higher healthcare and informal care costs, and greater lost lifetime earnings than the general population (Santomauro et al., 2021). The rise in EDs has also mirrored a general increase in the estimated numbers of persons with a mental health disorder across the world. According to Public Health England, in 2016 mental and substance misuse disorders accounted for 21.3 percent of the total morbidity burden in England (GOV.UK, 2018). Mental distress is not an individual concern; rather, it is aligned with social inequities including poverty, migration, extreme stress, exposure to violence (domestic, sexual, and gender-based), emergency and conflict situations, natural disasters, trauma, and low social support. Eating disorders appear to be no different in that they are multifaceted, with the expansion of categories meaning that they are likely to be part of a wider picture of intersectionality[7], that has yet to be fully understood. In the face of these caveats, it seems important to gain some appreciation of current discourse around eating disorders in terms of their classification and distribution, and this is the topic of the following section.

[7] Intersectionality relates to the way in which different types of discrimination and unfair treatment based on sex, race, social class, etc., are interconnected to each other.

ED Classification and Distribution

In recent years, the number of diagnoses for an eating disorder (ED) is said to have reached alarming, and global proportions (Erskine et al., 2016). According to the National Eating Disorders Association (NEDA, 2022), an estimated 20 million women and 10 million men in the US will experience a clinically significant eating disorder at some point in their lives. These figures do not simply equate to a greater prevalence of disordered eating patterns, they illustrate how diagnostic categorization and detection strategies have evolved. DSM-V (APA, 2013) and ICD-10 (WHO, 2019)[8] are considered the main repositories of information on the recognized feeding and eating disorders. DSM-V defines these as "characterized by a persistent disturbance of eating or eating related behavior that results in the altered consumption or absorption of food, and that significantly impairs, physical health or psychosocial functioning" (APA, 2013, p. 326). Anorexia nervosa (AN), the oldest recognized eating disorder, is characterized by deliberate weight loss, intense fear of gaining weight, and distorted body image. Individuals with AN typically use one or more of three strategies for weight loss: food restriction, purging and vomiting, use of laxatives, and excessive exercise (Fisher et al., 2010). DSM-V did away with the amenorrhea (absence of menstruation) criterion for AN, and the weight threshold was marginally increased (Jenkins et al., 2021).

Bulimia nervosa (BN) is characterized by frequent binge eating followed by purging to prevent weight gain (APA, 2013). Unlike anorexia nervosa (AN), individuals with BN may not be underweight, but they can transition between conditions. Purging by vomiting or use of laxatives can lead to severe dehydration and gastrointestinal problems (Zhao & Encinosa, 2011), increasing the risk of hospitalization and even death. First included as a full diagnostic entity in DSM-V (APA, 2013), binge eating disorder (BED) involves regular binge eating episodes during

[8] The ICD is a diagnostic classification system published by the World Health Organization. It is used to collect and compare morbidity and mortality statistics across the world. Chapter V *Mental and Behavioural Disorders* contains a subsection F50 on eating disorders. ICD-10 (2019) categories largely mirror those in DSM-V, although atypical categories for anorexia and bulimia are also listed.

which individuals ingest comparably large amounts of food and experience loss of control over their eating behavior. Body mass index (BMI) of people with BN and BED may be within the normal range, yet both conditions are associated with a host of psychological, physiological, and social complications. Mortality rates in those with BN are considered significant relative to the general population (Chesney et al., 2014), while studies suggest that BED can considerably impair quality of life and in the longer-term lead to obesity and Type II Diabetes (Giel et al., 2022).

The category Eating Disorders Not Otherwise Specified (EDNOS) first appeared in DSM-IV-TR (APA, 2000) to incorporate cases which fail to fulfill the diagnostic criteria for AN or BN. Described as a "broad hodgepodge that includes many heterogeneous and not well-defined ED cases" (Riesco et al., 2018), EDNOS rapidly became the most common disorder among those seeking treatment at ED facilities (Machado & Rodrigues, 2019). DSM-V reconfigured and renamed this broad category as Other Specified Feeding and Eating Disorder (OSFED). OSFED includes more borderline categories such as atypical anorexia nervosa (atypical-AN), purging disorder (PD), subthreshold bulimia nervosa (Sub-BN), subthreshold binge eating disorder (Sub-BED), and night eating syndrome (NES). Avoidant Restrictive Food Intake Disorder (ARFID) was another addition to DSM-V. Its main diagnostic feature is avoidance or restriction of food intake manifested by significant failure to meet requirements for nutrition and insufficient energy oral intake of food with consequent weight loss or failure to gain weight, without a preoccupation with body weight or body image distortion (Claudino et al., 2019). A high percentage of children and adults diagnosed with autism are also diagnosed with ARFID (Yule et al., 2021).

The distribution of the different EDs over time and the expansion of diagnoses are inextricably linked. Data from surveys suggest that the occurrence of AN has remained relatively consistent over recent decades (Santomauro et al., 2021), while BED and OSFED now make up by far the bulk of cases (Hay et al., 2017; Santomauro et al., 2021). The distribution of EDs across age groups and locations has also notably shifted, with the number of cases of AN and BED in persons under 15 years of age having increased (Santomauro et al., 2021; Smink et al., 2012). Eating disorders are still largely identified in young women; however, the gender gap may be diminishing and is potentially overestimated (Hoek, 2016). Recent studies suggest that approximately a quarter of identified cases are now found in males (Sweeting et al., 2015), with men representing up to 36 percent of BED cases (NEDA, 2023). Of the male cases ascertained by NEDA, 15 percent identified as gay or bisexual. A history of dieting or obesity and participation in a sport or occupation that emphasizes muscularity or thinness were all associated with a subsequent ED diagnosis in male patients (Murray et al., 2016). Risk factors in men included a history of military service or being in prison (Tyler et al., 2019), while disordered eating in older males often goes unreported and is still a scantly researched area (Murray et al., 2016). The prevalence of comorbidity in those with eating disorders has been emphasized in many studies. Research around unspecified eating disorders remains in its infancy; however, around 80 percent of those with OSFED and BED are considered as qualifying for at least one other DSM listed disorder (Kessler et al., 2013).

Since DSM-I first described anorexia nervosa as a "psychophysiologic gastro-intestinal reaction," and placed it alongside other gastrointestinal disorders considered as emotional in origin, the gastric element of eating disorders has continued to be recognized as an element of the patient's psychopathology. In Salvioli et al.'s study (2013), gastrointestinal disturbances were reported in 96 percent of those diagnosed with an eating disorder. The authors concluded that digestive symptoms in these patients were signs of the "neurotic hysteric" which implied a "lack of insight" but improved following an appropriate "psycho-nutritional rehabilitation cycle" program (p. 643). This account of gastric complaints by Salvioli et al. might reflect the fact that many patients had been diagnosed with Irritable Bowel Syndrome (IBS), a condition which has often been met with disbelief or treated as a minor issue in patient encounters with their healthcare professionals (Björkman et al., 2016). Other recent studies have uncovered a connection between immunobiological gastric conditions and having a diagnosis for an ED. A review by Sato and Fukudo (2015) indicated that individuals with EDs present with a variety of gastrointestinal complaints including severe constipation, bowel obstruction, acute gastric dilatation, gastric perforation, and dyspepsia. Not only are gastric symptoms commonly reported in people diagnosed with virtually every type of eating disorder (Wiklund et al., 2021), these gastric symptoms may be far from minor. Yelencich et al.'s (2022) study of people with Crohn's disease, ulcerative colitis, and other forms of inflammatory bowel disease (IBD) illustrates how likely it is that patients with serious gastrointestinal diseases would also fit the criteria for avoidant restrictive food intake disorder (ARFID). Far from being "neurotic," based on their pain history, a fear of eating certain food groups might seem a perfectly rational choice for some in this group. In addition to the DSM/ICD diagnostic categories, attempts have been made to classify longstanding and severe EDs as "severe and enduring eating disorders", or "SEED" (Robinson et al., 2015). This is partly in recognition that some people with an ED such as anorexia nervosa may experience persisting, unresolved symptoms, with varying severity and impact on quality of life, which may not respond to treatment. Nevertheless, studies suggest that the long-term prognosis for AN patients need not be dire; over 50 per cent of hospitalized AN patients made a full recovery in one 21-year prospective study (Zipfel et al., 2000).

Treatment and Support

According to Strober (2010), the one uncontroversial fact about anorexia nervosa is that it very rarely resolves quickly. Eating disorders as an illness category are considered very difficult conditions to treat for many reasons, including because individuals may be of a young age, they may conceal the severity of their condition or may hold a belief that they are not sick enough to need treatment. An underlying fear of gaining weight can be a significant barrier to treatment, particularly in anorexia nervosa. Of all the psychiatric conditions, EDs have the highest rate of mortality (Zhao & Encinosa, 2011). Stigma still overshadows EDs, with misconceptions about their causes hampering knowledge advancements, misdirecting lay perceptions of these conditions, and preventing those in need from seeking help (Ali et al., 2017). BED appears to carry the greatest stigma, meaning that sufferers are thought to considerably under-utilize available healthcare services (Mond et al., 2007). Individuals with EDs frequently display multiple forms of distress with the risk of self-harm estimated to be over seven times higher in those with eating disorders in comparison to the general population (John et al., 2021). Alcohol and substance use are also thought to commonly coexist with eating disorders (Franko et al., 2008; Root et al., 2010), while suicide remains a leading cause of death in individuals diagnosed with AN (Goldstein & Gvion, 2019). Treatment failure and relapse are common after completing treatment, and a substantial proportion of patients develop severe and enduring symptoms. Given the importance attached to early intervention, the usual time from the start of an eating disorder and treatment initiation may seem unreasonably long, and many people will not receive any treatment (Griffiths et al., 2018; Kazdin et al., 2017).

The treatment decision made by a psychiatrist or practitioner is seen as crucial and as directly impacting on a patient's care and outcomes. Typically, the doctor or GP (general practitioner) is the first point of contact; however, GPs may, in their patient's estimation, lack sufficient understanding of this area or come across as pessimistic concerning the outcomes of treatment. In several studies of patient experiences of AN treatments, participants found their health practitioners over-focused on weight and food, with an overemphasis on rigid, short-term CBT treatment and offering insufficient "holistic" care (Escobar-Koch, et al., 2010; Rance et al., 2017). The traditional model of treatment delivery for eating disorders is based on a psychotherapeutic intervention delivered by a trained professional in a treatment setting context (e.g., clinic, private office, or hospital). Cognitive behavioral therapy (CBT), dialectical behavior therapy (DBT), and family based treatment (FBT) have shown degrees of efficacy in studies of various eating disorder populations (Fisher et al., 2010; NICE, 2021). Medical and nutritional interventions are also required to address the physiological consequences of malnutrition and to restore physical health. However, access to specialized care, financial constraints, and societal stigma continue to impede the delivery of timely and appropriate treatment. Comprehensive school-based programs and community outreach campaigns are considered to play a pivotal role in raising awareness and promoting early intervention (NEDA, 2023).

In-patient care is considered more disruptive, more costly, and usually involves a longer time on a waiting list than outpatient care (Frostad & Benz, 2022). Hospitalization for an eating disorder is relatively rare, and admission to the acute medical setting is often said to be done to save a life. Typically, this involves medical treatments including electrolyte replacement, electrocardiograph monitoring, oral tube feeding, and monitoring of refeeding syndrome (see also Chap. 3). The odds of being hospitalized increased in one study with younger age, lower BMI percentile, a diagnosis of anorexia nervosa, higher number of social risk factors, and a diagnosis of self-harm (Kemp et al., 2023). The unique needs of males, such as increased stigmatization, gender role conflicts, and feelings of emasculation, also need to be factored into long-term treatment and support plans. According to Robinson et al. (2013), hospitalizations of male patients with eating disorders saw an increase of 53 percent from 1999 to 2009 in the US.

For patients themselves, hospitalization for an eating disorder can be a deeply distressing experience and can exacerbate existing trauma or lead to new trauma. A range of factors contribute to this experience including loss of autonomy, invasion of privacy, disruption of routines and rituals, the stigma and shame of hospitalization (Troop et al., 2008), and previous experiences of mental health treatments (Kazdin et al., 2017). Men in studies appear to hold particularly negative views of health interventions (Vogel & Heath, 2016). In one study, involuntary treatment for an ED was perceived as traumatic and punitive, with practitioners regarded as lacking understanding/education, blaming patients, and overemphasizing the physical dimensions of the illness (Bannatyne & Stapleton, 2018). Nevertheless, not everyone's experiences of hospitalization will be negative, and in retrospect patients may be grateful for the care they received when they were in crisis. Holmes (2016), in her autoethnography, describes her time in the clinic as "not only overwhelmingly positive, but one of the best times of my life." She notes, however, that it was not just the medical and psychiatric interventions that she found helpful but "rather the wonderful simplicity of female company, community, laughter, and empathy—and a place to *be*—which provided the foundations for recovery" (Holmes, 2016, p. 206).

Following the emphasis on remote and self-help treatment of mental health issues, online therapy platforms for EDs have become common practice. Studies of Internet-mediated treatment suggest they can be an effective means of delivering psychological treatment for an ED (Machado

& Rodrigues, 2019). Findings from recent studies of self-help interventions in the treatment of bulimic disorders have been promising and support its use across the stages of the care pathway (Yim & Schmidt, 2019). A systematic review and multiregression analysis of manualized self-help for BN and BED concluded that treatments for these conditions were effective in cases where all aspects of the delivery were considered carefully (Beintner et al., 2014). However, these positive findings on online interventions are largely based on ease of use and lower delivery costs, while their long-term efficacy and utility compared to traditional face-to-face treatments for eating disorders has yet to be established.

Support and treatment are not synonymous. While acute treatment for eating disorders is inevitably focused on medical stabilization, a sustained, holistic, and individualized approach to support, with the social, emotional, and relational aspects of care, is highlighted in studies involving both ED patients and health professionals (Corral-Liria et al., 2022). The assumption is often that the more avenues of support the better, but for those diagnosed with an ED this may not necessarily be the case. Peer support is a complex issue, especially as advice given by peers can conflict with medical opinion (Keski-Rahkonen et al., 2009). Conflicting and alternative advice is especially common on the so-called pro-ED social media forums, where "tips and tricks" on how to achieve further weight loss or purge more effectively are exchanged (Martin, 2004), and seeking professional help is often actively discouraged (Roulea & von Ranson, 2011; Tragantzopoulou et al., 2024). In the absence of other forms of emotional support or ones not treated with suspicion, millions of young people with disordered eating are drawn to these sites, either as silent browsers or active participants (Fairplay, 2022).

Continued support beyond clinical "recovery" is vitally important, as the lives of people with disordered eating may continue to be blighted by the effects of past trauma, difficult life circumstances, and the longer-term effects of treatment. People with a history of disordered eating frequently suffer from experiences of isolation, related to a lack of social support, and a history of toxic relationships (Bray et al., 2022). Many of those subsequently diagnosed with an ED have suffered sexual and/or childhood abuse (Feldman & Mayer, 2007; Mangweth-Matzek & Hoek, 2017) with disordered eating sometimes spanning a lifetime (Micali et al., 2017). One study examining the recovery status in people diagnosed with bulimia nervosa (BN) found they had significantly fewer friends and family members available to provide emotional support and that support provided by relatives was considered unsatisfactory (Rorty et al., 1999). Participants in another study of recovery from BN pointed out the difficulties and importance of being able to accept the help and support being offered. Social support was seen as different from going into treatment because treatment could take a long time and was not seen as synonymous with "help" (Lindgren et al., 2015). Many of those who have "clinically recovered" from BN in terms of abstaining from bingeing and purging continue to experience psychological distress for a long time (Keski-Rahkonen et al., 2009). In a study by Copperman (2000), men reported difficulty discussing their disordered eating with peers but also lacked recognition from GPs, support from family and friends, and experienced poor access to services. Better treatments and public awareness campaigns may be slowly improving this situation; nevertheless, relatively few studies have paid attention to actual availability and utility of informal support mechanisms.

Experiences and Perceptions of ED Professionals

In recent years there has been a growing interest in studying how health professionals and those in allied sectors experience and cope with the stresses and dilemmas of work in the ED sector. Health professionals are expected to act as both care providers and gatekeepers for patients, balance out short- and long-term goals, liaise with family members, keep up to date with education and training, and generally play the part of the "good doctor" or health provider. Studies of healthcare professionals suggest that even experienced staff can have difficulties in accurately identifying complications of disordered eating behaviors and can misattribute their causes (Currin et al., 2007, 2009). In 2017, the UK Parliamentary and Health Service Ombudsman presented a report addressing the gaps of ED services in the country, pointing out the lack of serious training that professionals working in healthcare receive. Similarly, Brelet et al. (2021) highlighted a low and insufficient knowledge of GPs of different countries across the world about diagnostic criteria and available treatments for ED patients.

Studying the views and lived experiences of professionals who work with people with eating disorders is important, both to understand the treatment gaps and the emotional and logistical challenges, and because the quality of the clinician-client relationship is considered to have a significant influence on patient outcomes (Graves et al., 2017). As part of a project on eating disorders, we (myself, students, and colleagues at a London university) conducted a series of qualitative studies exploring professionals' attitudes to, and experiences of, working with patients or clients with an eating disorder (Fixsen et al., 2023). The findings described in this chapter come from a secondary analysis of 40 one-to-one semi-structured interviews with professionals with various health qualifications who had worked in the ED field for at least two years in the UK, the US, and Italy. Analysis focused on work context, treatment approaches, views on eating disorder development, and attitudes toward psychiatric labeling. Emerging concepts were cross-referenced with existing theory and literature (Strauss & Corbin, 1990). Themes relating to fragmented services, patient resistance, and professionals' views of the utility of psychiatric labeling are explained below.

Fragmented ED Services

Problems with adequate service provision for eating disorders have already been touched upon in this chapter. In a similar manner, the professionals we interviewed noted a high volume of ED cases, with mental health provision more overstretched since the Covid pandemic. Professionals also noted a diversifying in cases, along with a big increase in ARFID, which was considered difficult to work with because "we haven't got a very good idea or clear therapy line to help support [ARFID] yet." Common challenges to state-funded care included uneven funding across regions, fragmented services, and long treatment delays. Inadequate staffing and the absence of medical professionals were observed in both the

UK and Italy, where public health sector funding and resource shortages compelled patients to transition between public and private sectors, further delaying treatment. One UK professional complained that even though ED services had the highest mortality rates of all the mental health services, NHS provision for ED services was completely inadequate, e.g., "I'm unable to do my job well due to high demands. The NHS system is currently the biggest hindrance." For psychologists working in hospitals, the physical absence of a psychiatrist and other medical professionals could make decision-making more difficult and was considered by this participant as potentially hazardous:

> The stress for therapists is because of the lack of psychiatrists and medical professionals- and you're then thinking, "God, I need to try and understand, and I have absolutely no clue!" It's dangerous and not safe for psychologists to give medical input.

Longer experience in the field has been associated with lower levels of stigma toward patients with EDs (Brelet et al., 2021); however, a sense of insufficient training and unsatisfactory experiences in the workplace were seen as encouraging staff to move out of the ED care sector.

Resistant Patients

Treatment resistance is a major issue for ED practitioners, with many individuals failing to respond to available treatments or dropping out of programs (Abbate-Daga et al., 2013; Halmi, 2013). This is especially the case for anorexia nervosa, where a patient's defense mechanisms may be directly activated by practitioners encouraging or even coercing them into weight gaining treatments (Abbate-Daga et al., 2013). The physical and psychological risks for their patients make this work challenging for professionals, who reportedly experience a range of emotional responses including feeling anxious, morally distressed, helpless, deskilled, emotionally drained by, and apathetic about, their work (Geller et al., 2012; Walker & Lloyd, 2011). In Katsounari and Andreou's (2020) study, professionals cited patients' indecisiveness, resistance, and denial as major hindrances to providing adequate treatment.

As two clinical psychologists in our study explained, "Trying to get them, an [ED] patient to move out of their patterns is absolute murder"; "The longer it goes on, the more rigid they become." These problems went beyond the professional-patient dynamic; a child with an ED posed difficulties for the whole family; hence, family therapist Emma would always involve parents or caregivers, while adding that the parents "often needed support in changing some of their own behaviors." Professionals agreed that the stigma surrounding EDs deterred individuals from seeking help, exacerbated by misunderstandings about the nature of their disorder. Stigmatization around mental health was seen as being particularly pronounced in minority and religious communities.

Professionals spoke of a wide variety of psychological models and strategies they used with their ED patients and clients. Dietician Lucy explained the centrality of relationship building to her work; "You go with them on a journey ... you worry about them ... you feel guilty when you aren't available for them," she said. Clinical psychologist Daniel said he would only use evidence-based approaches such as CBT to treat EDs but still favored a patient-centered approach, in which you meet the client, "where they are, and not the other way around." Transitioning from in-patient care to normal life was seen as posing significant challenges, as the disorder fundamentally alters patients' identities and behaviors.

The Utility of ED Labels

Professional's views on the utility of psychiatric diagnoses or labels were decidedly mixed. The existing psychiatric taxonomy was generally portrayed as reductive and in the US was designed to fit the requirements of insurance companies so they could say, "Yes, we will cover it." The act of labeling also felt contrary to the person-centered approach, which for psychotherapist Sophie was her "route to understanding the world." The existing DSM system simply did not reflect the complexity of what professionals saw in everyday practice: "They [the clients] don't just fit into a box, the NHS structure, I don't see somebody as needing treatment just because of their size, it's not always relevant" (Sophie). David, the one psychiatrist in our sample, thought medical practitioners should not become "slaves" to the diagnostic system: "I think it's a bit like rearranging the chairs on the Titanic at times … making sure you get the diagnostic label right, but [you] forget to look at the patient."

It was also recognized that ascribing certain mental disorder labels carried elements of stigma and shame in society. Even after recovery a label remained hard to shed: "I guess it's called a label because it sticks," Lauren surmised. A diagnostic treatment hierarchy for eating disorders existed within the system, which prevented some clients from receiving free treatment or getting well. For example, despite changes in criteria, a body mass index of below 17.5 was often needed to gain immediate access to NHS care in the UK. According to dietician Lucy, very few NHS services were provided for EDs such as binge eating, because "people aren't actually dying" from these conditions:

> I think that patients that don't just have anorexia … for example [those who] are deemed atypical anorexia … they don't feel as worthy of treatment because they maybe are not as underweight and things like that. *Ellie*

Professionals also spoke about the competitive nature of eating disorders among patients, with the anorexia nervosa label described as a "badge of honor" among peers. Being diagnosed with an ED could be "self-justifying," or worse, could encourage some people to starve themselves to the point where they were entitled to the AN label. This could lend itself to an attitude of "I have to do even better than that, which means I have to be sicker." The hierarchy of diagnostic labels could also result in some patients feeling unworthy of treatment, particularly those with atypical presentations or with those diagnosed with binge eating disorder (BED).

However, there were two sides to the argument concerning the utility of an ED label. "It depends which way you look at it," hospital manager Catherine stated. "I've had many conversations on both sides; sometimes labeling can be extremely beneficial." From a treatment pathway perspective, the existence of common psychiatric diagnostic criteria had practical advantages. Diagnostic terminology was like a common language, which could aid communication between practitioners and other professionals:

> I'm not able to diagnose psychiatric conditions, but if I have a referral saying its anorexia nervosa that is useful, that's helpful [in] the initial stage of understanding. What is less helpful is that it leaves less room for other areas to be considered. *Sophie*

For those involved in commissioning, "putting a name" (Jutel, 2011) to a condition could be the best way of securing resources from the public and private sector, including charitable bodies. For a diagnosis to be of any real value, however, it needed to be seen as "part of a full treatment package." Having different ED categorizations allowed for standardization of procedures, but, on the other hand, they failed to account for possible underlying factors:

> I think in these [hospital] settings, they do need a high intervention of care. And so, I think labeling then is necessary to follow … the NICE guidelines on how to treat them and making sure that that's kind of being followed … I think sometimes labels might be tricky in these settings because for example, they might stop eating for a period.

As well as understanding the experiences of those who undergo treatment for ED, studying the experiences and perceptions of those who work closely with ED patients or clients can also be extremely revealing concerning such things as the challenges of working with resistant patients, the strong emotional reactions elicited by such encounters (Graham et al., 2020), and the competition over ED labels. Our findings suggest that labels help to inform the array of approaches used in ED treatment, navigating patients toward certain treatment pathways and often determining who has access and who is denied immediate treatment. For professionals themselves, knowledge of diagnoses represents a form of professional and cultural capital which carries the power to make decisions about other people's bodies.

In another study of mental health professionals, staff depicted themselves as advocates for their clients and called for more holistic care approaches, while also tacitly or explicitly endorsing the language of the DSM or ICD (Lakeman & Cutcliffe, 2016). Similarly, members of our cohort were prepared to compromise their ideals about patient centeredness and use what was ultimately deemed as reductionist terminology for practical reasons. Those who work in private systems must also deal with insurance companies and funding bodies, and these may only support persons with specific named conditions. Paradoxically, the labeling of eating disorders and their medicalization creates further expectations on individuals in terms of achieving specific weight levels and diagnostic labels, which mirrors hierarchical treatment waiting lists within the public health system (Vollert et al., 2020). This raises interesting questions about the meaning and value of ED labels to lay people, the answer to which we are seeking in further studies.

Summary

Our own and other studies highlight the challenges of establishing practical goals which are acceptable to patients (O'Connell, 2023), while also trying to establish which kinds of healthcare interventions work best for whom and in which situations (Austin et al., 2023). They also confirm that labels for EDs function, not as sets of stable diagnoses, but as ongoing human, social processes, which are received differently and are acted on by players in diverse situations. In practical terms, accurate diagnosis remains a significant challenge in the field of eating disorders due to the complexity of symptom presentation and the overlap with other mental health conditions. Labels can help to determine and navigate different treatment pathways, yet inevitably they oversimplify the complex nature of eating disorders. Diagnostic categories fail to capture the individual nuances and personal experiences of those affected, leading to a one-size-fits-all approach in treatment. The diverse manifestations of disordered eating cannot be fully encompassed by rigid diagnostic categories, and inevitably this can result in misdiagnosis or inadequate treatment. Moreover, what constitutes disordered eating can vary across cultures, and a label that is meaningful in one cultural context might not be applicable or understood in another. As new research emerges, definitions and criteria may change, but the lingering effects of old labels may persist in clinical practice and societal perceptions. Whatever the difficulties of doing so, it remains important to make a distinction between what society assumes to be a problem because it has been defined by others as such, and the nature of personal and social ills as evidenced from narrative and historical perspectives.

In addition to their diagnostic and therapeutic frameworks, the construction of EDs and disordered eating rests upon the changing landscapes of food production and distribution, the epidemiology of EDs, theories around cultural and social change, and public health policy and its messages relating to diet and health. These topics are examined in the following chapter, "Chapter 5: Disordered Eating, Food Landscapes, and Public Health."

References

Abbate-Daga, G., Amianto, F., Delsedime, N., De-Bacco, C., & Fassino, S. (2013). Resistance to treatment in eating disorders: A critical challenge. *BMC Psychiatry, 13*, 294.

Ali, K., Farrer, L., Fassnacht, D. B., Gulliver, A., Bauer, S., & Griffiths, K. M. (2017). Perceived barriers and facilitators towards help-seeking for eating disorders: A systematic review. *International Journal of Eating Disorders, 50*(1), 9–21.

American Psychiatric Association. (2000). Diagnostic and Statistical Manual of Mental Disorders: DSM-IV-TR. Fourth Edition. American Psychiatric Association Publishing.

American Psychiatric Association. (2013). *Diagnostic and statistical manual of mental disorders: DSM-V* (5th ed.). American Psychiatric Association Publishing.

Austin, A., De Silva, U., Ilesanmi, C., Likitabhorn, T., Miller, I., Fialho, M. D. L. S., et al. (2023). International consensus on patient-centred outcomes in eating disorders. *The Lancet Psychiatry, 10*(12), 966–973.

Bannatyne, A., & Stapleton, P. (2018). Eating disorder patient experiences of volitional stigma within the healthcare system and views on biogenetic framing: A qualitative perspective. *Australian Psychologist, 53*(4), 325–338.

BEAT. (2023). *How many people have an eating disorder in the UK?* Retrieved August 22, 2024, from https://www.beateatingdisorders.org.uk/get-information-and-support/about-eating-disorders/how-many-people-eating-disorder-uk/

Becker, H. S. (1963). *Outsiders: Studies in the sociology of deviance*. The Free Press.
Beintner, I., Jacobi, C., & Schmidt, U. H. (2014). Participation and outcome in manualized self-help for bulimia nervosa and binge eating disorder- a systematic review and metaregression analysis. *Clinical Psychology Review, 34*(2), 158–176.
Björkman, I., Simrén, M., Ringström, G., & Jakobsson Ung, E. (2016). Patients' experiences of healthcare encounters in severe irritable bowel syndrome: An analysis based on narrative and feminist theory. *Journal of Clinical Nursing, 25*(19–20), 2967–2978.
Bray, B., Bray, C., Bradley, R., & Zwickey, H. (2022). Binge Eating Disorder is a social justice issue: A cross-sectional mixed-methods study of Binge Eating Disorder experts' opinions. *International Journal of Environmental Research and Public Health, 19*(10), 6243. MDPI AG.
Brelet, L., Flaudias, V., Désert, M., Guillaume, S., Llorca, P. M., & Boirie, Y. (2021). Stigmatization toward People with Anorexia Nervosa, Bulimia Nervosa, and binge eating disorder: A scoping review. *Nutrients, 13*(8), 2834.
Brinkmann, S. (2016). *Diagnostic cultures: A cultural approach to the pathologization of modern life*. Routledge.
Bullitt-Jonas, M. (2000). *Holy hunger: A woman's journey from food addiction to spiritual fulfillment*. Vintage.
Chesney, E., Goodwin, G. M., & Fazel, S. (2014). Risks of all-cause and suicide and mortality in mental disorders: A meta-review. *World Psychiatry., 2014*(13), 153–160.
Claudino, A. M., Pike, K. M., Hay, P., Keeley, J. W., Evans, S. C., Rebello, T. J., et al. (2019). The classification of feeding and eating disorders in the ICD-11 results of a field study comparing proposed ICD-11 guidelines with existing ICD-10 guidelines. *BMC Medicine, 17*, 1–17.
Cohen, B. M. Z. (2016). *Psychiatric hegemony: A Marxist theory on mental illness*. Palgrave Macmillan.
Conrad, B., & Barker, K. K. (2010). The Social construction of illness: Key insights and policy implications. *Journal of Health and Social Behavior, 51*(1_suppl), S67–S79.
Conrad, P., & Schneider, J. W. (1980). Looking at levels of medicalization: A comment on Strong's critique of medical imperialism. *Social Science & Medicine, 14*(1), 75–78.
Copperman, J. (2000). *Eating disorders in the United Kingdom: Review of the provision of health care services for men with eating disorders*. Eating Disorders Association.

Corral-Liria, I., Alonso-Maza, M., González-Luis, J., Fernández-Pascual, S., Becerro-de-Bengoa-Vallejo, R., & Losa-Iglesias, M. (2022). Holistic nursing care for people diagnosed with an eating disorder: A qualitative study based on patients and nursing professionals' experience. *Perspectives in Psychiatric Care, 58*(2).

Corrigan, P. W., & Watson, A. C. (2002). The paradox of self-stigma and mental illness. *Clinical Psychology: Science and Practice, 9*(1), 35.

Currin, L., Schmidt, U., & Waller, G. (2007). Variables that influence diagnosis and treatment of the eating disorders within primary care settings: A vignette study. *International Journal of Eating Disorders, 40*(3), 257–262.

Currin, L., Waller, G., & Schmidt, U. (2009). Primary care physicians' knowledge of and attitudes toward the eating disorders: Do they affect clinical actions? *International Journal of Eating Disorders, 42*(5), 453–458.

D'Abundo, M., & Chally, P. (2004). Struggling with recovery: Participant perspectives on battling an eating disorder. *Qualitative Health Research, 14*(8), 1094–1106.

Darmon, M. (2008). *Devenire anorexique: Une approache sociologue. La Découverte*. Poche/Sciences humaines et sociales.

Dellwing, M., & Harbusch, M. (2022). Conclusion. In M. Harbusch (Ed.), *Troubled Persons Industries: The expansion of psychiatric categories beyond psychiatry*. Springer International Publishing.

Durso, L. E., & Latner, J. D. (2008). Understanding self-directed stigma: Development of the weight bias internalization scale. *Obesity, 16*(S2), S80–S86.

Erskine, H. E., Whiteford, H. A., & Pike, K. M. (2016). The global burden of eating disorders. *Current Opinion in Psychiatry, 29*(6), 346–353.

Escobar-Koch, T., Banker, J. D., Crow, S., Cullis, J., Ringwood, S., Smith, G., et al. (2010). Service users' views of eating disorder services: An international comparison. *International Journal of Eating Disorders, 43*(6), 549–559.

Fairplay. (2022). *Designing for Disorder: Instagram's Pro-eating Disorder Bubble*. Fairplay. Retrieved August 22, 2024, from https://fairplayforkids.org/wp-content/uploads/2022/04/designing_for_disorder.pd

Feldman, M. B., & Meyer, I. H. (2007). Childhood abuse and eating disorders in gay and bisexual men. *International Journal of Eating Disorders, 40*(5), 418–423.

Fisher, C. A., Hetrick, S. E., & Rushford, N. (2010). Family therapy for anorexia nervosa. *Cochrane Database of Systematic Reviews*, (4).

Fixsen, A., Ridge, D., Ponsford, O., Holder, M., & Saran, G. (2023). Battles over 'unruly bodies': Practitioners' interpretations of eating disorders and the utility of psychiatric labeling. *Sociology of Health & Illness, 45*(3), 560–579.

Franko, D. L., Dorer, D. J., Keel, P. K., Jackson, S., Manzo, M. P., & Herzog, D. B. (2008). Interactions between eating disorders and drug abuse. *The Journal of Nervous and Mental disease, 196*(7), 556–561.

Frostad, S., & Bentz, M. (2022). Anorexia nervosa: Outpatient treatment and medical management. *World Journal of Psychiatry, 12*(4), 558.n.

Geller, J., Srikameswaran, S., Zelichowska, J., & Williams, K. D. (2012). Working with severe and enduring eating disorders: Enhancing engagement and matching treatment to client readiness. In J. Fox & K. Goss (Eds.), *Eating and its disorders* (pp. 412–426). Wiley Blackwell.

Giel, K. E., Bulik, C. M., Fernandez-Aranda, F., Hay, P., Keski-Rahkonen, A., Schag, K., et al. (2022). Binge eating disorder. *Nature Reviews Disease Primers, 8*(1), 16.

Goffman, E. (1963). *Stigma: Notes on the management of spoiled identity*. Simon & Schuster.

Goldstein, A., & Gvion, Y. (2019). Socio-demographic and psychological risk factors for suicidal behavior among individuals with anorexia and bulimia nervosa: A systematic review. *Journal of Affective Disorders, 245*, 1149–1116.

GOV.UK. (2018). *Research and analysis. Chapter III. Tends in morbidity and risk factors.* Retrieved August 22, 2024, from https://www.gov.uk/government/publications/health-profile-for-england-2018/chapter-3-trends-in-morbidity-and-risk-factors#mental-health

Graham, M. R., Tierney, S., Chisholm, A., & Fox, J. R. E. (2020). *The lived experience of working with people with eating disorders: A meta-ethnography.* Cardiff University | Prifysgol Caerdydd. https://orca.cardiff.ac.uk/id/eprint/127249/

Graves, T. A., Tabri, N., Thompson-Brenner, H., Franko, D. L., Eddy, K. T., Bourion-Bedes, S., et al. (2017). A meta-analysis of the relation between therapeutic alliance and treatment outcome in eating disorders. *International Journal of Eating Disorders, 50*(4), 323–340.

Griffiths, S., Rossell, S. L., Mitchison, D., Murray, S. B., & Mond, J. M. (2018). Pathways into treatment for eating disorders: A quantitative examination of treatment barriers and treatment attitudes. *Eating Disorders, 26*(6), 556–574.

Halmi, K. A. (2013). Perplexities of treatment resistance in eating disorders. *BMC Psychiatry, 13*(1), 1–6.

Hay, P., Mitchison, D., Collado, A. E. L., González-Chica, D. A., Stocks, N., & Touyz, S. (2017). Burden and health-related quality of life of eating disorders, including Avoidant/Restrictive Food Intake Disorder (ARFID), in the Australian population. *Journal of Eating Disorders, 5*, 1–10.

Hazell, C. M., Fixsen, A., & Berry, C. (2022). Is it time to change the approach of mental health stigma campaigns? An experimental investigation of the effect of campaign wording on stigma and help-seeking intentions. *PLoS ONE, 17*(8), e0273254.

Hoek, H. W. (2016). Review of the worldwide epidemiology of eating disorders. *Current Opinion in Psychiatry, 29*(6), 336–339.

Holmes, S. (2016). Between feminism and anorexia: An autoethnography. *International Journal of Cultural Studies, 19*(2), 193–207.

Horwitz, A. (2012). Social constructions of mental illness. In *Oxford handbook of philosophy of the social sciences* (pp. 1–23).

Horwitz, A. V. (2021). *DSM. A history of psychiatry's bible*. JHU Press.

Jenkins, Z. M., Mancuso, S. G., Phillipou, A., & Castle, D. J. (2021). What is OSFED? The predicament of classifying 'other' eating disorders. *BJPsych Open, 7*(5), e147.

Jeske, M., James, J., & Joyce, K. (2024). Diagnosis and the practices of patienthood: How diagnostic journeys shape illness experiences. *Sociology of Health & Illness, 46*(S1), 225–241.

John, A., Marchant, A., Demmler, J., Tan, J., & DelPozo-Banos, M. (2021). Clinical management and mortality risk in those with eating disorders and self-harm: e-cohort study using the SAIL databank. *BJPsych Open, 7*(2), e67.

Jutel, A. M. (2011). *Putting a name to it: Diagnosis in contemporary society*. Johns Hopkins University Press.

Katsounari, I., & Andreou, S. (2020). Perspectives of professionals on the treatment and service delivery of eating disorders in Cyprus. *The European Journal of Counselling Psychology, 8*(1), 78–92.

Kazdin, A. E., Fitzsimmons-Craft, E. E., & Wilfley, D. E. (2017). Addressing critical gaps in the treatment of eating disorders. *The International Journal of Eating Disorders, 50*(3), 170–189.

Kemp, A. F., Bentz, M., Olsen, E. M., Moslet, U., Plessen, K. J., & Koch, S. V. (2023). Predictors for and duration of hospitalization among children and adolescents with eating disorders. *International Journal of Eating Disorders, 56*(10), 1866–1874.

Kendell, R., & Jablensky, A. (2003). Distinguishing between the validity and utility of psychiatric diagnoses. *American Journal of Psychiatry, 160*(1), 4–12.

Keski-Rahkonen, A., Hoek, H. W., Linna, M. S., Raevuori, A., Sihvola, E., Bulik, C. M., Rissanen, A., & Kaprio, J. (2009). Incidence and outcomes of bulimia nervosa: A nationwide population-based study. *Psychological Medicine, 39*(5), 823–831.

Kessler, R. C., Berglund, P. A., Chiu, W. T., Deitz, A. C., Hudson, J. I., Shahly, V., et al. (2013). The prevalence and correlates of binge eating disorder in the World Health Organization World Mental Health Surveys. *Biological Psychiatry, 73*(9), 904–914.

Kirkbride, J. B., Anglin, D. M., Colman, I., Dykxhoorn, J., Jones, P. B., Patalay, P., Pitman, A., Soneson, E., Steare, T., Wright, T., & Griffiths, S. L. (2024). The social determinants of mental health and disorder: Evidence, prevention and recommendations. *World Psychiatry, 23*(1).

Lakeman, R., & Cutcliffe, J. (2016). Diagnostic sedition: Re-considering the ascension and hegemony of contemporary psychiatric diagnosis. *Issues in Mental Health Nursing, 37*(2), 125–130.

Lindgren, B. M., Enmark, A., Bohman, A., & Lundström, M. (2015). A qualitative study of young women's experiences of recovery from bulimia nervosa. *Journal of Advanced Nursing, 71*(4), 860–869.

Link, B. G., Cullen, F. T., Struening, E., Shrout, P. E., & Dohrenwend, B. P. (1989). A modified labeling theory approach to mental disorders: An empirical assessment. *American Sociological Review*, 400–423.

Link, B. G., Wells, J., Phelan, J. C., & Yang, L. (2015). Understanding the importance of "symbolic interaction stigma": How expectations about the reactions of others adds to the burden of mental illness stigma. *Psychiatric Rehabilitation Journal, 38*(2), 117–124.

Machado, P. P. P., & Rodrigues, T. F. (2019). Treatment delivery strategies for eating disorders. *Current Opinion in Psychiatry, 32*(6), 498–503.

Mangweth-Matzek, B., & Hoek, H. W. (2017). Epidemiology and treatment of eating disorders in men and women of middle and older age. *Current Opinion in Psychiatry, 30*(6), 446–451.

Martin, A. K. (2004). Stick a toothbrush down your throat: An analysis of the potential liability of pro-eating disorder websites. *Texas Journal of Women and the Law, 14*, 151.

McGann, P. J., Hutson, D., & Rothman, B. K. (Eds.). (2011). *Sociology of diagnosis*. Emerald Group Publishing.

Micali, N., Martini, M. G., Thomas, J. J., Eddy, K. T., Kothari, R., Russell, E., et al. (2017). Lifetime and 12-month prevalence of eating disorders amongst women in mid-life: A population-based study of diagnoses and risk factors. *BMC Medicine, 15*, 1–10.

Mond, J. M., Hay, P. J., Rodgers, B., & Owen, C. (2007). Health service utilization for eating disorders: Findings from a community-based study. *International Journal of Eating Disorders, 40*(5), 399–408.

Moreno, R., Buckelew, S. M., Accurso, E. C., & Raymond-Flesch, M. (2023). Disparities in access to eating disorders treatment for publicly insured youth and youth of color: A retrospective cohort study. *Journal of Eating Disorders, 11*(1), 10.

Murray, S. B., Griffiths, S., & Mond, J. M. (2016). Evolving eating disorder psychopathology: Conceptualising muscularity-oriented disordered eating. *The British Journal of Psychiatry, 208*(5), 414–415.

National Eating Disorders Association (NEDA). (2022). *Eating disorders statistics.* Retrieved August 22, 2024, from https://www.nationaleatingdisorders.org/statistics/

National Eating Disorders Association (NEDA). (2023, June 14). *Men and eating disorders.* https://www.nationaleatingdisorders.org/men-eating-disorders

National Institute for Clinical Excellence (NICE). (2021). *Eating disorders recognition and treatment.* Retrieved August 22, 2024, from https://www.nice.org.uk/guidance/ng69/chapter/Recommendation

O'brien, K. S., Latner, J. D., Halberstadt, J., Hunter, J. A., Anderson, J., & Caputi, P. (2008). Do antifat attitudes predict antifat behaviors? *Obesity, 16*(S2), S87–S92.

O'Connell, L. (2023). Being and doing anorexia nervosa: An autoethnography of diagnostic identity and performance of illness. *Health (London, England: 1997), 27*(2), 263–278.

Parsons, T. (1975). The sick role and the role of the physician reconsidered. *The Milbank Memorial Fund Quarterly. Health and Society*, 257–278.

Puhl, R., & Suh, Y. (2015). Stigma and eating and weight disorders. *Current Psychiatry Reports, 17*, 1–10.

Rance, N., Moller, N. P., & Clarke, V. (2017). 'Eating disorders are not about food, they're about life': Client perspectives on anorexia nervosa treatment. *Journal of Health Psychology, 22*(5), 582–594.

Riesco, N., Agüera, Z., Granero, R., Jiménez-Murcia, S., Menchón, J. M., & Fernández-Aranda, F. (2018). Other Specified Feeding or Eating Disorders (OSFED): Clinical heterogeneity and cognitive-behavioral therapy outcome. *European Psychiatry, 54*, 109–116.

Robinson, K. J., Mountford, V. A., & Sperlinger, D. J. (2013). Being men with eating disorders: Perspectives of male eating disorder service-users. *Journal of Health Psychology, 18*(2), 176–186.

Robinson, P. H., Kukucska, R., Guidetti, G., & Leavey, G. (2015). Severe and enduring anorexia nervosa (SEED-AN): A qualitative study of patients with 20+ years of anorexia nervosa. *European Eating Disorders Review, 23*(4), 318–326.

Roehrig, J. P., & McLean, C. P. (2010). A comparison of stigma toward eating disorders versus depression. *International Journal of Eating Disorders, 43*(7), 671–674.

Root, T. L., Pisetsky, E. M., Thornton, L., Lichtenstein, P., Pedersen, N. L., & Bulik, C. (2010). Patterns of co-morbidity of eating disorders and substance use in Swedish females. *Psychological Medicine, 40*(1), 105–115.

Rorty, M., Yager, J., Buckwalter, J., & Rossotto, E. (1999). Social support, social adjustment, and recovery status in bulimia nervosa. *The International Journal of Eating Disorders, 26*(1), 1–12.

Rouleau, C. R., & von Ranson, K. M. (2011). Potential risks of pro-eating disorder websites. *Clinical Psychology Review, 31*(4), 525–531.

Saguy, A. C., & Gruys, K. (2010). Morality and health: News media constructions of overweight and eating disorders. *Social Problems, 57*(2), 231–250.

Salvioli, B., Pellicciari, A., Iero, L., Di Pietro, E., Moscano, F., Gualandi, S., et al. (2013). Audit of digestive complaints and psychopathological traits in patients with eating disorders: A prospective study. *Digestive and Liver Disease, 45*(8), 639–644.

Santomauro, D. F., Melen, S., Mitchison, D., Vos, T., Whiteford, H., & Ferrari, A. J. (2021). The hidden burden of eating disorders: An extension of estimates from the Global Burden of Disease Study 2019. *The Lancet Psychiatry, 8*(4), 320–328.

Sato, Y., & Fukudo, S. (2015). Gastrointestinal symptoms and disorders in patients with eating disorders. *Clinical Journal of Gastroenterology, 8*(5), 255–263.

Scheff, T. (1966). *Being mentally ill: A sociological theory*. Aldine.

Sedgwick, P. (1982). *Psychopolitics*. Pluto Press.

Sikorski, C., Luppa, M., Kaiser, M., Gkemsmer, H., Schomerus, G., König, H. H., & Riedel-Heller, S. G. (2011). The stigma of obesity in the general public and its implications for public health—A systematic review. *BMC Public Health*.

Smink, F. R., Van Hoeken, D., & Hoek, H. W. (2012). Epidemiology of eating disorders: Incidence, prevalence and mortality rates. *Current Psychiatry Reports, 14*(4), 406–414.

Strauss, A., & Corbin, J. (1990). *Basics of qualitative research*. Sage.

Strober, M. (2010). The chronically ill patient with anorexia nervosa: development, phenomenology, and therapeutic considerations. In C. Grilo C & J.E. Mitchell (Eds.), *The Treatment Of Eating Disorders* (pp. 225–238). A Clinical Handbook.

Sweeting, H., Walker, L., MacLean, A., Patterson, C., Räisänen, U., & Hunt, K. (2015). Prevalence of eating disorders in males: A review of rates reported in academic research and UK mass media. *International Journal of Men's Health, 14*(2), 1.

Szasz, T. S. (1960). The myth of mental illness. *American Psychologist, 15*(2), 113.

Tragantzopoulou, P., Fixsen, A., Ridge, D., & Cheshire, A. (2024). 'You are not alone, we've got you': Power plays, devotion, and punishment on Healthy Eating and Pro-Eating Disorder websites. *Qualitative Health Research*. https://doi.org/10.1177/10497323241238628

Troop, N. A., Allan, S., Serpell, L., & Treasure, J. L. (2008). Shame in women with a history of eating disorders. *European Eating Disorders Review: The Professional Journal of the Eating Disorders Association, 16*(6), 480–488.

Tyler, N., Miles, H. L., Karadag, B., & Rogers, G. (2019). An updated picture of the mental health needs of male and female prisoners in the UK: Prevalence, comorbidity, and gender differences. *Social Psychiatry and Psychiatric Epidemiology, 54*, 1143–1152.

van Eeden, A. E., van Hoeken, D., & Hoek, H. W. (2021). Incidence, prevalence and mortality of anorexia nervosa and bulimia nervosa. *Current Opinion in Psychiatry, 34*(6), 515–524.

Vogel, D. L., & Heath, P. J. (2016). Men, masculinities, and help-seeking patterns. In Y. J. Wong & S. R. Wester (Eds.), *APA handbook of men and masculinities* (pp. 81–104). American Psychological Association.

Vollert, B., von Bloh, P., Eiterich, N., Beintner, I., Hütter, K., Taylor, C. B., & Jacobi, C. (2020). Recruiting participants to an Internet-based eating disorder prevention trial: Impact of the recruitment strategy on symptom severity and program utilization. *International Journal of Eating Disorders, 53*(5), 746–754.

Walker, S., & Lloyd, C. (2011). Barriers and attitudes health professionals working in eating disorders experience. *International Journal of Therapy and Rehabilitation, 18*(7), 383–390.

Weinberg, D. (2021). Diagnosis as topic and as resource: Reflections on the epistemology and ontology of disease in medical sociology. *Symbolic Interaction, 44*(2), 367–391.

Wiklund, C. A., Rania, M., Kuja-Halkola, R., Thornton, L. M., & Bulik, C. M. (2021). Evaluating disorders of gut-brain interaction in eating disorders. *International Journal of Eating Disorders, 54*(6), 925–935.

World Health Organization. (2019). *International Classification of Diseases 10th Revision: Ch. 5 Mental and Behavioural Disorders.* https://icd.who.int/browse10/2019/en#/F50.0

Wright, A., Jorm, A. F., & Mackinnon, A. J. (2011). Labeling of mental disorders and stigma in young people. *Social Science & Medicine, 73*(4), 498–506.

Yelencich, E., Truong, E., Widaman, A. M., Pignotti, G., Yang, L., Jeon, Y., et al. (2022). Avoidant restrictive food intake disorder prevalent among patients with inflammatory bowel disease. *Clinical Gastroenterology and Hepatology, 20*(6), 1282–1289.

Yim, S. H., & Schmidt, U. (2019). Self-help treatment of eating disorders. *The Psychiatric clinics of North America, 42*(2), 231–241.

Yule, S., Wanik, J., Holm, E. M., Bruder, M. B., Shanley, E., Sherman, C. Q., et al. (2021). Nutritional deficiency disease secondary to ARFID symptoms associated with autism and the broad autism phenotype: A qualitative systematic review of case reports and case series. *Journal of the Academy of Nutrition and Dietetics, 121*(3), 467–492.

Zhao, Y., & Encinosa, W. (2011). *An update on hospitalizations for eating disorders, 1999 to 2009.* https://www.ncbi.nlm.nih.gov/books/NBK65135/

Zipfel, S., Löwe, B., Reas, D.L., Deter, H. C., & Herzog, W. (2000). Long-term prognosis in anorexia nervosa: lessons from a 21-year follow-up study. *The Lancet, 355*(9205), pp. 721–722.

5

Disordered Eating, Food Landscapes, and Public Health

In recent years, the interplay between food ecology, public health, and disordered eating has garnered more attention. This is in recognition that, in addition to their diagnostic and therapeutic frameworks, disordered eating and eating disorders (EDs) must be considered alongside wider concerns including changes to food systems and their influence on consumer choice and behavior. Intercultural dietary practices, new avenues of communication, and variable responses to official advice concerning "healthy" and "unhealthy" foods, all confound the ED picture. This chapter explores the complex and often contentious relationship between food landscapes, food policy, and disordered eating. Understanding the complexities of food environments—the physical, economic, and sociocultural contexts in which food choices are made—seems crucial for addressing present and future challenges related to diet and nutrition (Li, 2017; Steel, 2020). The chapter also critically examines the role of epidemiology in the framing of the prevailing narratives concerning ED prevalence and distribution. It then takes a broad sweep approach to consider some of the non-biological discourses which purport to explain the "what, when and why's" of disordered eating and

A. Fixsen, *The Construction of Eating Disorders*, The Politics of Mental Health and Illness, https://doi.org/10.1007/978-3-031-70318-8_5

eating disorders (EDs). Finally, government-endorsed digital platforms designed to support those with eating disorders are discussed.

Changing Food Landscapes

The term "food landscapes" is used to describe the wide array of factors involved in food consumption, including the availability and affordability of food, cultural norms, marketing practices, and governmental policies. These elements shaping individual's and community's eating behaviors are considered to have significant implications in terms of health outcomes. The landscapes of food have always been politically charged because the stakes involved in food production, distribution, and marketing are high, while a regular and sufficiently nutritious diet lies at the heart of human survival. Modern food policy is embedded within complex international structures, with overlapping and competing mechanisms operating within the commercial sector. Public health initiatives, as reported, aim to create supportive environments that foster healthy eating habits and reduce the incidence of disordered eating. Global food governance and regulations are of concern not only to governments but to the multiplicity of private actors and international organizations seeking to make profits out of food and commerce.

Changes in dietary and food systems are influenced by a host of factors, including the movement of foodstuffs (plants and animals), people and their cultures, and the concentration of power and resources. Global sourcing of food has created new types of risks within the supply chain. Foods are now subject to greater degrees of transformation and transportation, along with fragmented supply chains across multiple enterprises, food production systems operating under diverse environmental conditions, different technological capacities, and variable regulatory frameworks (Havinga et al., 2015). The post-World War II era saw a decided shift from the public to private, and national to international governance (Havinga et al., 2015). International bodies including UNESCO, the World Health Organization, and the European Commission were set up to address pressing global issues, which—in the field of nutrition—now include food insecurity, recurrent food safety crises, the spread of obesity, the negative impact of climate change, and environmental degradation (Candel & Pereira, 2017). Despite decades of "welfare" capitalism, hunger and malnutrition persist, with food insecurity prevalent in both developing and developed nations (Richards et al., 2016).

One major challenge for addressing food issues at the international level is institutional fragmentation (Mathieu-Bolh & Wendner, 2020). Associated with this are divergencies of political and economic interests and differing ontological views among governments and their representatives, which can make the translation of discussion into action fraught with problems. Concentration of power, along with increasing privatization, generally ensures the supremacy of "rich world" interests. The pursuit of profit in the food industry often comes at the expense of workers, especially in developing countries. Many agricultural workers face poor working conditions, low wages, and exposure to harmful chemicals. In some cases, workers are subjected to exploitative practices such as child labor and forced labor. Corporate control over food production often involves squeezing suppliers and farmers for lower prices, which can trap them in cycles of poverty and force them to cut corners, sometimes compromising the safety and quality of the food produced.

The global supply chain, controlled by a few large corporations, often leaves little room for smaller producers to compete, leading to further consolidation and reduced competition. Welfare organizations must coexist with neoliberal economics, which supports the idea that food choices should be individual decisions rather than governed by restrictive food and fiscal policies. The neoliberal argument holds that public health bodies should not be overly didactic and unnecessarily interfering in personal choices regarding diet and health, as given sufficient choice, consumers will make wise decisions about what they buy and eat (Lang et al., 2009). However, this individualistic perspective is contradicted by evidence such as that showing wealthy individuals in affluent countries to be less obese due to their consumption of a lower-calorie, high-quality diet, while those with lower economic status in the same economy can only afford a less nutrient-rich but higher-calorie diet (Mathieu-Bolh & Wendner, 2020). According to the Food and Agriculture Organization of the United Nations (FAO, 2024), 40 percent of the global diet still consists of starchy foods such as cassava, rice, and potatoes.

A further issue for food policy lies in the way in which messages around health are received by consumers. Food messages and the mediated foodscapes that co-produce them are now omnipresent (Goodman et al., 2017), but how they are subsequently acted upon by different sections of the public is far less predictable. Some discourses, like "too much sugar is bad for you," are so entrenched that thinking or acting outside of them may seem virtually impossible or risks being labeled as "bad" or "mad." Nevertheless, studies suggest that food guidelines from governments and health agencies—such as consuming a variety of items from different food groups and limiting high-calorie, high-fat, and high-sugar foods and beverages—are chiefly followed by more motivated, educated, and better-resourced individuals (Darmon & Drewnowski, 2008; Guertin et al., 2020; Reid & Hammersley, 2016).

Not all sectors of the population are equally affected by the fast food market. Higher income and education have consistently been associated with healthier eating choices and lower caloric intake, including more whole grains, low-fat dairy, and fresh fruits and vegetables (Darmon & Drewnowski, 2008; Mathieu-Bolh & Wendner, 2020). While education plays a part, these stark social disparities between middle class and lower income food choices has a lot to do with positioning of fast food outlets and supermarkets selling relatively cheap ultra processed foods in lower income neighbourhoods (FFCC, 2024). As illustrated by five years of a Soft Drinks Industry Levy in the UK, taxes on items such as sugar can influence consumer consumption, where the onus falls on manufacturers themselves to reformulate products and reduce sugar content. Yet many health policies continue to overlook or underplay the importance of social and environmental influences on health and eating patterns, preferring to portray diet as a matter of individual choice. For instance, widespread availability of nutritious free school meals, fruit, and easy access to water fountains could do a great deal to reduce children's consumption of sugar and other processed foods (O'Mara & Vlad, 2023), yet implementing these measures is still far from a universal policy.[1]

[1] Some of the countries that do provide free school meals are India, Brazil, Finland, and Estonia. Some states in the US and parts of the UK have also implemented a free school meals policy.

Pedagogies of Food and Diet

Modern technology has provided unique opportunities and ways to promote certain social facts and encourage the adoption of health behaviors based on them. Adherence to this type of public health information is seen as essential for health promotion; some might say that it has replaced the injection of funding into physical health services (Lambert & Loiselle, 2007). "Biopedagogy" is a term sometimes used to describe the multifarious news-bites which help to shape what it means to be fit and healthy, along the lines of neoliberal public health imperatives (Bernstein, 2001). Slogans such as "avoid fat," "stop smoking," and "eat your 5 a day" (portions of fruit and vegetables) are brought to our notice almost daily (Tinning & Glasby, 2002) but can also change at a whim. "Nudging"—now a branch of behavioral science—is one such "biopedagogic" tool, that is expressly designed to improve citizens' decisions about "health, wealth, and happiness" (Thaler & Sunstein, 2008). The influence of nudge theory on corporate culture and government health strategy has been immense, with "algorithmic nudging" now aiming to change decision-making and behaviors on a vast scale (Vlaev et al., 2016). The thinking seems to be that without these pro-health messages and incentives, the advances of science and technology could be for nothing.

In the promotion of health messages there is invariably more at stake than simply keeping others well. Governments and other agencies recognize the potential to train people in self-directed health behaviors and activities to maintain social order. It has become common to stress the subversive aspects of the media (fake news, misogyny, etc.), but the capacity of the media to activate citizens' responses via "biopedagogies" remains very powerful. For example, even with political inconsistencies, it was surprising to some just how law-abiding most people were during the chaotic lockdown period of the Covid pandemic.[2] Citizens in the UK

[2] In Peter May's dystopian crime novel *Lockdown*, written round 15 years before the Covid pandemic (but only published in 2020), civil chaos reigns during a flu epidemic in London in the early years of this century. Similar scenarios are played out during major pandemics in disaster films such as *Contagion*. In fact, there was surprisingly little looting of shops and civil disorder during the time of enforced closure of commercial properties in the UK and most other cities. The public's seemingly worst "crime" was to buy up shelves of toilet paper and other products, fearing that they might be quarantined in their homes for months.

and many countries were instructed to stay in their homes for extended periods of time with virtually no contact with others and with leisure areas and most shops closed. Access to medical treatment became limited and many services were overwhelmed or unable to function. Governments and commercial institutions looked to the media to circulate new and repurposed instructions on how to find or purchase ways of looking after themselves, such as online shopping apps, and various self-help activities to pursue at home. Disobedience came about in other, more self-directed ways. Overall compliance to the UK's government recommendations for healthy eating is said to be poor. According to one study, people in Britain were the biggest lockdown bingers in Europe (Smithers, 2020).

Part of the problem is that messages about bodies and health designed to help prevent eating disorders land differently on different bodies. The thinking behind many health education policies is that certain groups of people who, for education, class, and cultural reasons, are presently ignorant of health measures such as calorie counting and BMI (body mass index) can be educated to achieve a more normative body. LaMarre and Rice (2016) cite the "anti-obesity biopedagogy" as hinging on the neoliberal assertion that everyone is responsible and accountable for their own health, such that fatness is viewed as a personal choice. Such measures mark out certain bodies as disordered and influence stereotypes around who is at risk for restrictive or binge-purge–type eating disorders and obesity. Those from middle and upper classes may be assumed to "know better" than to engage in behaviors assumed to result in fatness (McPhail, 2013). Others from lower socioeconomic classes or from minority ethnic groups may be considered more prone to ignorance and unruliness, while other social circumstances and beliefs are not considered.

As mediated food landscapes have diversified, so the politics and pedagogies around food have grown more contentious. Different factions now compete over so-called food facts. The term "post-truth" society (Heinrich, 2020; Iyengar & Massey, 2019) has recently entered popular vocabulary, implying that the notion of universally accepted facts is being replaced by a more subjective and fragmented understanding what counts as "truth." If, as Foucault (1972) states, discursive practice is an exercise in power, it has become a matter of who shouts loudest and/or pursues the most aggressive advertising strategy. Allied to this are notions about the erosion of trust in institutions, the proliferation of "misinformation" on social media (Sismondo, 2017), an emphasis on emotion over fact, and the division of society along polarized lines. How these divisions play out in relation to diet and health is illustrated by the vociferous debates concerning the production and consumption of meat. One study followed news items on this topic, from the fallout of the bovine encephalopathy (BSE) crisis, the Atkins Diet craze, the Avian Flu episode of 2007, to the 2015 International Agency for Research report on Cancer. The authors found many conflicting news items whereby, at moments of crisis, the potential hazards of meat-eating were vividly depicted, swiftly followed by counter messages stressing the benefits of meat as a rich source of nutrients (Leroy et al., 2018).[3] Meanwhile, more arguments have emerged concerning the environmental benefits of a non-meat diet (Marrone et al., 2021). It is also posited that the potent mixture of ethical claims, meat scares, and body anxieties have led some people to adopt what might be considered obsessively health-oriented eating behaviors, sometimes to the detriment of their health (Barthels et al., 2018; Brytek-Matera, 2021) (see Chap. 9 on Orthorexia Nervosa).

Many endeavors over the years have been made to amalgamate theory and data stemming from various disciplinary realms, aiming for more cohesive consensus on the factors contributing to health and illness. Policymakers have sought guidance from academic and scientific perspectives, particularly in understanding the intersection between psychological and social influences (Culbert et al., 2015). These segments inform not only strategic decisions but the public narratives told to substantiate such policies (Cairney, 2019). In the area of mental health policy, psychiatry, psychology, social work, and educational science all provide materials to support administrative solutions, so that social control can be applied to widening populations (Dellwing & Harbusch, 2022). Neither should we overlook the governance implications of virtual, mediated food messaging, from figures like Jamie Oliver and his *#FoodRevolution*.[4] More and more people are deriving inspiration from

[3] These arguments possibly incited the big meat and dairy lobbyists to turn up in record numbers at Cop28 (Sherrington et al., 2023).

[4] See, for example, the article in *Huffington Post* (2017) in which Jamie Oliver celebrates the introduction of a sugar tax in the UK. He went on to launch his anti-sugar campaign in the US.

these celebrity cooks, along with the marketers of semi-prepared "fresh food" menu plans available for home delivery. Given the popularity of "healthy eating" broadcasts, one could be left asking why it is that disordered eating still haunts public health policy.

The Epidemiology of Eating Disorders

A 2016 editorial in the *Journal of Eating Disorders* made the following announcement: "Eating disorders, like mass communications are now global" (Hay & Touyz, 2016). The authors point to the invitation from the World Health Organization's Global Clinical Practice Network for readers to contribute their expertise in eating and feeding disorders to the current revisions to the ICD-11, so that it can be modified to account for global and cultural diversity. In adopting the idea of globalization, the journal follows the increasing acceptance of this term in political sciences, sociology, and epidemiology. The basic argument around globalization is that, in contemporary times, people commonly engage with others in different parts of the world and communicate readily across space due to cheaper, faster travel, and now digital media. However, the language of globalization is politically charged (Rosenberg, 2005). It can be used positively for mutual benefit or to fuel moral and social panics, including concerning health matters. When terms such as "health epidemic" become jaded, stronger adjectives are employed to emphasize these developments. For example, a 2021 *Guardian* article cited a psychiatrist describing the "tsunami" of patients needing support for eating disorders since the Covid pandemic. Their use of this terminology is then explained: "The bottom line is that there has been a year-on-year increase in hospital admissions since 2000, so before the pandemic … We don't have a very good understanding of why that surge has happened, but the chances are that it's going to be multiple factors" (Addley, 2023).

This kind of language sells newspapers but may also serve to induce alarm, and it fails to address questions about such escalating numbers. Meanwhile, the study of eating disorders has proliferated in different disciplines. Research in the fields of genetics (Bulik et al., 2021)[5] and neuroscience (Steinglass et al., 2019) has been moving on rapidly, while multiple biological and psychological disciplines have proposed their specific epistemological and methodological approaches to EDs and disordered eating. Yet, with identification of multiple causes of illness increasingly occupying researchers, efforts have been made to bring together knowledge from different disciplinary areas, to reach a better consensus concerning factors underlying EDs and disordered eating.[6] Many of these revolve around the statistical evidence gathered from epidemiological studies, at both population and local level.

Epidemiologically, EDs are now high up in the global burden of disease (Erskine et al., 2016; Santomauro et al., 2021). While medical epidemiologists agree on a correlation between sociopolitical determinants and health determinants (Kickbusch, 2015; Marmot et al., 2018), no apparent agreement exists around these in connection with EDs, nor how any such intersectional inequalities should be addressed in the future. Instead, a variety of personal, social, cultural, psychological, and biological reasons for ED development have been put forward, supporting a multi-causative model of eating disorders (Culbert et al., 2015). The distribution of EDs across continents appears to mirror the patterns observed in the US and western Europe in terms of high prevalence in the younger age group (Silén & Keski-Rahkonen, 2022). In other studies, rising numbers of EDs in Asian and Arab nation countries have been linked to industrialization, globalization, and urbanization (Hoek, 2016). These figures produced by epidemiological studies are important in establishing the distribution and growth of eating disorders. Statistics are nevertheless recognized as being open to manipulation and abuse. Accusations have been made about hoodwinking by epidemiologists of ordinary citizens, with even epidemiologists admitting that their science is not perfect (Ness & Rothenberg,

---

[5] The paper by Bulik et al. (2021) concerns the Eating Disorders Genetics Initiative (EDGI): an international investigation exploring the role of genes and environment in anorexia nervosa, bulimia nervosa, and binge eating disorder.

[6] An example is the "Nine Truths about Eating disorders" statements crafted by the Academy for Eating Disorders in collaboration with international patient, advocacy, and parental organizations (Schaumberg et al., 2017). These statements are backed up by selected empirical studies and assume a largely biomedical but non-judgmental approach to eating disorders.

2007). Statistical studies can ignore important features or discard dimensions or observations, use samples which suit with a bias, misreport, underestimate figures, or deduce causality where it does not really exist. The adage that correlation does not constitute causality may be overlooked by statisticians eager to come up with interesting data around social and medical problems, as well as politicians and media staff searching out figures to substantiate eye-catching headlines. For example, critics point to how alarmist claims about the "obesity time-bomb" are continually being recycled in policy reports, reviews, and white papers, each beginning with the assumption that fatness is fundamentally unhealthy and damaging to national economies (Monaghan & Evans, 2014).

Epidemiology is not a standalone science; it needs to be studied as part of the apparatus of biopower concerned with the control of health at population level, which uses technology to measure things in society. As Foucault (1973) states, from early on, the collective phenomena of diseases as epidemics required a "multiple gaze" and presented unique opportunities for the study of social dynamics between individuals. This multiple lens continues to formulate policy. What has been called "surveillance medicine" has led to the fundamental remapping of spaces of illness. Armstrong (1995) describes this institutionalization effect as constituting, "the problematisation of normality, the redrawing of the relationship between symptoms, signs and illness and the localization of illness outside of the corporeal body" (p. 393). The actions of surveillance medicine begin pre-birth with ultrasound screening of the fetus, followed by charting of weight and height, with each line marking the normal experience of a child and then adult within the context of the general population trajectory. While some of this is centuries-old, in our era of digitalization, surveillance medicine has rapidly progressed, and what this means for those classified with an eating disorder is considered in this and subsequent chapters.

Eating Disorders and Social Change

Over the years, different authorities have put forward their own conjectures concerning what they see as the key sociocultural factors driving disordered eating. As discussed before, a factor frequently cited as instrumental is the radical change in people's relationship to food. With a global market now replacing more localized food production, the long chain of events that precede acts of eating, including the sowing, growing, collecting, and distribution of edible products through an elaborate market, and the processes and human relationships underpinning them, remains a mystery to the average consumer. We live in an age of food plenty, in which mountains of food are wasted. We also live in times of staggering wealth inequality. Natural, political, and economic fluctuations contribute to food scarcity and hunger, and of the eight or so billion people on the planet around one billion are estimated to be malnourished. Several million die each year of easily preventable hunger-related conditions (Barnhill, 2018).

In both rich and poor nations, inequalities in food production and consumption apply. Forced out of business by economies of scale, many people have abandoned traditional methods of food production, resulting in far greater consumption of mass-produced, branded foods. Unequal profits arising from food production have promoted both hunger and obesity in those lower down the income scale. Albritton's (2013) essay on obesity and hunger explains how the industrial food system manipulates the price of commodity goods to shape the diet of Americans within a global capitalist food system that is cheap and addictive. The author points to the huge disparities in prices paid to local producers and the massive profits made by the multinational food industries. The expansion of takeaway meals and the online food delivery channels are said to constitute one of the main physical obstacles to healthy eating in the UK (D'angelo et al., 2020). There is also the issue of when and how health information is released and how it is altered to fit the goals of the commercial sector. After many decades of supermarkets flooding their shelves with ultra-processed foods, news headlines are only now warning of the dangers of these foods to long-term health (Gregory, 2023).

Western culture often takes center stage in discussions surrounding the development of disordered eating. One line of thought suggests that the culture's emphasis on consumption and materialism fosters personal dissatisfaction, driving individuals to seek fulfillment through consumerism. This view posits that individualism and profit-making, both integral to western culture, unnaturally raise personal expectations and desires

(Eckersley, 2006). Another perspective highlights the influence of Judeo-Christian morality, which underpins capitalist ideology (Ryan, 2012). Historically, as food production and distribution improved in the nineteenth century, efforts emerged to curb excessive consumption, framing it as a moral and economic matter. What came to be termed the "civilizing of appetite" (Mennell, 1987) initially responded to external constraints on food availability and later evolved into internalized constraints through personal choices in diet, hygiene, and exercise. Gracia-Arnaiz (2010) identifies five interconnected outcomes of this process: the establishment of ideal body norms and dietary standards, the association of thinness with health, the promotion of self-discipline and social distinction, the recognition of obesity as an illness, and the commercialization of dietary health. These phenomena are adapted across different political and economic systems worldwide.

Others have pointed to a giving way of classic liberal values to neoliberalism and its prioritization of individualism as a deliberate move to limit the role of state intervention and expand private markets in the direction of health (Harvey, 2005; Rose, 1998). From this perspective, the rise in disordered eating can be viewed as resulting from a contradiction between neoliberal ideals of individual responsibility and the mass consumption patterns promoted by market-driven food systems. Public health policies stress individual responsibility, yet deregulated markets promote consumption patterns which are at odds with self-care, while replacing traditional food practices (Pirie, 2016). As a result, regardless of widespread awareness of the negative impacts of processed foods, confusion persists among consumers regarding specific healthy choices (Santomauro et al., 2021). Lacking the stabilizing influence of traditional institutions, such as community and religion, culinary traditions on food consumption and dietary practices are done away with, to be replaced by atomized eating, accompanied by generalized anxiety about the quality of food and its impact on personal health (Nicolosi, 2006). Conflicting messages about "healthy" foods alongside advertisements promoting comfort foods serve to exacerbate this confusion (Graham et al., 2022). The constant search for accurate information within an increasingly contradictory food system, alongside changeable expert advice, leaves participants feeling doubly anxious about food choices (Rangel et al., 2012). This search for the perfect food combination is compounded, by other factors such as the media's emphasis on body shape and image (Silén & Keski-Rahkonen, 2022)—as discussed later in Chap. 7 on disordered eating and the media industry.

With eating disorders recorded in places such as Africa (van den Heuvel et al., 2023; van Hoeken et al., 2016), scholars have been wondering how, beyond ideas of westernization, they can account for the rise of EDs in non-western societies. Theories put forward for the growth of EDs in the non-western world include a prevailing fear of fatness; internalization of western concepts of individualism associated with ideas of romantic love; modifications of existing local patterns of dieting and self-denial; and the prevalence of body dissatisfaction among young women, largely due to pervasiveness of western body ideals promoted on mass media (Thornborrow et al., 2022). Yet not all these theories have proven to be cast-iron, and an emphatic association between AN and a cultural focus on dieting and thinness ideals has long been cast into doubt (Banks, 1992). Research carried out in the 1990s in Hong Kong by Lee et al. (1993) involving Chinese females indicated that the element "fat phobia" was frequently absent from clinical assessments of anorexia nervosa in these patients. When Nasser et al. (2001) reported on "the remarkable emergence of eating in areas that were once thought to be culturally incompatible with them" (p. 11), including South Africa, Argentina, Hong Kong, and Rumania, it seemed clear to the authors that the politics of gender and female oppression extended beyond matters of body weight. Writing in the same volume, Gordon (2001) noted the development of EDs within societies witnessing rapid market changes associated with an impact on the status of women. Meehan and Katzman (2001) interpreted the rise of EDs among girls and women in Argentina as arising from a clash of cultures, which has left women "feeling confused, hungry for success, but frustrated by false opportunities" (p. 148). The eating disordered woman, they conclude, will turn to food for solace, while relying on her appearance for approval.

Capitalism and Colonialism

To answer some of the "what, why and when" questions around the construction of disordered eating, we must look to the role of capitalism and colonialism in directing people's eating practices. Turner (2008) writes of how under traditional capitalism, discipline and restriction prevented excessive gluttony among the elite, while sufficient nutrition kept the workers productive. Yet, as Karl Marx asserted, capitalism is marked by contradictory forces; individual capitalists have a strong interest in health, reliability, and discipline of their own workers, but they do not want the burden of welfare taxation. One solution for early capitalists was to educate the working classes in the principles of health and hygiene. For example, in the US, representatives of *New Nutrition*—a group of nutritionist social reformers and specialists in home economics in the 1890s—attempted to organize workers food expenditure by changing their cooking habits (although their "fortifying" New England dishes were met with a lack of enthusiasm among workers from European immigrant communities) (Levenstein, 1980). In time, nutrition became an integral part of the US culture and economy (Turner, 2008). The operations of private markets have had the effect of creating both a glut of foods available to the public and a proliferation of dietary trends and programs to cope with the growing problems of weight gain and obesity.

Apparatus run by the state have continued to capitalize on nutritional claims to promote and corner certain markets. Gracia-Arnaiz (2010) points out the lack of coincidence between a broad approval of biomedical claims regarding items within traditional diets (such as olive oil, avocado, quinoa) and economic interests in protecting local agricultural products to export these high value products to international markets. This confluence of interests has led to the celebration of the "Mediterranean diet," proposed in 2009 as a candidate for UNESCO's Intangible Cultural Heritage status with support from the governments of Spain, Greece, Italy, and Morocco (Gracia-Arnaiz, 2010, p. 220). On the other side, capitalism has produced and continues to feed and grow, a massive ultra processed market controlled by a handful of companies, some of whom have a strong co-dependancy with the manufacturers of weight and diet related pharmaceuticals (FFCC, 2024). Reflecting on these types of changes and developments, medical anthropologist Van Esterik (2002) called for a complete rethinking about EDs in the context of social and economic factors so that we could begin to map the relationship between people and their social environment.

Statistics suggesting that incidences of EDs in different countries are rising should not lead to the assumption that eating patterns or body size must be interpreted in the same manner in non-western societies. EDs are principally western conceptualizations that have been transported and sometimes imposed elsewhere under post-colonialism. For example, the "problems" of unhealthy eating as linked with overweight and obesity in non-western societies are also associated with radical changes in the conditions in which people live and work. The growth of commercial food production networks has altered peoples' eating patterns in the developing world, along with decreased physical activity and other corresponding changes to ways of life. Among the top ten countries ranked as the most obese, nine are in the Pacific Islands (World Health Organization, 2023). Much of this has been put down to a combination of poor diet, lack of exercise, and genetic predisposition. Less spoken about are the ill-effects of colonialism, the medicalization of obesity, combined with traditional western ideas about gluttony and guilt which are exported across the globe (de Zwaan, 2001). The new food environment in which local people have found themselves has, along with other ways in which indigenous people's lives have been disrupted, led to an increased consumption of cheap imported foods and alcohol. Since binge eating disorder (BED) is medically linked to obesity, people in non-white countries may find themselves doubly stigmatized, not just for being overweight but for their lack of psychological order. Meanwhile the exportation of western health strategies and ideals is proving to be hugely profitable to the multinational medical and health companies (like *Roche* and *Eli Lilly and Co.*). The countries of Southeast Asia are predicted to see the biggest growth in the eating disorder market in the next few years, largely due to BED (InnoScope Insights, 2024).

In addition to blatant profiteering, there are moral issues about the way that western health ideas are superimposed onto the eating practices of other places and cultures. What Braidotti (2013) refers to as the "European Enlightenment project" holds up affluent white embodiment as a norm against which to judge who qualifies as a human and as a citizen. The western medical field intersects with post-colonialism, adhering to a practice of medicine that is exclusive in its examination of pathology and distress through a western lens. Western medicine looks at disease from a particular perspective; more than a science, it is an ideology. For example, the body mass index (BMI) has become a normalization measurement considered applicable across the world (World Health Organization, 2023). Some also consider that the developments in biogenetics around weight and eating have allowed for a form of racism in scientific circles, which might be considered profoundly unethical in the social sciences. These "racializing narratives" concerning genetic differences are held up as necessary because ethnic groups—such as African Americans, Latinos, Native Americans, Asian Americans in the US and "non-white" populations in their own countries—are considered as being in the at-risk category for Type II Diabetes, obesity, and other weight-associated conditions. Other racialized discourses such as the "thrifty gene hypothesis"[7] (which poses that certain individuals could easily store extra energy having an evolutionary advantage during famines) now cause scientists themselves discomfort (Fee, 2006).

Such racialized discourses concerning weight and eating fail to account for either historical famines in societies or the dire effects of white colonization on food production and availability over hundreds of years. Chronic malnutrition was relatively prevalent in preindustrial society, not simply because of crop failure but failure to distribute food equitably among populations. The "delocalization" of food and diet means the processes through which food production and distribution occur have been disseminated throughout the world in an ever-increasing and intensified network of socioeconomic and political interdependency. This has benefited those in wealthier economies but has been at the expense of local food producers and consumers in the developing world (FAO, 2024; Pelto & Pelto, 1983). Climate change is also contributing to the way that food production is being shaped for western markets. For example, it was predicted that the rain-fed agriculture yield would fall by 50 percent from 2020 at the present rate of global warming (Gomez-Zavaglia et al., 2020). This and other changes in climate and in climate variability are having an impact on the prevalence of undernutrition, with the likelihood of severe

[7] The phrase "thrifty genotype" was first used by JV Neel in 1962. His thesis was that in times of food surplus, adaptations that allow an organism to rapidly lay down fat would have a survival advantage in times of food shortages and famine (Neel, 1962).

stunting in south Asia and East and South Africa in the following decades (Lloyd et al., 2011). Machine learning has been proposed as a means of predicting and warning of catastrophic climactic events, but this is a late and partial solution to a climate crisis brought about by the rich countries of the world. In the meantime, people are compelled to abandon their traditional ways of producing food and eating as they fall under the ambit of the cheap, fast-food conglomerates.

Afflicting both developed and developing worlds, crises generated by such things as illness and inflation have also been cited as factors in disordered or unhealthy eating. During the Covid pandemic, numbers suffering from eating disorders are thought to have increased (Spigel et al., 2021). Various reasons have been posited for this, including travel restrictions, limited access to healthcare services and grocery stores, sedentary behaviors, greater use of social media, emotional eating, and social isolation (Gao et al., 2022; Naja & Hamadeh, 2020; Madali et al., 2021; McAtamney et al., 2021). At least some of the changes in eating habits can be attributed to food insecurity. A UK household food security survey estimated that over 16 percent of participants have experienced food insecurity since the lockdown, while nearly 22 percent worried about the availability of food (Loopstra, 2020). Food insecurity has continued post-pandemic, suggesting that factors other than social disruption and isolation need to be considered, especially among lower income groups. In 2023, more than one in six households reported experiencing recent food insecurity in the UK, including eating less, skipping meals, or fasting even when hungry, because they could not afford or access food (Page & Marshall, 2023). In the light of this, Shanks et al. (2020) argue that too much attention has been focused on influencing individuals' dietary choices and insufficient attention paid to the food system as an upstream determinant of health. The pandemic simply exposed the fundamental structural weaknesses and inequalities, and the fragility of food and medical systems in countries such as the UK. One pre-Covid study looked at the incidence of, and risk factors for, binge eating by socioeconomic class status (SES) in US adolescents (West et al., 2019). Food insecurity was not mentioned in adolescents from higher SES but was a relatively significant predictor of binge eating risk in those from low SES. These kinds of issues come to light when, faced with a crisis, fragile social and welfare systems break down further.

Digital Solutions

In recent years, digital technologies, including artificial intelligence (AI), have assumed a major role in public and private health strategy, and have been widely hailed as positive developments. This argument states that for some time healthcare systems have been struggling with increasing costs and worsening outcomes, leading policymakers, politicians, clinical entrepreneurs, and data scientists to regard technologies such as machine learning (ML) and AI as integral to future healthcare, enhancing the accuracy of detection, diagnosis, and operational efficiency, and supporting drug discovery and personalized medicine (Morley et al., 2019; Schijven & Kroh, 2023). Social media data, for instance, can be analyzed using natural language processing and machine learning techniques to detect signs of mental disorders that need attention, such as depression and suicidal ideation (Skaik & Inkpen, 2020). There are clearly cost and time benefits to online therapeutic interventions, which can be carried out in the subject's own home, with minimum interruption to their daily activities, potentially increasing their sense of autonomy as agents of their own mental healthcare.

Yet, the delivery of digital interventions for mental health and eating disorders is not without disadvantages, including in terms of the implications of mass health data collection and infringement on people's minds and lives (Han, 2014). Parties have noted the considerable ethical, normative, and accountability issues inherent in both the use and design of machine learning and advanced technologies (Marx, 2019; Morley et al., 2019). Commenting on cloud geographies and their role in social surveillance, Amoore (2018) notes how the computer cloud can render "perceptible and actionable" things which would otherwise be "beyond the threshold of human observation." Besides their potentially intrusive nature, inbuilt racial, gender, and social prejudices in biometric surveillance tools exist, which are hard to eradicate (Gates, 2011; Wachter, 2018). In the area of mental health, the acquisition and utilization of extremely sensitive patient information throw up issues around privacy, targeting, and stigmatization. Digital media also adds to a situation in which the proliferation of psychiatric vocabulary across people's life-worlds cannot be controlled (Dellwing & Harbusch, 2022; Han, 2014). The assumptions underlying technologies aimed at detecting mental health and eating disorders rest on the characteristics drawn up by powerful institutions, such as the American Psychiatric Association and the World Health Organization, who have considerable interests invested in these categories. The expanding list of mental disorder categories narrows down both the perimeters of normality and serves the interests of traditional and emerging markets, including pharmaceutical, health provision, and medical insurance industries, whose expansion hinges on more people being labeled with some disorder or another.

There are also practical limitations to digital technologies which are evident to those who have been following the progress of the online mass screening of people's mental health. In the UK, policymakers were quick to seize on the opportunities for better mental health surveillance and cost cutting, with a shifting of services online resulting in the now well-established Improving Access to Psychological Therapies (IAPT) program. When introduced by the UK government in 2007, IAPT was hailed as a real step forward, which could provide effective therapy to thousands of people experiencing depression and anxiety. Critics of the service however point to its roots in the model promoted by Professor Richard Layard, an economist who regarded psychological conditions such as anxiety and depression as naturalistic, concrete, and quantifiable (Rizq, 2019). From its inception, the program content was based around certain "evidence-based" therapeutic modalities, primarily cognitive behavioral therapy (CBT), which favors a technical and measurable understanding of mental health problems and solutions. The present IAPT model has been described as a "factory system of care," and an individualistic, medicalized, and industrialized solution to mental health, which ignores issues such as marginalization, abuse, homelessness, and enforced migration, or deals with these as separate issues (Rizq, 2019). Its individualistic understanding of care, Thomas (2019) argues, is part of a wider cultural shift that has led to the erosion of the fundamental human values of compassion, solidarity, and connectedness. Furthermore, this approach perpetuates the idea of mental illness as a disease. A recent article in the *Economist* (2023) described Britain's mental health system as a "mess." The authors point out how the British were more likely than people in any other rich country to think that mental health is a disease like any other. The article argues for the social causes of mental health to receive more attention, with an end to the mass medicalization of mild forms of distress and the funneling of people into overstretched health-care systems.

Despite all the theorizing and research, serious gaps in good practice remain, with mental health services seemingly unable to process the numbers of people being put forward for treatment. A WHO report on access to mental health services in 14 countries found that 35–50 percent of serious cases in developed countries, and a far greater number in less developed countries, had received no medical treatment in the last 12 months (Demyttenaere et al., 2013). According to sources, multilevel treatment barriers are preventing up to 80 percent of individuals experiencing eating disorders from accessing care (Schleider et al., 2023). For individuals in the UK, digital health solutions may be the only option. Access to other kinds of low cost or no cost treatment for mental health is often unavailable (Rose, 2019). In the meantime, medical legal jurisdiction has seen an inexorable expansion. In UK and other countries, statutory law continues to be the ultimate authority over those considered unable, or unwilling, to assess their own health and provide their own self-care, including those with eating disorders. Although differing from other forms of deviance such as criminality or antisocial actions that pose immediate harm or threat to others, DSM eating disorders fall under the same type of punitive legislation. Compulsory in-patient treatment is enforceable in the UK under the Mental Health Act 2007 and the Children's Act 1989 (NICE, 2021).

In conclusion, the co-existence of food poverty and disordered eating suggest that neither state-sponsored initiatives nor the actions of private businesses have properly addressed the socioeconomic disparities and issues of food quality and sustainability which are central to the development of unhealthy eating patterns. With healthy diets remain unaffordable for a third of the world's population (FAO, 2024), it is evident that much more needs to be done in the direction of ending huge global food inequalities. Furthermore, many of the existing theories concerning disordered eating and the genesis of EDs still ignore or fail to recognize the socially constructed nature of disordered eating. As a result, the "macro" factors of colonialism, capitalism, food conglomerates, and medical imperialism are largely hidden in favor of a continued focus on the individual psychology and singular solutions.

Just as the settings in which eating disorders exist are dynamic, so too are the wider narratives which determine the way we live and how we measure ourselves against another, including those related to eating practices. Scientific and social discourses are constantly being modified, updated, and even refuted as conditions change and new types of discourse are introduced. As discussed in Chap. 8, "Disordered Eating in the Virtual World," narratives running counter to "official" food biopedagogies are constantly being generated by users of ED services themselves (Sparks, 2017). Meanwhile, dietary interventions, and theories around them, continue to underscore individual behavioral change without introducing the economic policies and sanctions, which might reshape food landscapes in more fundamental and egalitarian ways.

Following on from these arguments, Chap. 6, "Biopolitics of Weight and Disordered Eating," will consider the operations of biopolitics in relation to the governance of weight and disordered eating. Topics explored include the permeation of fat stigma deep into societies marked by social and economic disparities, the theories concerning the obesogenic environment, and the debatable role of body positivity in deconstructing mainstream discourses around weight and body normativity.

References

Addley, E. (2023, August 4). *Friday briefing: Eating disorders are soaring in the UK, and so awaiting times for vital support.* The Guardian. Retrieved August 22, 2024, from https://www.theguardian.com/world/2023/aug/04/first-edition-eating-disorders-nhs-support

Albritton, R. (2013). Between obesity and hunger: The capitalist food industry. In P. Counihan & P. Van Esterik (Eds.), *Food and Culture: A reader* (pp. 342–355). Routledge.

Amoore, L. (2018). Cloud geographies: Computing, data, sovereignty. *Progress in Human Geography, 42*(1), 4–24.

Armstrong, D. (1995). The rise of surveillance medicine. *Sociology of Health & Illness, 17*(3), 393–404.

Banks, C. G. (1992). 'Culture' in culture-bound syndromes: The case of anorexia nervosa. *Social Science & Medicine, 34*(8), 867–884.
Barnhill, A. (2018). Introduction. In A. Barnhill, M. Budolfson, & T. Doggett (Eds.), *The Oxford handbook of food ethics*. Oxford University Press.
Barthels, F., Meyer, F., & Pietrowsky, R. (2018). Orthorexic and restrained eating behaviour in vegans, vegetarians, and individuals on a diet. *Eating and Weight Disorders-Studies on Anorexia, Bulimia and Obesity, 23*, 159–166.
Bernstein, B. B. (2001). From pedagogies to knowledges. In I. Neves, A. Morais, B. Davies, & H. Daniels (Eds.), *Towards a sociology of pedagogy: The contribution of Basil Bernstein to research* (pp. 363–378). Peter Lang.
Braidotti, R. (2013). *Patterns of dissonance: A study of women and contemporary philosophy*. Wiley.
Brytek-Matera, A. (2021). Vegetarian diet and orthorexia nervosa: A review of the literature. *Eating and Weight Disorders-Studies on Anorexia, Bulimia and Obesity, 26*, 1–11.
Bulik, C. M., Thornton, L. M., Parker, R., Kennedy, H., Baker, J. H., MacDermod, C., Guintivano, J., Cleland, L., Miller, A. L., Harper, L., Larsen, J. T., Yilmaz, Z., Grove, J., Sullivan, P. F., Petersen, L. V., Jordan, J., Kennedy, M. A., & Martin, N. G. (2021). The Eating Disorders Genetics Initiative (EDGI): Study protocol. *BMC Psychiatry, 21*(1), 1–9.
Cairney, P. (2019). *Understanding public policy: Theories and issues* (Vol. 2). Bloomsbury Publishing.
Candel, J. J., & Pereira, L. (2017). Towards integrated food policy: Main challenges and steps ahead. *Environmental Science & Policy, 73*, 89–92.
Culbert, K. M., Racine, S. E., & Klump, K. L. (2015). Research Review: What we have learned about the causes of eating disorders–a synthesis of sociocultural, psychological, and biological research. *Journal of Child Psychology and Psychiatry, 56*(11), 1141–1164.
D'angelo, C., Gloinson, E. R., Draper, A., & Guthrie, S. (2020). *Food consumption in the UK: Trends, attitudes and drivers*. Retrieved August 22, 2024, from www.randeurope.org
Darmon, N., & Drewnowski, A. (2008). Does social class predict diet quality? *The American Journal of Clinical Nutrition, 87*(5), 1107–1117.
de Zwaan, M. (2001). Binge eating disorder and obesity. *International Journal of Obesity, 25*(1), S51–S55.
Dellwing, M., & Harbusch, M. (2022). Conclusion. In M. Harbusch (Ed.), *Troubled Persons Industries: The expansion of psychiatric categories beyond psychiatry*. Springer International Publishing.

Demyttenaere, K., Bruffaerts, R., Posada-Villa, J., Lepine, J. P., Angermeyer, M. C., Bernert, S., et al. (2013). Prevalence, severity, and unmet need for treatment of mental disorders in the World Health Organization World Mental Health Surveys. *Journal of the American Medical Association, 291*(21), 2581–2590.

Eckersley, R. (2006). Is modern Western culture a health hazard? *International Journal of Epidemiology, 35*, 252–258.

Erskine, H. E., Whiteford, H. A., & Pike, K. M. (2016). The global burden of eating disorders. *Current Opinion in Psychiatry, 29*(6), 346–353.

Fee, M. (2006). Racializing narratives: Obesity, diabetes and the "Aboriginal" thrifty genotype. *Social Science & Medicine, 62*(12), 2988–2997.

Food and Agriculture Organization of the United Nations (FAO). (2024). *Statistics*. Retrieved August 16, 2024, from https://www.fao.org/statistics/en

Food, Farming, and Countryside, Commission (2024, November 15). *The False Economy of Big Food*. Retrieved 23 November from https://ffcc.co.uk/publications/the-false-economy-of-big-food

Foucault, M. (1972). *The archaeology of knowledge and the discourse of language*. Tavistock.

Foucault, M. (1973). *The birth of the clinic: An archaeology of perception*. Routledge.

Gao, Y., Bagheri, N., & Furuya-Kanamori, L. (2022). Has the COVID-19 pandemic lockdown worsened eating disorders symptoms among patients with eating disorders? A systematic review. *Journal of Public Health, 30*(11), 2743–2752.

Gates, K. A. (2011). *Our biometric future: Facial recognition technology and the culture of surveillance* (Vol. 2). NYU Press.

Gomez-Zavaglia, A., Mejuto, J. C., & Simal-Gandara, J. (2020). Mitigation of emerging implications of climate change on food production systems. *Food Research International, 134*, 109256.

Goodman, M. K., Johnston, J., & Cairns, K. (2017). Food, media and space: The mediated biopolitics of eating. *Geoforum, 84*, 161–168.

Gordon, R. (2001). Eating disorders East and West: A culture bound syndrome unbound. In M. Nasser, M. A. Katzman, & R. A. Gordon (Eds.), *Eating disorders and cultures in transition* (pp. 1–24). Brunner- Routledge.

Gracia-Arnaiz, M. (2010). Fat bodies and thin bodies. Cultural, biomedical and market discourses on obesity. *Appetite, 55*(2), 219–225.

Graham, L., Friedman, J., & Vega, X. (2022). Forbidding your cake and eating it too: Health performance strategies in U.S. middle class families. *Social Theory of Health, 20*, 237–259.

Gregory, A. (2023). *Ultra-processed food raises risk of heart attack and stroke, two studies show.* The Guardian. https://www.theguardian.com/science/2023/aug/27/ultra-processed-food-raises-risk-of-heart-attack-and-stroke-two-studies-show

Guertin, C., Pelletier, L., & Pope, P. (2020). The validation of the Healthy and Unhealthy Eating Behavior Scale (HUEBS): Examining the interplay between stages of change and motivation and their association with healthy and unhealthy eating behaviors and physical health. *Appetite, 144*, 104487.

Han, B.-C. (2014). *Psychopolitics: Neoliberalism and new technologies of power.* Verso.

Harvey, D. (2005). *A brief history of neoliberalism.* Oxford University Press.

Havinga, T., van Waarden, F., & Casey, D. (2015). *The changing landscape of food governance: Public and private encounters.* Edward Elgar Publishing.

Hay, P., & Touyz, S. (2016). Globalisation and the journal of eating disorders. *Journal of Eating Disorders, 4*, 1–2.

Heinrich, S. (2020). Medical science faces the post-truth era: A plea for the grassroot values of science. *Current Opinion in Anesthesiology, 33*(2), 198–202.

Hoek, H. W. (2016). Review of the worldwide epidemiology of eating disorders. *Current Opinion in Psychiatry, 29*(6), 336–339.

InnoScope Insights. (2024, March 20). *Latest size binge eating disorder treatment market to see huge growth [with CAGR of %] by 2032.* Linkedin. Retrieved August 22, 2024, from https://www.linkedin.com/pulse/latest-size-binge-eating-disorder-treatment-market-92kpc

Iyengar, S., & Massey, D. S. (2019). Scientific communication in a post-truth society. *Proceedings of the National Academy of Sciences, 116*(16), 7656–7661.

Kickbusch, I. (2015). The political determinants of health—10 years on. *BMJ, 350.*

LaMarre, A., & Rice, C. (2016, March). Embodying critical and corporeal methodology: Digital storytelling with young women in eating disorder recovery. In *Forum Qualitative Sozialforschung/Forum: Qualitative Social Research* (Vol. 17, No. 2).

Lambert, S. D., & Loiselle, C. G. (2007). Health information—Seeking behavior. *Qualitative Health Research, 17*(8), 1006–1019.

Lang, T., Barling, D., & Caraher, M. (2009). *Food policy: Integrating health, environment and society.* Oxford University Press.

Lee, S., Ho, T. P., & Hsu, L. G. (1993). Fat phobic and non-fat phobic anorexia nervosa: A comparative study of 70 Chinese patients in Hong Kong. *Psychological Medicine, 23*(4), 999–1017.

Leroy, F., Brengman, M., Ryckbosch, W., & Scholliers, P. (2018). Meat in the post-truth era: Mass media discourses on health and disease in the attention economy. *Appetite, 125*, 345–355.

Levenstein, H. (1980). The New England Kitchen and the origins of Modern American eating habits. *American Quarterly, 32*(4), 369–386.

Li, A. M. (2017). Ecological determinants of health: Food and environment on human health. *Environmental Science and Pollution Research International, 24*(10), 9002–9015.

Lloyd, S. J., Kovats, R. S., & Chalabi, Z. (2011). Climate change, crop yields, and undernutrition: Development of a model to quantify the impact of climate scenarios on child undernutrition. *Environmental Health Perspectives, 119*(12), 1817–1823.

Loopstra, R. (2020). *Vulnerability to food insecurity since Covid Lockdown. A preliminary report.* Retrieved August 22, 2024, from https://foodfoundation.org.uk/sites/default/files/2021-10/Report_COVID19FoodInsecurity-final.pdf

Madali, B., Alkan, Ş. B., Örs, E. D., Ayrancı, M., Taşkın, H., & Kara, H. H. (2021). Emotional eating behaviors during the COVID-19 pandemic: A cross-sectional study. *Clinical Nutrition ESPEN, 46*, 264–270.

Marrone, G., Guerriero, C., Palazzetti, D., Lido, P., Marolla, A., Di Daniele, F., & Noce, A. (2021). Vegan diet health benefits in metabolic syndrome. *Nutrients, 13*(3), 817.

Marmot, M. (2018). An inverse care law for our time. *BMJ, 362.*

Marx, G. T. (2019). *Windows into the soul: Surveillance and society in an age of high technology.* University of Chicago Press.

Mathieu-Bolh, N., & Wendner, R. (2020). We are what we eat: Obesity, income, and social comparisons. *European Economic Review, 128*, 103495.

McAtamney, K., Mantzios, M., Egan, H., & Wallis, D. J. (2021). Emotional eating during COVID-19 in the United Kingdom: Exploring the roles of alexithymia and emotion dysregulation. *Appetite, 161*, 105120.

McPhail, D. (2013). Resisting biopedagogies of obesity in a problem population: Understandings of healthy eating and healthy weight in a Newfoundland and Labrador community. *Critical Public Health, 23*, 289–303.

Meehan, O., & L., & Katzman, M. (2001). Argentina: The social body at risk. In M. Nasser, M. A. Katzman, & R. A. Gordon (Eds.), *Eating disorders and cultures in transition* (pp. 148–171). Brunner-Routledge.

Mennell, S. (1987). On the civilizing of appetite. *Theory, Culture & Society, 4*(2–3), 373–403.

Monaghan, C. R., & Evans, B. (2014). *Obesity discourse and fat politics: Research, critique and interventions* (Monaghan, R. Colls, & B. Evans, Eds.). Routledge.

Morley, J., Machado, C., Burr, C., Cowls, J., Taddeo, M., & Floridi, L. (2019). The debate on the ethics of AI in health care: A reconstruction and critical review. *Available at SSRN 3486518.*

Naja, F., & Hamadeh, R. (2020). Nutrition amid the COVID-19 pandemic: A multi-level framework for action. *European Journal of Clinical Nutrition, 74*(8), 1117–1121.

Nasser, M., Katzman, M., & Gordon, R. A. (Eds.). (2001). Eating disorders and cultures in transition. Psychology Press.

Neel, J. V. (1962). Diabetes mellitus: A "thrifty" genotype rendered detrimental by "progress"? *American Journal of Human Genetics, 14*(4), 353.

Ness, R. B., & Rothenberg, R. (2007). Critique of epidemiology: Changing the terms of the debate. *Annals of Epidemiology, 17*(12), 1011–1012.

NICE. (2021). *Eating disorders recognition and treatment.* Retrieved August 22, 2024, from https://www.nice.org.uk/guidance/ng69/chapter/Recommendations

Nicolosi, G. (2006). Biotechnologies, alimentary fears and the orthorexic society. *Tailoring Biotechnologies, 2*(3), 37–56.

O'Mara, J. & Vlad, I. (2023). Looking back at 5 years of UK Soft Drinks Industry Levy. *World Cancer Research Fund International.* https://www.wcrf.org/looking-back-at-5-years-of-the-uk-soft-drinks-industry-levy/

Oliver, J. (2017, March 30). We need a global food revolution. *Huffpost.* Retrieved August 22, 2024, from https://www.huffingtonpost.co.uk/jamie-oliver/jamie-oliver-sugar-food-revolution_b_9565484.html

Page, B., & Marshall, M. (2023). Briefing: Food, insecurity: What can local government do? *The Health Foundation.* https://health.org.uk

Pelto, G. H., & Pelto, P. J. (1983). Diet and delocalization: Dietary changes since 1750. *The Journal of Interdisciplinary History, 14*(2), 507–528.

Pirie, I. (2016). Disordered eating and the contradictions of neoliberal governance. *Sociology of Health & Illness, 38*(6), 839–853.

Rangel, C., Dukeshire, S., & MacDonald, L. (2012). Diet and anxiety. An exploration into the Orthorexic Society. *Appetite, 58*(1), 124–132.

Reid, M., & Hammersley, R. (2016). Is the British diet improving? *Nutrition Bulletin, 41*(4), 360–364.

Richards, C., Kjærnes, U., & Vik, J. (2016). Food security in welfare capitalism: Comparing social entitlements to food in Australia and Norway. *Journal of Rural Studies, 43*, 61.

Rizq, R. (2019). Introduction: The modern myths of IAPT. In C. Jackson & R. Rizq (Eds.), *The industrialisation of care: Counselling, psychotherapy and the impact of IAPT* (pp. 1–23). PCCS Books.

Rose, N. (1998). *Inventing our selves: Psychology, power, and personhood.* Cambridge University Press.

Rose, N. (2019). Forward. In C. Jackson & R. Rizq (Eds.), *The industrialisation of care: Counselling, psychotherapy and the impact of IAPT* (pp. v–x). PCCS Books.

Rosenberg, J. (2005). Globalization theory: A postmortem. *International Politics, 42*, 2–74.

Ryan, A. (2012). *The making of modern liberalism*. Princeton University Press.

Santomauro, D. F., Melen, S., Mitchison, D., Vos, T., Whiteford, H., & Ferrari, A. J. (2021). The hidden burden of eating disorders: An extension of estimates from the Global Burden of Disease Study 2019. *The Lancet Psychiatry, 8*(4), 320–328.

Schaumberg, K., Welch, E., Breithaupt, L., Hübel, C., Baker, J. H., Munn-Chernoff, M. A., et al. (2017). The science behind the academy for eating disorders' nine truths about eating disorders. *European Eating Disorders Review, 25*(6), 432–450.

Schijven, M. P., & Kroh, M. (2023). Harnessing the power of AI in health care: Benefits, risks, and preparation. *Surgical innovation, 30*(4), 417–418.

Schleider, J. L., Smith, A. C., & Ahuvia, I. (2023). Realizing the untapped promise of single-session interventions for eating disorders. *International Journal of Eating Disorders, 56*(5), 853–863.

Shanks, S., van Schalkwyk, M. C., & McKee, M. (2020). Covid-19 exposes the UK's broken food system. *BMJ (Clinical research ed.), 370*, m3085. https://doi.org/10.1136/bmj.m3085

Sherrington, R., Carlile, C., & Healy, H. (2023, December 9). *Big meat and dairy lobbyists turn out in record numbers at Cop28.* The Guardian. Retrieved August 22, 2024, from https://www.theguardian.com/environment/2023/dec/09/big-meat-dairy-lobbyists-turn-out-record-numbers-cop28#:~:text=Meat%20and%20dairy%20are%20particularly,since%202022%20to%20reach%20340

Silén, Y., & Keski-Rahkonen, A. (2022). Worldwide prevalence of DSM-V eating disorders among young people. *Current Opinion in Psychiatry, 35*(6), 362–371.

Sismondo, S. (2017). Post-truth? *Social Studies of Science, 47*(1), 3–6.

Skaik, R., & Inkpen, D. (2020). Using social media for mental health surveillance: A review. *ACM Computing Surveys (CSUR), 53*(6), 1–31.
Smithers, R. (2020, December 1). *Britons were the lockdown bingers of Europe, finds study.* The Guardian. Retrieved August 22, 2024, from https://www.theguardian.com/society/2020/dec/01/britons-were-the-lockdown-bingers-of-europe-finds-study
Sparks, M. (2017). Promoting health in a post-truth world. *Health Promotion International, 32*(4), 599–602.
Spigel, R., Lin, J. A., Milliren, C. E., Freizinger, M., Vitagliano, J. A., Woods, E. R., et al. (2021). Access to care and worsening eating disorder symptomatology in youth during the COVID-19 pandemic. *Journal of Eating Disorders, 9*(1), 1–9.
Steel, C. (2020). *Sitopia: How food can save the world.* Random House.
Steinglass, J. E., Berner, L. A., & Attia, E. (2019). Cognitive neuroscience of eating disorders. *Psychiatric Clinics, 42*(1), 75–91.
Thaler, R., & Sunstein, C. (2008). *Nudge: Improving decisions about health, wealth and happiness.* Yale University Press.
The Economist. (2023, July 12). *How to stop over medicalising mental health. What the world could learn from Britain's flawed approach.* Retrieved August 22, 2024, from https://www.economist.com/leaders/2023/12/07/how-to-stop-over-medicalising-mental-health
Thomas, P. (2019). Neoliberalism what it is, and why it matters. In I. C. Jackson & R. Rizq (Eds.), *The Industrialisation of care: Counselling, psychotherapy and the impact of IAPT* (pp. 23–44). PCCS Books.
Thornborrow, T., Evans, E. H., Tovee, M. J., & Boothroyd, L. G. (2022). Sociocultural drivers of body image and eating disorder risk in rural Nicaraguan women. *Journal of Eating Disorders, 10*(1), 1–16.
Tinning, R., & Glasby, T. (2002). Pedagogical work and the 'cult of the body': Considering the role of HPE in the context of the 'new public health'. *Sport, Education and Society, 7*(2), 109–119.
Turner, B. S. (2008). *The body and society: Explorations in social theory.* Sage.
van den Heuvel, L. L., Van der Merwe, C. A., Jordaan, G. P., & Szabo, C. P. (2023). Eating disorders in Africa. In *Eating disorders: An international comprehensive view* (pp. 1–22). Springer International Publishing.
Van Esterik, P. (2002). Contemporary trends in infant feeding research. *Annual Review of Anthropology, 31*(1), 257–278.

van Hoeken, D., Burns, J. K., & Hoek, H. W. (2016). Epidemiology of eating disorders in Africa. *Current Opinion in Psychiatry, 29*(6), 372–377.

Vlaev, I., King, D., Dolan, P., & Darzi, A. (2016). The theory and practice of "nudging": Changing health behaviors. *Public Administration Review, 76*(4), 550–561.

Wachter, S. (2018). Normative challenges of identification in the Internet of Things: Privacy, profiling, discrimination, and the GDPR. *Computer Law & Security Review, 34*(3), 436–449.

West, C. E., Goldschmidt, A. B., Mason, S. M., & Neumark-Sztainer, D. (2019). Differences in risk factors for binge eating by socioeconomic status in a community-based sample of adolescents: Findings from Project EAT. *International Journal of Eating Disorders, 52*(6), 659–668.

World Health Organization. (2023). *The Global Health Observatory. Body Mass Index among Adults.* Retrieved August 22, 2024, from https://www.who.int/data/gho/data/themes/topics/topic-details/GHO/body-mass-index

6

Biopolitics of Weight and Disordered Eating

So far in this book I have made several references to the biopolitical nature of disordered eating but have yet to give a clear explanation of the concept of biopolitics. Broadly, biopolitics involves the ways in which modern states and institutions manage the bodies and lives of populations through various regulatory mechanisms related to risk management, health and welfare. Although biopolitics permeates contemporary society, it is so widespread and internalized that it largely goes unnoticed. It is only when new forms of biopolitical power emerge—such as during the Covid pandemic, when governments implemented measures like mass vaccinations, mask mandates, and movement restrictions to control the spread of the virus—that the operations of biopolitics become the subject of serious scrutiny. These debates often revolve around concerns about the restriction of personal freedoms and conflicts between public health goals and economic interests. This chapter explores the role of biopolitics in the regulation of weight and disordered eating. In everyday life, diet and weight are essential aspects of both biological and social existence, heavily influenced by societal norms and policies. For example, for over half a century, a government-driven "war on fat" has been waged through public information campaigns, weight monitoring, efforts to

A. Fixsen, *The Construction of Eating Disorders*, The Politics of Mental Health and Illness, https://doi.org/10.1007/978-3-031-70318-8_6

modify individual dietary behaviors, and the penalization of obesity (Wright & Harwood, 2012). Simultaneously, food corporations and other commercial forces have continued to promote high-calorie processed foods, such that the war on obesity seems never to be won.

As I argue in this chapter, overweight and obesity are, in developed societies, closely tied to structural socioeconomic inequalities, such as limited access to healthy food, spaces for exercise and nutritional education. Obesity is associated with negative moral judgments and social stigma, which in turn shape the development and implementation of policies. Consequently, weight is a not just an individual concern but a political issue that intersects with policies related to poverty, education, and social welfare. The chapter begins with a detailed explanation of biopolitics, which readers in a hurry may choose to skim, but which is important in understanding the construction of disordered eating, such as through the ubiquitous use of BMI (body mass index) to distinguish normal from unhealthy bodies. The chapter then examines the measures taken to reduce obesity, from changing individual behaviors and eating practices to interventions aimed at tackling the "obesogenic environment." Finally, the controversial role of body positivity in challenging mainstream narratives around weight and body norms is considered. Regardless of society's apparent liberalization concerning body image, weight continues to dominate debates around political, economic, medical, and moral governance of disordered eating. Furthermore, with the advent of new biotechnologies, arguments around the obesogenic environment may be overshadowed by individual pharmaceutical solutions.

The Concept of Biopolitics

Pinpointing any precise starting point for the existence of biopolitics in society appears elusive (Prozorov, 2022). Some regard biopolitics as a force existing since antiquity (Agamben, 1998), while others argue that what counts as biopolitics requires some technological invention. Many regard the term itself as originating from the writings of Michel Foucault (1926–1984) who attempted to trace its genealogy. For Foucault, biopolitics or biopower (the operational arm of biopolitics) signifies a transition from sovereign power to liberalism, wherein governmental control is achieved with minimal intervention yet exerts maximum impact on populations (Foucault, 1976, 2003; Foucault et al., 2008). In *The Birth of the Clinic*, Foucault (1973) delineates two streams of medical discourse made possible due to institutionalization and technical progress: the medicine of the species, concerned with disease classification, posology, and individual patient care; and the medicine of social spaces, which directly addresses population health on a national scale, aimed at preventing and controlling infectious diseases and epidemics. It is interesting to note how the language of infectious disease control has since been appropriated to describe non-infectious issues such as in the term "obesity epidemic."

Campbell and Sitze (2013) explain biopolitics as representing the juncture where life (bios) intersects with the political sphere which, they add, is not the same as saying that life and politics are one. Biopolitics extends beyond conventional notions of citizenry, political affiliations, and democratic processes to involve the regulation and management of health of both state (polis) and populace (Dewey-Hagborg, 2023). It involves the rendering of a population and its health visible, traceable, and measurable, and entrusting chosen professionals to deliver services and improve health outcomes. In essence, biopolitics operates to permeate and exert control over every aspect of life, aiming to infiltrate and dominate all facets of existence. The notion of managing population health is often associated with notions of welfare, yet its connotations carry darker undertones. Historians have pointed out how the concept of "biopolitics" came to prominence in Nazi Germany,[1] and was later adopted by a 1960s US "naturalist" movement with questionable objectives (Lemke, 2012).[2] Present-day realms of biopolitics encompass issues ranging from population control, climate change, and social security breakdowns to retirement age, immigration, unequal access to medicine, and abortion rights. These areas, while heavily influenced by science, statistics, and economics, are also matters of public morality and political judgment.

[1] The regulation of life and through race took a prominent role in Nazi Germany (Lemke, 2012).

[2] The Anglo-US movement in political science is based on the idea that political action rests on biological laws.

Part of the brilliance of Foucault's thesis was in explaining how modernity assumes a hold on people's bodies via taken-for-granted biological thresholds within a social order. Biopower—a term used by Foucault for the operational side of biopolitics—permeates every aspect of our daily lives, through the various mechanisms designed to facilitate tasks aimed at sustaining life and promoting health, largely at the behest of subjects themselves. Hence, biopower reflects not so much a societal shift toward altruism but a recognition that healthy human capital, from a cost-benefit perspective, operates more efficiently when it is largely self-sustaining.[3] Inevitably, biopower extends to governance over minds, and another feature emphasized by Foucault is that of truth telling or confession (Foucault et al., 2008). Confessional discourse takes various forms we can recognize, such as health surveys, psychotherapy sessions, or personal online journals. Practically all forms of non-physiological health assessments, whether somatic or psychological, rely on individuals providing truthful responses about their health. That people will relate truthful responses is an assumption made by numerous scientific researchers, and one upon which many health statistics are based.

The operations of biopolitics and biopower can be broadly understood as proceeding in two interconnected ways. First, individuals engage in various techniques and self-care practices to maintain their health and well-being (Foucault, 1988). While the pursuit of self-care has a long history, under neoliberalism these practices have become increasingly economic and self-conscious. Many of us feel compelled to devote time and resources each day or week to sustain our physical and mental health, whether through activities like yoga, running, dieting programs, or cognitive exercises such as quizzes or book clubs. We often invest in apps that meticulously track our progress in these areas, both for personal satisfaction and to meet social expectations that self-monitoring can help relieve pressure on overburdened healthcare and social systems. Within this framework, disordered eating is seen as either a failure of self-care or an extreme manifestation of it. This perspective has been used to explain the rise of new eating disorders, such as binge eating disorder (BED) and,

[3] Foucault's lecture on the Birth of Biopolitics (Foucault et al., 2008) was mostly a treatise on the history of liberalism, the creation of *homoœconomicus* and neoliberalism.

more recently, orthorexia nervosa (ON), characterized by an obsessive focus on healthy eating.

A second mode of biopower, which is more central to this chapter, involves the management and regulation of the health of entire populations. Medicine and psychiatry have expanded into technological realms where individuals are encouraged to monitor and evaluate their physical health, aiming to meet "normative" biological standards—such as normal blood pressure or typical eating habits. For instance, body mass index (BMI) serves as a prime example of how a simple tool has not only normalized the routine measurement of bodies but has become a predictor of long-term health outcomes. This metric, which originated from the concept of social averages introduced by Belgian astronomer and statistician Lambert Adolf Jacques Quetelet (1796–1874), calculates a person's weight in kilograms divided by the square of their height in meters. According to the World Health Organization (2023a), overweight is defined as having a BMI of 25 or higher, while obesity is defined as having a BMI of 30 or more. However, critics argue that BMI overlooks the social and economic factors contributing to health disparities, such as the accumulation of risks and disadvantages from early life and their transmission across generations (Schoon et al., 2002, 2003). Additionally, BMI has been criticized for failing to account for factors like sedentary lifestyles, occupational activities, and changing consumer and dietary habits (Ebbeling et al., 2002). Its inability to consider cultural and ethnic diversity in body types and biosocial variations may contribute to the significant disparities in average BMI levels observed among children and adults across different countries (WHO, 2023a). On a fundamental level, the instruments of biopower have led to fresh conceptions of what it means to be human, with the body increasingly viewed as a fragmented, biotechnologically manipulated object (Halse, 2012). People nowadays are expected to manage their bodily state and identity through adopting pro-health behaviors, purchasing pro-health products, and adopting a language based on biological and psychological factors which places them in a category with certain fellow citizens, while distinguishing them from others (Rose & Novas, 2005)—for instance those with "normal" BMI or abnormal BMI.

One sociological concept which helps to shed light on the framing and acceptance of terms such as BMI as a defining categories in contemporary society is that of "social facts." Originating from Durkheim's writings in the late nineteenth century, social fact theory explains how individuals within a society internalize external phenomena as inherent aspects of their own reality. We are victims of an illusion, Durkheim argued, which leads us to believe we have produced what has been imposed upon us externally (Durkheim & Lukes, 1982). When social engineering fails to work or to act in people's favor, individuals and families are called out by institutions and others in society as lacking or even deviant. We can see this in the attitudes to parental upbringing and food and weight control of children. Ever since clinicians like Hilde Bruch (1982) and Arthur Crisp (1980) published case studies linking poor food habits and childhood obesity with anorexia nervosa development, parent blaming has continued in education, social, and health services. Both overweight and underweight in children have been inferred as forms of parental abuse, leading to the removal of obese children and the use of bariatric surgery—with all its negative implications in terms of discomfort, nutritional deficiencies, and the emergence of ED pathologies post-surgery (Beamish & Reinehr, 2017; Calcaterra et al., 2021; Conceição et al., 2013). Even though numerous studies have emphasized the link between economic deprivation and obesity (Béghin et al., 2014; Fernández et al., 2021; Kelly et al., 2019), individuals deemed as overweight are seen as bypassing or breaking normal and accepted dietary rules, and as such are classed as socially and morally deviant.

Weight as a Discourse of Power

In everyday life, diet and weight are central aspects of biological and social life, which are heavily regulated and influenced by societal norms and policies. Primarily, attention has been directed toward addressing the perceived "obesity epidemic" through measures such as information dissemination, food industry regulations, weight monitoring, and individual sanctions and interventions in dietary habits (Wright & Harwood, 2012). The influence of health education in schools has played a crucial role in shaping this narrative by advocating for food policies and pedagogies that operate as directives, demanding compliance from individuals irrespective of age or circumstance (Fernández et al., 2021; Leahy, 2014). The discourse around the psychology of diet and weight has also gained much prominence and serves as a pivotal means of distinguishing between normal and pathological states of body and mind. The incorporation of lifestyle-focused classifications into the DSM and ICD has extended their reach into bodily domains like binge eating and muscle body dysmorphia. Developments in genetics (Bulik et al., 2021), neuroscience (Steinglass et al., 2019), AI modeling (Haynos et al., 2021), and the tracking technologies allowing individuals to monitor their own health have together led to a shift in focus away from sociocultural constructs, such as the "obesogenic"[4] environment, toward a biochemical conception of "disease." Together, these technologies and taxonomies have amounted to a new type of governmentality, which is aimed at medicalizing, tracking, and controlling "oversize" bodies both locally and globally.

Beyond the physiological and ethical implications associated with weight, there exists significant overlap between bodies categorized as above or below normal BMI and those classified as having mental disorders. Although obesity itself is not considered an eating disorder but rather a metric calculation, it is often construed in a manner that lends itself to psychiatric classification (Brewis, 2010). The emergence of binge eating disorder (BED) as a category (APA, 2013) has accelerated the connection between physical appearance and a perceived disordered psyche, leading to a rise in official diagnoses of eating disorders. When an individual with a larger body, especially from a lower socioeconomic status or marginalized background, presents with distress, there is a tendency to assume that overeating is the primary issue, despite research showing that most diets fail in body mass terms (Gotovac et al., 2020). The general view is that dietary programs and medications can produce no more than 10 percent weight loss (Waseem et al., 2007).

The biopolitics of food production has been one of an elaborate interplay between governmental power, societal norms and the production, marketing, and consumption of edible items. For example, the

[4] Swinburn et al. (1999) describe the obesogenic environment as the collective effects exerted by surroundings, opportunities, and life circumstances and conditions that contribute to the promotion of obesity among individuals or populations.

biopolitics of sugar is deeply tied in with a grossly unequal and racist system of food production and distribution. Historically, the cultivation and trade of sugarcane played a pivotal role in shaping global economies and societies, fueling colonial expansionism, racialism, labor and sexual exploitation, and the rise of industrial capitalism. Along with these often abhorrent features of the sugar trade were the earlier idealized portrayals of migration and colonization and more recently the interweaving of biomedical knowledge around displaced bodies and colonized land (Bastos, 2008). In contemporary times, the politics of sugar still dominates political, medical, and social debate (Doucet-Battle, 2021). Government policies such as agricultural subsidies and trade agreements influence sugar production and distribution, and impact both local economies and global dynamics, for example, by cultivating technologies and markets for alternative sweeteners like the intensely sweet-tasting plant, stevia.

While public health initiatives and regulatory measures seek to address the consequences for health of excessive sugar consumption, including obesity, diabetes, and other disorders, the sugar industry continues to significantly influence governance through its lobbying efforts, marketing strategies, and sponsor deals. Debates around sugar taxes, food labeling requirements, and advertising restrictions highlight the contested terrain of sugar regulation, and how deeply tied in it is with the politics of weight and size. In the meantime, African Americans and those from African descent have found themselves primary subjects and customers of Type II Diabetes drugs and treatments (Doucet-Battle, 2021). Not only are African Americans the subjects of aggressive pharmacological marketing, but as geonomics moves from calculating risk probabilities to calculating complex traits in individuals, they are prime subjects for genetic counseling (Jabloner, 2021).

The "War on Fat"

The western campaign against obesity is built upon certain presumptions and narratives of normalization. Firstly, there is the belief that obesity and being overweight are illnesses necessitating regulation due to their substantial economic burden on nations. The sheer volume and breadth of obesity statistics are staggering, with a wealth of literature detailing the risks and detriments associated with excessive adiposity,[5] not just for the health of a nation but its moral character. Governmental efforts to control various aspects of public health—including personal hygiene, weight, and exercise—hinge on the willingness of individuals to adopt alternative practices and behaviors. To convey these narratives effectively, authorities often resort to using alarming language such as "epidemic," "burden," "scourge," and "terror" to depict perceived surges in physical or moral aberrations. A recent Google Scholar search yielded over 500,000 results for the term "burden of eating disorders" and 244,000 for "epidemic of eating disorders," underscoring the shifting focus of health discourse toward these maladies. The World Health Organization adopts such epidemiological language when they describe obesity as a "global killer" (WHO, 2023b).

The fear of fat and its moral and physical consequences have gone hand in hand with capitalist economics. Cohen (1972) wrote how moral panics are driven by "moral entrepreneurs" who, through their interest-based claims making, continue to play a key role in defining crises such as the one concerning obesity (Boero, 2016). Nineteenth-century righteous food reformers Drs Graham[6] and Kellogg capitalized on this effect in their outcries against gluttony (along with masturbation). The former called on all "good American mothers" to act as moral bulwarks by ensuring that his whole meal products featured on the table of every US home. For these capitalist evangelists, wheat symbolized not only domestic order, civic health, and moral prosperity but a flourishing and civilized nation due to the crop's upright, uniform, and colonizing attributes (Tompkins, 2009). Ironically, the rise of mass food production, including wheat, was later blamed for the surge in obesity during the post-World War II era, leading to widespread societal disapproval of both fat bodies and carbohydrate-rich foods. It was as though the scientific community and media had belatedly the impact of food capitalism on the dietary

[5] According to WHO statistics, in 2016, more than 1.9 billion adults over 18 years were overweight and 250 million of these adults were obese (WHO, 2023b).

[6] Dr Graham's health mission was both religious and colonialist. According to Tompkins (2009), Graham imagined an ideal Americanness founded upon an imperial fantasy and indigeneity, regulated through the daily consumption of farinaceous foods. Others like Kellogg followed in his wake.

habits of entire generations. By the 1960s, mainstream media coverage of obesity had reached unprecedented levels, "solidifying" fat as one of the most pressing issues confronting both North America and the global community (Boero, 2016).

The term "war on fat" first gained traction in biopolitical discourse within the United States (US), drawing from a historical link between military fervor and anti-gluttony sentiments amidst population growth, cultural shifts, and societal fractures (Greenhalgh, 2012). Fatness has since evolved beyond an issue of individual discipline to a perceived burden of chronic disease on society at large (Williams, 2014), with obese individuals facing blame for various societal issues, including increased fuel and travel costs (Boero, 2012). The conspicuous presence of the obese contrasted with the invisibility of corporate actors working for mega companies promoting high-fat, low-cost fast food in underserved communities, most with interested and investments in medical and pharmaceutical solutions for obesity (FFCC, 2024). The medicalization of obesity in post-World War II America, coupled with the spread of western diets and sedentary lifestyles, facilitated its emergence in regions where it was previously rare (McCullough & Hardin, 2013), fueling a global panic amplified by sensationalized portrayals of overweight individuals in the media (Campos et al., 2006). These narratives often highlight rankings of nations by obesity rates and physical inactivity levels (McCullough & Hardin, 2013). Governments, besides taxing high-fat and high-sugar foods, have targeted parents of obese children through written or financial penalties. In England and some US states, families have received warning letters if their children are overweight, eliciting varied responses ranging from shock and self-blame to relief and self-congratulation (Nnyanzi et al., 2016). Some countries have gone further, proposing fines for parents of obese children, as seen in Puerto Rico in 2015 (Parkinson, 2015),[7] drawing criticism for stigmatizing children and inadequately addressing economic disparities and access to healthy food options. Given the high price of fresh food and prevalence of fast-food restaurants in low-income areas, eating out is often the cheaper

[7] In 2015, the Puerto Rican government sought to introduce the policy of fining parents of obese children up to $800 if, after a warning, no improvement was seen in a year (Parkinson, 2015).

option for big families. In summary, addressing obesity requires a multi-faceted approach, including efforts to reduce obesogenic environments and promote healthy behaviors in young people (Swinburn et al., 1999; Lipek et al., 2015). Central to this is the reduction of disparities in access to nutritious food and community amenities (Larson et al., 2009; Rosi et al., 2017), although such policies inevitably face opposition rooted in resistance to wealth taxation and efforts to mitigate residential segregation by class and ethnicity.

Fat Stigma and Social Inequality

Fat stigma has permeated deeply into societies marked by social and economic disparities. In recent western history, obese individuals have been subjected to ridicule and shock, with pervasive negative attitudes portraying them as lazy, lacking willpower, and non-compliant (Puhl & Heuer, 2010). Such perceptions contribute to weight stigma and body dissatisfaction, framing obesity as a global scourge to be swiftly eliminated (McCullough & Hardin, 2013; Swinburn et al., 2011) and associating biological deviation with social and psychiatric deviance (Farrell, 2011). Overweight individuals are shamed for occupying more physical and societal space, leading to diminished self-esteem, psychological distress, self-harming behaviors, and avoidance of medical care (Puhl & Heuer, 2010). Stigma, rooted in discrimination and prejudice, erects barriers for obese individuals across various spheres, including healthcare, employment, sport, and education (Forhan & Salas, 2013; Hunger et al., 2015). In explaining the high rates of obesity in adolescent youth from less privileged social backgrounds, Von Kardorff and Ohlbrecht (2008) reject individualistic explanations of health, arguing that personality traits, genetic determinants, and family histories fail to explain how such an increase in adolescent obesity could occur within a relatively short timeframe. Instead, they draw on the concept of the "obesogenic environment" to examine eating disorders as specific socio-somatic reactions linked to social change. Cultural and social perceptions of adolescence have, for a very long time, been seen to embody fitness, mobility, spontaneity, and a focus on the future. Under present social and economic conditions, the critical transition from adolescence to adulthood is one of immense pressure to find a suitable job in the face of an inadequate training market and increased demands of knowledge, social competence, and self-presentation. The result is often maladaptive behaviors, including mental illness and obesity in this age group:

> Overweight adolescents symbolically "withdraw" from these aspirations in the face of increased demands and fiercer competition when it comes to maintaining or gaining in status and in view of a developing social exclusion. Bulimia sufferers, on the other hand, try symbolically but in vain to aspire to these status gains by working constantly on their own body's diet. (von Kardorff & Ohlbrecht, 2008, p. 433)

While weight is often viewed as solely within individual control, disparities in healthcare and self-care accessibility persist across economic and geographical divides. Mass-produced cheap food, often the only option for low-income families, exacerbates issues of chronic illness and reduced lifespan (Marmot, 2018; WHO, 2023a). The "inverse law of care" perpetuates disadvantage for those in lower socioeconomic status areas, highlighting the need for equitable access to physical activity and healthier dietary options, particularly for the poorest individuals (WHO, 2023a). However, health policies often focus on monitoring and surveillance, neglecting systemic solutions and widening the gap between the rich and poor, complicating the paradoxical link between obesity and poverty (Żukiewicz-Sobczak et al., 2014).

The cultural crusade against fat in the US has exacerbated societal weight anxieties and resulted in widespread socioemotional suffering, particularly among marginalized groups (Greenhalgh, 2012). Ethnographic research reveals instances of fat-shaming directed at non-white teenagers, exacerbating feelings of moral deficiency and marginalization (Greenhalgh, 2012). Similar observations have been corroborated by studies documenting systematic exclusion of overweight individuals from educational and employment opportunities (Forhan & Salas, 2013; Hunger et al., 2015). "Fat talk" has remained an important way of distinguishing between productive and deviant individuals. Obese people can experience discrimination in many parts of their lives, with the workplace being no exception. According to a recent study published in *The Economist* (2023), despite anti-discriminatory legislation, fat stigma in workplaces continues to negatively impact the earnings of people of all genders. In the fields of education and healthcare, weight stigmatization may be justified on the basis that shame can motivate individuals to adopt healthier behaviors. Fat people are no longer merely "lazy" and "ugly," they are biologically abnormal, at risk of disease, and in need of medical treatment. Politicians and celebrities in the media (such as Oprah Winfrey) have taken up the cause of "remaking overweight and obese subjects into thin, fit, proper Americans" (Greenhalgh, 2012, p. 473).

As a discourse, fat talk moves attention away from more insidious and pervasive structural problems in society, such as poverty, inequality, and deprivation (Boero, 2013). Yet, fat stigma draws on the authority of scientific experts, doctors, physical education teachers, and others, such that making challenges to their assertions may appear reckless and fool hardy. These kinds of stigmatizing discourses rub off on young people, not just those who are stigmatized but those who wish to avoid stigma by any means. In one study in the US, over 90 percent of the three hundred and two adolescents scored high on weight stigma and anti-fat bias, with 20 percent describing adopting disordered eating behaviors, 15 percent fasting, 5 percent taking pills, and 5.3 percent vomiting or using laxatives to avoid weight gain. The authors concluded that obesity was seen as an identity threat by young people and as associated with negative collective representations of obesity in US society (Hunger et al., 2015).

Weight, Gender, and Ethnicity

Among those scholars challenging assertions about obesity are those who do so based on gender discrimination. Arguments that weight gain and fatness are deviant and maladaptive behaviors have been contested by feminists for decades. In *Fat is a Feminist Issue*, Susie Orbach wrote of how fat was the external result of women's compulsive eating, which was itself a coping mechanism for gender inequality (Orbach, 1978). Binge eating entered the DSM in 1987; however, this type of erratic, emotionally driven overeating in women, is, according to Orbach, driven by an unconscious desire to hide from male sexual objectification and trivialization, and competition with other women. Thin women are not taken seriously; hence, some women put on weight as an unconscious protest at the gender divide. Research has found that obesity in women remains discriminated against in both society and workplace to a greater degree than their male counterparts (Puhl et al., 2008; Puhl & Heuer, 2009). In one recent study looking at work resumes sent out to employers in Mexico, where a job application requires a photograph of the candidate, statistically, an obese woman would need to send out 37 percent more resumes to obtain the same number of callbacks as the non-obese candidate (Campos-Vazquez & Gonzalez, 2020).

Orbach's seminal work has been critiqued for appearing to support the idea that fatness itself signifies a form of disordered eating (Cooper, 1998; Saguy, 2012). Yet, Orbach must be credited for highlighting the politics around women and weight norms. Reflecting on her book 40 years later, Orbach (2018) considers how little has changed, except that eating has become far more medicalized and women's relationship to food and bodies more pathologized. Beauty work, she argues, has become a relentless task, and the ubiquity of judgment and failures creates insecurities that hurt women's minds. "Obesity Inc" has set about creating so-called disease entities which medicalize and pathologize people's relationship to food and body so successfully that vast industries have emerged to treat the very problems that these industries have instigated. "If we weren't continually assaulted by the merchants of body hatred, we would not be as vulnerable to the assaults," Orbach (2018) states.

Fikkan and Rothblum (2012) agree that fat is a feminist issue because fat women are subjugated to bias, discrimination, and abuse, simply based on their size. The authors signal the importance of examining how the social experiences of fat people vary by sex and social class. Their work is substantiated by statistical studies which show women to be at greater risk of weight/height discrimination than men. These effects may be aided by the propulsion of scientific studies on eating disorders in the direction of genetics and neuroscience (Steinglass et al., 2019). A flaw in these feminist studies, however, is the assumption that the fear and disgust of fatness is something only women experience, with patriarchy posed as the central cause of women's fat oppression. Writing in the

1980s, Chernin (1981) acknowledged that some men did wish to lose weight, but overall, fat men were spared the burden of negative symbolic meaning attached to fatness that the fat woman had taken on. More recent studies refute this idea; men of today are concerned about the shape and look of their bodies and are just as likely to feel stigmatized by being over or underweight as women (Gilman, 2004; Dworkin & Wachs, 2009).

While it is important to examine why women continue to be penalized for their weight such as women over a certain BMI level being denied in vitro fertilization treatment (Campbell, 2012), feminist scholars would be wrong to dismiss fat men's experiences with weight stigma. The public condemnation of criticism of women based on their body size and weight (e.g., on the television show *Australian idol*) has, according to Bell and McNaughton (2007), become more common place. It reflects the extent to which popular feminist interpretations that link gender, patriarchy, body image, and weight have been taken up by those in touch with media. Moreover, fat has long been portrayed as feminizing, devaluing to the male body (Bell and McNaughton, 2007; Gilman, 2004), and leading to ridicule from derogatory terms such as "man boobs." Whereas once larger size in men might have signified wealth, it now represents underproductivity. Fat talk buys into the "culture of lack" (Dworkin & Wachs, 2009), through which consumer capitalism first points out people's body flaws, then sells them the means to improve their bodies. This leads to a culture in which younger man are embarrassed or feel discouraged from help seeking (Nagata et al., 2020).

The portrayal of obesity as a "self-inflicted health risk" by various institutions such as governments, medicine, and media has significantly impacted the experiences of black and Colored communities in the US and beyond. This perspective, generally framed as resulting from personal lifestyle choices lacking in morality and self-discipline, has largely dominated obesity debates. Saguy and Gruys (2010) cite examples of the ways that the media negatively constructs eating disorders as individual moral deficits and examine how these attitudes may rub off on health professionals, affecting how they view and treat their patients with eating disorders. These attitudes, along with anti-obesity measures which target individuals, mean that attempts to challenge or change social and market policies contributing to the obesogenic environment are confined to the margins of sociology and equal rights campaigns. In the US, obesity rates have risen much faster among minority groups compared to white populations, worsening existing racial and ethnic disparities, and leading to numerous negative psychosocial consequences for these communities (Sanders, 2019).

The discourse surrounding anti-obesity often targets marginalized groups, including indigenous populations, and those who are poor or otherwise disadvantaged (Gotovac et al., 2020). Statistics from the Centers for Disease Control and Prevention (CDC) indicate that the highest rates of self-reported obesity are found among non-Hispanic black adults (41 percent), compared to a figure of 31 percent in non-Hispanic white adults and 11.7 percent in non-Hispanic Asian adults. Similar disparities exist among black and Latino children compared to their white counterparts (Sanders, 2019). The CDC (2013) emphasizes the role of neighborhood design, access to healthy food and beverages, and opportunities for physical activity in influencing obesity rates. They stress the importance of addressing social determinants of health such as poverty, education, and housing to eliminate barriers to good health. However, scholars, including Sanders (2019), argue that framing obesity as a racialized epidemic serves to maintain racial hierarchies and uphold white norms. This construction of obesity as a threat to health is one way in which dominant groups define both health risks and marginalized identities, thus preserving their own privilege. Sympathetic portrayals of obesity as a medical condition often target black and Latina/o women and children, perpetuating racial injustices and justifying discriminatory practices that reinforce structural racial inequalities. Regardless of all the rhetoric used in health policy discussions, portraying obesity as a condition linked to ethnicity has failed to reduce the stigma faced by people of color. The media's tendency to highlight obesity statistics and stories involving black and Latino families may shed light on why, in a 2013 public survey, only 33 percent of whites, compared to 66 percent of blacks and 69 percent of Hispanics, thought that the government needed to play a significant role in reducing obesity (The Pew Centre, 2013).

Weight Loss and Healthism

The selling of weight-loss products goes back centuries and remains one of the least regulated of health sectors. Many prescription and nonprescription drugs for weight loss developed from 1960s were subsequently withdrawn from the US market because of adverse effects, while there is little evidence of the efficacy of "natural" and herbal dietary supplements for weight loss (Lenz & Hamilton, 2004). The millions of people who enroll in commercial and self-help weight-loss programs know little about what to expect from them. One review of supervised weight-loss treatment programs found that while patients who completed could lose from up to 15–25 percent of their initial weight, the long-term outcomes of programs were far less evident. Most of these programs were associated with high costs, high attrition rates, and a probability of regaining half or more of ones lost weight in one or two years. In other studies, commercial interventions available over the Internet and organized self-help programs have produced minimal weight loss. Aside from one *Weight Watchers* trial, evidence supporting the use of the major commercial and self-help weight-loss programs was concluded to be suboptimal (Tsai & Wadden, 2005).

Despite these issues, the weight-loss industry continues to grow exponentially and is expected to be worth around \$54bn (£45bn) by 2033 (Das & Ungoed-Thomas, 2023a). One of the major players in the slimming market is Novo Nordisk, whose sales of obesity treatments include the semiglutide drug *Wegovy*—an appetite suppressor hailed as a "weight-loss magic bullet." Writing in the *Guardian* newspaper, Das and Ungoed-Thomas (2023b) revealed an orchestrated publicity campaign to boost the UK sales of *Wegovy* and see it established as the NHS drug of choice. Academics and health organizations who backed the "skinny jab" *Wegovy* were being paid millions of pounds by the company. This included a paid clinical expert describing the slimming injection as a "game changer" to the National Institute for Health and Care Excellence (NICE) and payments made to MPs, obesity charities, and Royal Colleges to promote the product (Das & Ungoed-Thomas, 2023b). Less publicised is the likelihood that once the drug is stopped, weight is likely to return relatively quickly without other health interventions. Moreover, semiglutides are not considered to be safe for long-term use, due to their potentially serious side-effects (NICE, 2023). Judging by the present flow of drug company money through the NHS and the publicity the drugs are receiving, these drawbacks are unlikely to deter their production by other companies and their use on an enormous scale in the next decades (Das & Ungoed-Thomas, 2023c).[8]

The close links between medical and nutritional experts and big drug and food companies appear to extend across continents and healthcare sectors. A recent US report published in Public Health Nutrition and cited in *Med Page Today* (DePeau-Wilson, 2022) found that several of those in key leadership posts in the Academy of Nutrition and Dietetics (AND) held important positions in multinational food and agri-business companies. AND had invested funds in corporations such as *Nestlé, PepsiCo*, and pharmaceutical companies and had accepted substantial corporate financial contributions. A subsequent official statement by AND described the report as "a calculated attack" which included misleading claims and figures (eatrightpro.org., 2022). Meanwhile a weight-loss tool that uses magnets cemented into the mouth to stop people from opening their mouths wide enough to eat solid food has been developed to tackle obesity. By only permitting users to open their mouths to 2mm wide, the device, *DentalSlim Diet Control*, enforces a liquid-only diet. Eating disorder charities have described the device as heinous, oversimplifying the issue of obesity and as potentially seriously damaging a person affected by binge eating disorder (Ng, 2021). Academics have similarly critiqued the jaw locking device for being "locked into the past" and the infamous history of jaw wiring while completely ignoring a nuanced and holistic analysis of obesity in the pursuit of commercial gains (Tu et al., 2021). Nevertheless, it is likely that these kinds of piecemeal solutions will continue to be recommended and sought after in the society which vilifies fat while failing to come up with policy solutions to the obesogenic environment.

[8] Writing about the association between multinational drug companies and the NHS, Das and Ungoed-Thomas (2023c) note how in 2022, the total value of drug company payments to healthcare organizations and professionals was more than £200m.

The weight normative approach to weight loss has also faced criticism for potentially contributing to unhealthy weight cycling. In a 15-year study by Rzehak et al. (2007) focusing on weight change and weight "cycling" (from losing weight to gaining weight) in middle-aged men, it was discovered that weight fluctuations significantly increased the risk of all-cause mortality in this demographic. On the other hand, stable obesity did not show a further rise in mortality in men aged 55–77 during long-term follow-up, suggesting that the emphasis on higher weight alone as a health risk factor may be overstated. Although evidence substantiates a correlation between weight gain and increased rates of chronic illnesses such as Type II Diabetes and a heightened risk of ischemic heart disease (Ebbeling et al., 2002), these risks seem to be especially associated with very high BMI.

Meanwhile, the crossover between "fast" food and "healthy" food remains a confusing area for consumers with constrained budgets. Since the 1960s, low-fat foods have been touted as the healthy choice, with reduced-fat convenience foods being among the most heavily advertised items in media commercials. As consumer awareness about health has increased, fast-food chains have introduced new "healthy option" products and adopted health-focused communication strategies. Food and beverage companies have actively positioned themselves as part of the solution, utilizing strategies like the International Food and Beverage Alliance—a coalition comprising multinational corporations such as *Pepsi, Coca-Cola, Nestlé, Mars,* and *Unilever*—assuring the WHO of their commitment to addressing childhood obesity (Commetric, 2019). Employing similar approaches, "better for you" brands like *Dig Inn* and *Sweet Green* aim to compete with *McDonald's* on aspects other than price by carving out their own niche and emphasizing locally sourced ingredients. Furthermore, long-standing players in this market include manufacturers of vitamins, protein shakes, and various sports supplements, which are now heavily promoted online, often accompanied by images of toned male and female bodies reminiscent of the "corporate athlete" (Kelly et al., 2007).[9] Jumping on the weight-loss bandwagon has been the

[9] Kelly et al. (2007) used the term the "corporate athlete" for the person who embodies their own and corporate goals. They are the embodiment of the pro-health market and its link with the work-

various televised weight-loss boot camps and "reality" shows about obesity, and public campaign and adverts featuring "headless fatties," supposedly cropped to protect people's identities, but effectively dehumanizing people and leaving them open to ridicule and abuse (Mayes, 2015, 2016).

The concept of "health" is laden with subjective assessments and unexamined assumptions, reflecting power dynamics and societal privileges as much as it does physical well-being (Metzl et al., 2010). Health is commonly perceived as an ideal condition, yet the methods of attaining health are deeply intertwined with economic and political factors (Fullagar, 2019). Ivan Illich (1975) famously criticized the medical establishment as a significant threat to health, while Skrabanek (1994) wrote about the rise of a coercive healthism resulting in the loss of body autonomy. Skrabanek, a radical libertarian, viewed the pursuit of health as ultimately counterproductive, serving to fill a void left by religion in secular societies (O'Mahony, 2019). Skrabanek's perspective has been criticized as dangerous (he disagreed with legislation against tobacco use as well as obesity); however, he was correct in noting medicine's shift toward targeting lifestyle choices. A 2016 report by the Royal College of Surgeons revealed that more than one in three Clinical Commissioning Groups (CCGs) in England were either refusing or delaying routine surgeries for smokers and obese patients.[10] The College cautioned against this trend, warning that these patients were being made "soft targets for NHS savings" (Senthilingham, 2017).

The tenets of healthism have been internalized by many consumers, which, by projecting health as a personal choice, exonerate weight bias (Walsh et al., 2023). Adding the term "healthy," "low fat," or "reduced sugar" to their product promotions is often a ploy by corporations to increase their prices or reduce their product size. Metzl et al. (2010) point to PepsiCo's marketing strategy to sell their low-fat version of *Naco-Cheese Doritos* to AfroAmerican customers at an increased cost (Metzl et al., 2010). Yet, studies suggest that weight-loss schemes work best when

place and neoliberal entrepreneurism. The corporate athlete has also been widely used in the business literature as an idealized state to achieve.

[10] One argument put forward for this practice has been that overweight patients are more at risk of health complications.

people are supported in other ways, for example, by situating parents as the agents of change and providing them with the skills to change the dietary practices of themselves and their families (Arredondo et al., 2018). Moreover, high-quality foods remain largely the property of the privileged, whereas disadvantaged neighborhoods are over-populated by fast-food outlets, with spaces for physical activity and large supermarkets often absent. The influence of low socioeconomic status on weight begins very early in life. Poverty in very early childhood (under two years) was a key indicator of obesity in teenage years (Lee et al., 2014). Attempts to turn healthism itself into psychiatric pathology are explored in Chap. 9 of this book.

Body Positivity

In the last few decades, a movement designed to promote diversity and inclusivity of bodies has emerged, which in essence can be viewed as a counterforce to capitalism and patriarchy. Stemming from the activism of individuals from fat, black, and Queer communities in response to the pervasive representation of only white, slim bodies as visible or valuable in discourses and visual media (such as fashion advertising), the body positivity movement is part of a broader discourse on intersectionality, championed by influential writers and activists such as bell hooks, Audre Lorde, and Patricia Hill Collins. The roots of body positivity can also be traced back to fat activism (Cooper, 1998), in North American movements such as the National Association to Aid Fat Americans (NAAFA) and the Fat Underground (FU). With the advent of social media, body positivity has gained traction by advocating for the acceptance of bodies of "all shapes, sizes, and appearances" (Downey, 2020, p. 8).

The body positivity movement has also faced criticism, especially regarding its ties to marketing and its co-option by a predominantly white-centered political agenda (Downey, 2020; Griffin et al., 2022). Body positivity itself has been turned into a form of "brand possibility" through which corporations can align themselves with social and medical issues. Online platforms have witnessed a rapid proliferation of body positivity discussions, with hashtags like #bodypositive and

#bodypositivity amassing over 13 million posts in 2020 (Gelsinger, 2021). Predictably, these hashtags and other symbols of body positivity have been appropriated by various media outlets. Advertisers, for instance, have recognized the potential novelty of featuring larger-bodied individuals performing dances or acrobatics, while plus-size models have increasingly garnered attention in headlines. There are the thorny questions about how body positivity fits within the discourses of medicine and eating disorders. Even within the body positivity movement, individuals may feel pressured to publicly disclose their struggles with disordered eating for the sake of authenticity and societal benefit. One notable figure is plus-size model Tess Holliday, who gained fame not only for showcasing images of her body but for sharing her experiences and diagnosis of "atypical anorexia" (Nied, 2022; O'Neill, 2023). Holliday has been vocal about her challenging upbringing marked by family dysfunction and its detrimental effects on her body image and eating habits. Her approach to addressing these issues has involved cutting ties with "toxic" family members and seeking therapeutic intervention, actions which have been shared with her extensive online audience (Nied, 2022).

These types of weight narratives become focal points of public attention, as seen in instances like Piers Morgan's interviews with plus-size women on daytime television, where the limits of body positivity are debated in terms of weight and health. Such media interactions often center around a narrative of redemption through candid self-disclosure. By publicly embracing and affirming their bodies, individuals may perceive an improvement in personal health and well-being. One might interpret these actions as ways in which individuals navigate life in an interconnected world, using their bodies and relationship with food to construct their identities (Watson & Caldwell, 2005). From another perspective, these actions reflect a societal paradigm wherein the body in modernity has come to be viewed as a project to be worked on autonomously, toward one's chosen identity construction (Giddens, 1991). Both viewpoints hint at a degree of freedom in thought and action that arguably contradicts the capitalist underpinnings of these discourses.

In summary, biopolitics has proved itself to be an enduring and adaptable tool of analysis (Salter & Waldby, 2011). Despite apparent advancements in societal discussions on gender, ethnicity, and body image, Foucault's foundational concept of biopolitics, and biopower as a form of governance over peoples' bodies, persist. These concepts encompass the influential institutions shaping individuals' lives, such as medicine, education, and the legal system; the authoritative knowledge these institutions claim as truth; and the mechanisms of power and technologies, that enforce institutional narratives. People continue to be assessed based on specific norms regarding bodies, perpetuated through notions of normality, deviance, health, and disorder. This mode of social control endures, despite evolving norms and regulations exploiting uncertainty by constantly shifting health paradigms. Meanwhile—as discussed in Chap. 10—non-human technologies are swiftly supplanting human biomedical interventions, with investment in these technologies becoming a focal point in the global competition between nation-states, emphasizing health surveillance as much as health provision.

Following on from this, Chap. 7 "Disordered Eating and the Media Industry," explores the considerable part that the media plays in both the representation and commodification of bodies, and in the construction of public narratives around EDs and disordered eating. This includes the line between what counts as public education and entertainment and the changing norms around the portrayal of bodies on screen in different eras. Examples of portrayals of bodies and individuals with eating disorders in drama, comedy, and documentary across eras are scrutinized, along with the industry's eagerness to portray a greater range of body sizes, and the potential for their employees to become the targets of media exploitation.

References

Agamben, G. (1998). *Homo sacer: Sovereign power and bare life*. Stanford University Press.

American Psychiatric Association (APA). (2013). *Diagnostic and statistical manual of mental disorders: DSM-V* (5th ed.). American Psychiatric Association Publishing.

Arredondo, E. M., Ayala, G. X., Soto, S., Slymen, D. J., Horton, L. A., Parada, H., et al. (2018). Latina mothers as agents of change in children's eating habits: Findings from the randomized controlled trial Entre Familia: Reflejos de Salud. *International Journal of Behavioral Nutrition and Physical Activity, 15*(1), 1–11.

Bastos, C. (2008). Migrants, settlers and colonists: The biopolitics of displaced bodies. *International Migration, 46*(5), 27–54.

Beamish, A. J., & Reinehr, T. (2017). Should bariatric surgery be performed in adolescents? *European Journal of Endocrinology, 176*(4), D1–D15.

Béghin, L., Dauchet, L., De Vriendt, T., Cuenca-García, M., Manios, Y., Toti, E., et al. (2014). Influence of parental socio-economic status on diet quality of European adolescents: Results from the HELENA study. *British Journal of Nutrition, 111*(7), 1303–1312.

Bell, K., & McNaughton, D. (2007). Feminism and the invisible fat man. *Body & Society, 13*(1), 107–131.

Boero, N. (2012). *Killer fat: Media medicine, and morals in the American "Obesity Epidemic"*. Rutgers University Press.

Boero, N. (2013). Obesity in the media: Social science weighs in. *Critical Public Health, 23*(3), 371–380.

Boero, N. (2016). Obesity in the US Media, 1990–2011: Broad Strokes, Broad Consequences. In *Obesity, eating disorders and the media* (pp. 37–48). Routledge.

Brewis, A. A. (2010). *Obesity: Cultural and biocultural perspectives*. University Press.

Bruch, H. (1982). Anorexia nervosa: Therapy and theory. *American Journal of Psychiatry, 139*, 1531.

Bulik, C. M., Thornton, L. M., Parker, R., Kennedy, H., Baker, J. H., MacDermod, C., Guintivano, J., Cleland, L., Miller, A. L., Harper, L., Larsen, J. T., Yilmaz, Z., Grove, J., Sullivan, P. F., Petersen, L. V., Jordan, J., Kennedy, M. A., & Martin, N. G. (2021). The Eating Disorders Genetics Initiative (EDGI): Study protocol. *BMC Psychiatry, 21*(1), 1–9.

Calcaterra, V., Cena, H., Pelizzo, G., Porri, D., Regalbuto, C., Vinci, F., et al. (2021). Bariatric surgery in adolescents: To do or not to do? *Children, 8*(6), 453.

Campbell, D. (2012, April 28). *Doctors back denial of treatment for smokers and the obese.* Guardian online. Retrieved August 22, 2024, from https://www.theguardian.com/society/2012/apr/28/doctors-treatment-denial-smokers-obese

Campbell, T., & Sitze, A. (2013). *Biopolitics. A Reader*. Duke University Press.

Campos, P., Saguy, A., Ernsberger, P., Oliver, E., & Gaesser, G. (2006). The epidemiology of overweight and obesity: Public health crisis or moral panic? *International Journal of Epidemiology, 35*(1), 55–60.

Campos-Vazquez, R. M., & Gonzalez, E. (2020). Obesity and hiring discrimination. *Economics & Human Biology, 37*, 100850.

CDC. (2013). *Overweight and obesity.* Retrieved August 22, 2024, from https://www.cdc.gov/obesity/data/obesity-and-covid-19.html#:~:text=Non%2DHispanic%20Black%20adults%20had,Hispanic%20Asian%20adults%20(11.7%25)

Chernin, K. (1981). *The Obsession: Reflections on the tyranny of slenderness.* Harper.

Cohen, S. (1972/2011). *Folk devils and moral panics.* Routledge.

Commetric. (2019, January 4). *Fast food in the media. The rise of the health-conscious consumer.* Retrieved August 22, 2024, from https://commetric.com/2019/01/04/fast-food-in-the-media-the-rise-of-the-health-conscious-consumer/

Conceição, E., Orcutt, M., Mitchell, J., Engel, S., LaHaise, K., Jorgensen, M., et al. (2013). Eating disorders after bariatric surgery: A case series. *International Journal of Eating Disorders, 46*(3), 274–279.

Cooper, C. (1998). *Fat and proud: The politics of size.* Women's Press.

Crisp, A. H. (1980). *Anorexia nervosa: Let me be.* Academic Press.

Das, S. & Ungoed-Thomas, J. (2023a, March 12). *Orchestrated PR campaign: How skinny jab drug firm sought to shape obesity.* The Guardian. Retrieved August 22, 2024, from https://www.theguardian.com/society/2023/mar/12/orchestrated-pr-campaign-how-skinny-jab-drug-firm-sought-to-shape-obesity-debate

Das, S., & Ungoed-Thomas, J. (2023b, March 12). *Revealed: Experts who praised new 'skinny jab' received payments from drug maker.* The Guardian. Retrieved August 22 2024, from https://www.theguardian.com/business/2023/mar/12/revealed-experts-who-praised-new-skinny-jab-received-payments-from-drug-maker#:~:text=A%20professor%20who%20promoted%20the,3.6m%20by%20the%20firm

Das, S., & Ungoed-Thomas, J (2023c, July 8). *'It's naïve to think this is in the best interest, the NHS.' How big Pharma's billions are influencing health care.* The Guardian. Retrieved August 22, 2024, from https://www.theguardian.com/business/2023/jul/08/its-naive-to-think-this-is-in-the-best-interests-of-the-nhs-how-big-pharmas-millions-are-influencing-healthcare

DePeau-Wilson, M. (2022). *Nutrition group has close links to Food, Pharma industries. Analysis reveals a 'symbiotic relationship' between nutrition group and industry.* Medpage Today. Retrieved August 22, 2024, from https://www.medpagetoday.com/special-reports/features/101396

Dewey-Hagborg, H. (2023). Biopolitics -An interview with Timothy Campbell. *Authorea Preprints.*

Doucet-Battle, J. (2021). *Sweetness in the blood: Race, risk, and Type 2 Diabetes.* University of Minnesota Press.

Downey, R. S. (2020). *The commodification of Body Positivity: Constructing a neoliberal fat citizenship.* Toronto Metropolitan University. Thesis. Retrieved August 22, 2024, from https://doi.org/10.32920/ryerson.14654322.v1

Durkheim, E., & Lukes, S. (1982). *The Rules of sociological method and selected texts on sociology and its method. Edited with an Introduction by Steven Lukes.* Macmillan. (Original work published 1895).

Dworkin, S. L., & Wachs, F. L. (2009). *Body panic: Gender, health, and the selling of fitness.* NYU Press.

eatrightpro.org. (2022, October 22). *Official statement. Academy responds to inaccurate and misleading report.* Academy of Nutrition and Dietetics. Retrieved August 22 2024, from https://www.eatrightpro.org/about-us/who-we-are/public-statements/academy-responds-to-inaccurate-misleading-report

Ebbeling, C. B., Pawlak, D. B., & Ludwig, D. S. (2002). Childhood obesity: Public-health crisis, common sense cure. *The Lancet, 360*(9331), 473–482.

Farrell, A. E. (2011). *Fat shame: Stigma and the fat body in American culture.* NYU Press.

Fernández, E., Kitching, K., & Horgan, D. (2021). Young girls' experiences of 'good' food imperatives in a working-class school community: Rethinking food desire? *Cambridge Journal of Education, 51*(5), 543–561.

Fikkan, J. L., & Rothblum, E. D. (2012). We agree: Fat is a feminist issue! Response to commentators. *Sex Roles, 66*, 632–635.

Food, Farming, and Countryside Commission (FFCC) (2024, November 15). *The False Economy of Big Food.* Retrieved 23 November from https://ffcc.co.uk

Forhan, M., & Salas, X. R. (2013). Inequities in healthcare: A review of bias and discrimination in obesity treatment. *Canadian Journal of Diabetes, 37*(3), 205–209.

Foucault, M. (1973). *The Birth of the Clinic. An archaeology of medical perception.* Routledge.

Foucault, M. (1976). Two lectures. In C. Gordon (Ed.), *Power/knowledge: Selected interviews and other writings 1972–1977* (pp. 78–108). Pantheon.

Foucault, M. (1988). Technologies of the self. In *Technologies of the self: A seminar with Michel Foucault* (Vol. 18, p. 170).
Foucault, M. (2003). *"Society must be defended": Lectures at the Collège de France, 1975–1976* (Vol. 1). Macmillan.
Foucault, M., Davidson, A. I., & Burchell, G. (2008). *The birth of biopolitics: Lectures at the Collège de France, 1978–1979*. Springer.
Fullagar, S. (2019). A physical cultural studies perspective on physical (in) activity and health inequalities: The biopolitics of body practices and embodied movement. *Revista Tempos e Espaços em Educação, 12*(28), 63–76.
Gelsinger, A. S. (2021). A critical analysis of the body positive movement on Instagram: How does it really impact body image. *Spectra Undergraduate Research Journal, 1*(1), 4.
Giddens, A. (1991). *Modernity and self-identity: Self and society in the late modern age*. Polity.
Gilman, S. L. (2004). *Fat boys: A slim book*. University of Nebraska Press.
Gotovac, S., LaMarre, A., & Lafreniere, K. (2020). Words with weight: The construction of obesity in eating disorders research. *Health, 24*(2), 113–131.
Greenhalgh, S. (2012). Weighty subjects: The biopolitics of the US war on fat. *American Ethnologist, 39*(3), 471–487.
Griffin, M., Bailey, K. A., & Lopez, K. J. (2022). #BodyPositive? A critical exploration of the body positive movement within physical cultures taking an intersectionality approach. *Frontiers in Sports and Active Living, 4*, 908580.
Halse, C. (2012). Bio-citizenship: Virtue discourses and the birth of the bio-citizen. In *Biopolitics and the 'Obesity Epidemic'* (pp. 53–67). Routledge.
Haynos, A. F., Wang, S. B., Lipson, S., Peterson, C. B., Mitchell, J. E., Halmi, K. A., et al. (2021). Machine learning enhances prediction of illness course: A longitudinal study in eating disorders. *Psychological Medicine, 51*(8), 1392–1402.
Hunger, J. M., Major, B., Blodorn, A., & Miller, C. T. (2015). Weighed down by stigma: How weight-based social identity threat contributes to weight gain and poor health. *Social and Personality Psychology Compass, 9*(6), 255–268.
Illich, I. (1975). *Limits to medicine. Medical nemesis: The expropriation of health*. Calder & Boyers.
Jabloner, A. (2021). Relative Risk: Measuring Kinship for Future Health in US Genetic Counseling. *Social Analysis, 65*(4), 111–130.
Kelly, P., Allender, S., & Colquhoun, D. (2007). New work ethics? The corporate athlete's backend index and organizational performance. *Organization, 14*(2), 267–285.

Kelly, C., Callaghan, M., Molcho, M., Gabhainn, S. N., & Thomas, A. A. (2019). Food environments in and around post-primary schools in Ireland: Associations with youth dietary habits. *Appetite, 132*, 182–189.

Larson, N. I., Story, M. T., & Nelson, M. C. (2009). Neighborhood environments: Disparities in access to healthy foods in the US. *American Journal of Preventive Medicine, 36*(1), 74–81.

Leahy, D. (2014). Assembling a health [y] subject: Risky and shameful pedagogies in health education. *Critical Public Health, 24*(2), 171–181.

Lee, H., Andrew, M., Gebremariam, A., Lumeng, J. C., & Lee, J. M. (2014). Longitudinal associations between poverty and obesity from birth through adolescence. *American Journal of Public Health, 104*(5), e70–e76.

Lemke, T. 2012. Biopolitics: Current issues and future challenges. *Conference on Biopolitics, Society and Performance,* Dublin, 31 October – 2nd November 2012. Retrieved August 22, 2024, from https://www.youtube.com/watch?v=GPTz0-cWDgs

Lenz, T. L., & Hamilton, W. R. (2004). Supplemental products used for weight loss. *Journal of the American Pharmacists Association, 44*(1), 59–68.

Lipek, T., Igel, U., Gausche, R., Kiess, W., & Grande, G. (2015). Obesogenic environments: Environmental approaches to obesity prevention. *Journal of Pediatric Endocrinology and Metabolism, 28*(5–6), 485–495.

Marmot, M. (2018). An inverse care law for our time. *BMJ, 362.*

Mayes, C. (2015). *The biopolitics of lifestyle: Foucault, ethics and healthy choices.* Routledge.

Mayes, C. (2016). *Headless fatty pics don't protect people, they dehumanise them.* Huff Post. Retrieved August 22, 2024, from https://www.huffpost.com/archive/au/entry/headless-fatty-pics-dont-protect-people-they-dehumanise-them_au_5cd36401e4b0ce845d8020ce

McCullough, M. B., & Hardin, J. A. (Eds.). (2013). *Reconstructing obesity: The meaning of measures and the measure of meanings* (Vol. 2). Berghahn Books.

Metzl, J., Kirkland, A., & Kirkland, A. R. (Eds.). (2010). Against health: How health became the new morality. NYU press.

Nagata, J. M., Ganson, K. T., & Murray, S. B. (2020). Eating disorders in adolescent boys and young men: An update. *Current Opinion in Pediatrics, 32*(4), 476.

Ng, K. (2021, June 29). *'Heinous': Eating disorder charities slam jaw-locking device aimed at weight loss.* The Independent. Retrieved August 22, 2024, from https://www.independent.co.uk/life-style/health-and-families/eating-disorder-charities-weight-loss-device-b1874162.html

NICE. (2023, March 8). *Semiglutide for overweight and obesity.* Retrieved, 24 November, from https://www.nice.org.uk/guidance/ta875/chapter/1-Recommendations

Nied, J. (2022, January 19). *Model Tess Holliday opens up about her anorexia: 'I've since taken a lot of steps backwards in my recovery.'* Women's Health. Retrieved August 22, 2024, from https://www.womenshealthmag.com/health/a36320281/tess-holliday-weight-loss-anorexia-recovery-instagram/

Nnyanzi, L. A., Summerbell, C. D., Ells, L., & Shucksmith, J. (2016). Parental response to a letter reporting child overweight measured as part of a routine national programme in England: Results from interviews with parents. *BMC Public Health, 16*(1), 1–13.

O'Mahony, S. (2019). Petr Skrabanek: The abominable no-man. *Journal of the Royal College of Physicians of Edinburgh, 49*(1), 65–69.

O'Neill, M. (2023). *Tess Holliday discusses the stigma behind an atypical anorexia diagnosis.* Self. Retrieved August 22, 2024, from https://www.self.com/story/tess-holliday-atypical-anorexia-weight-bias#:~:text=Holliday%20first%20announced%20her%20diagnosis,say%20it%20out%20loud%20anymore

Orbach, S. (1978). *Fat is a feminist issue: The anti-diet guide to permanent weight loss.* Paddington Press.

Orbach, S. (2018, June 24). *Forty years since Fat is a feminist issue.* The Guardian. Retrieved August 22, 2024, from https://www.theguardian.com/society/2018/jun/24/forty-years-since-fat-is-a-feminist-issue

Parkinson, J. (2015, February 15). *Could fining parents cut childhood obesity?* BBC News. Retrieved August 22, 2024, from https://www.bbc.co.uk/news/magazine-31417102

Prozorov, S. (2022). When did biopolitics begin? Actuality and potentiality in historical events. *European Journal of Social Theory, 25*(4), 539–558.

Puhl, R. M., & Heuer, C. A. (2009). The stigma of obesity: A review an update. *Obesity, 17*(5), 941.

Puhl, R. M., & Heuer, C. A. (2010). Obesity stigma: Important considerations for public health. *American Journal of Public Health, 100*(6), 1019–1028.

Puhl, R. M., Andreyeva, T., & Brownell, K. D. (2008). Perceptions of weight discrimination: Prevalence and comparison to race and gender discrimination in America. *International Journal of Obesity, 32*(6), 992–1000.

Rose, N., & Novas, C. (2005). Biological citizenship. *Global assemblages: Technology, politics, and ethics as anthropological problems, 1*, 439–63.

Rosi, A., Zerbini, C., Pellegrini, N., Scazzina, F., Brighenti, F., & Lugli, G. (2017). How to improve food choices through vending machines: The importance of healthy food availability and consumers' awareness. *Food Quality and Preference, 62*, 262–269.

Rzehak, P., Meisinger, C., Woelke, G., Brasche, S., Strube, G., & Heinrich, J. (2007). Weight change, weight cycling and mortality in the ERFORT Male Cohort Study. *European Journal of Epidemiology, 22*, 665–673.

Saguy, A. (2012). Why fat is a feminist issue. *Sex Roles, 66*, 600–607.

Saguy, A. C., & Gruys, K. (2010). Morality and health: News media constructions of overweight and eating disorders. *Social Problems, 57*(2), 231–250.

Salter, B., & Waldby, C. (2011). Biopolitics in China: An introduction. *East Asian Science, Technology and Society: An International Journal, 5*(3), 287–290.

Sanders, R. (2019). The color of fat: Racializing obesity, recuperating whiteness, and reproducing injustice. *Politics, Groups, and Identities, 7*(2), 287–304.

Schoon, I., Bynner, J., Joshi, H., Parsons, S., Wiggins, R. D., & Sacker, A. (2002). The influence of context, timing, and duration of risk experiences for the passage from childhood to mid adulthood. *Child Development, 73*, 1486–1504.

Schoon, I., Sacker, A., & Bartley, M. (2003). Socio-economic adversity and psychosocial adjustment: A development-contextual perspective. *Social Science and Medicine, 57*, 1001–1015.

Senthilingham, M. (2017, October 31). *No surgery for smokers all the advice. Policy in UK stirs debate*. CNN. Retrieved August 22, 2024, from https://edition.cnn.com/2017/10/31/health/smokers-obese-no-surgery-nhs-uk/index.html

Skrabanek, P. (1994). *The death of humane medicine and the rise of coercive medicine*. St Edmundsbury Press Ltd..

Steinglass, J. E., Berner, L. A., & Attia, E. (2019). Cognitive neuroscience of eating disorders. *Psychiatric Clinics, 42*(1), 75–91.

Swinburn, B., Egger, G., & Raza, F. (1999). Dissecting obesogenic environments: The development and application of a framework for identifying and prioritizing environmental interventions for obesity. *Preventive Medicine, 29*(6), 563–570.

Swinburn, B. A., Sacks, G., Hall, K. D., McPherson, K., Finegood, D. T., Moodie, M. L., & Gortmaker, S. L. (2011). The global obesity pandemic: Shaped by global drivers and local environments. *The Lancet, 378*(9793), 804–814.

The Economist. (2023, November 23). *The obesity pay gap is worse than previously thought.* Retrieved August 22, 2024, from https://www.economist.com/finance-and-economics/2023/11/23/the-obesity-pay-gap-is-worse-than-previously-thought#

The Pew Centre. (2013, November 12). *Public agrees on obesity's impact, not government's role*. Retrieved August 22, 2024, from https://www.pewresearch.org/politics/2013/11/12/public-agrees-on-obesitys-impact-not-governments-role/

Tompkins, K. W. (2009). Sylvester Graham's imperial dietetics. *Gastronomica, 9*(1), 50–60.

Tsai, A. G., & Wadden, T. A. (2005). Systematic review: An evaluation of major commercial weight loss programs in the United States. *Annals of Internal Medicine, 142*(1), 56–66.

Tu, L., Bajaj, S. S., & Stanford, F. C. (2021). Locking ourselves into the past: The DentalSlim Diet Control device and an incomplete understanding of obesity. *International Journal of Obesity (2005), 45*(12), 2513–2514.

von Kardorff, E., & Ohlbrecht, H. (2008). Overweight, obesity and eating disorders in adolescents-a socio-somatic reaction to social change? *Journal of Public Health, 16*, 429–438.

Walsh, E. G., Rogalski, K., & Hibbler, L. (2023). Weight bias and healthism: An integrative health perspective. *Journal of Integrative and Complementary Medicine, 29*(5), 271–275.

Waseem, T., Mogensen, K. M., Lautz, D. B., & Robinson, M. K. (2007). Pathophysiology of obesity: Why surgery remains the most effective treatment. *Obesity Surgery, 17*, 1389–1398.

Watson, J. L., & Caldwell, M. L. (2005). *The cultural politics of food and eating: A reader*. Blackwell Publishing.

Williams, C. (2014, November 20). Obesity rivals smoking and war among self-inflicted health risk *Los Angeles Times*. Retrieved January 12, 2023, from https://www.latimes.com/world/europe/la-fg-global-obesitycosts-20141120-story.html

World Health Organization. (2023a). *The Global Health Observatory. Body Mass Index among Adults*. Retrieved August 22, 2024, from https://www.who.int/data/gho/data/themes/topics/topic-details/GHO/body-mass-index

World Health Organization. (2023b). *Obesity and overweight*. Retrieved August 22, 2024, from https://www.who.int/news-room/fact-sheets/detail/obesityand-overweight

Wright, J., & Harwood, V. (Eds.). (2012). *Biopolitics and the 'obesity epidemic': Governing bodies* (Vol. 3). Routledge.

Żukiewicz-Sobczak, W., Wróblewska, P., Zwoliński, J., Chmielewska-Badora, J., Adamczuk, P., Krasowska, E., et al. (2014). Obesity and poverty paradox in developed countries. *Annals of Agricultural and Environmental Medicine, 21*(3).

7

Disordered Eating and the Media Industry

The murky ground covered by cultural representations of individuals with disordered eating and their bodies has been of abiding interest and intrigue to scholars and public alike. The entertainment value of transgressive bodies is evident, not only in fiction but extends to media forms that, by presenting themselves as scientifically grounded, are generally deemed reliable. These representations include both "real-life" and fictional tales involving ordinary individuals and celebrities, which oscillate between glorifying and pathologizing dietary and body modification trends and attempts, designed to capture maximum consumer attention (Brechan & Kvalem, 2015). Media representations often contrast body sizes and sensationalize eating offenses, although some can claim to perform a public service by shining a spotlight on mental health issues. Due to its pervasive influence on societal norms and ideals, the media industry is widely believed as playing a pivotal role in shaping public perceptions of body image, beauty, and health. From the glorification of thinness in fashion magazines to the relentless promotion of diet culture, the media industry constructs and perpetuates narrow, often unattainable standards of physical appearance. Ultimately, the goal of mass media and its marketing arm is to ensure that we become more dissatisfied with not just

A. Fixsen, *The Construction of Eating Disorders*, The Politics of Mental Health and Illness, https://doi.org/10.1007/978-3-031-70318-8_7

what we have, but who we are and what we look like (Eckersley, 2006; Widdows, 2018). Within this context, disordered eating emerges not merely as an individual pathology but as a widespread social phenomenon deeply intertwined with the cultural and social messages disseminated by various media platforms.

This chapter takes a critical look at the relationship between mass media and disordered eating from a range of perspectives. It explores how media representations intersect with gender politics, medicine, psychology, and commerce, and what feminists have to say about the media's reinforcement of society's patriarchal pressures. Portrayals of bodies and individuals with eating disorders in through comedy, drama, and documentary are then scrutinized, through analysis of various depictions of disordered eaters on television and film. Finally, there are the implications of the film industry's treatment of its employees over the years, including its recent eagerness to feature a greater range of body sizes and more use of plus-size actors, in terms of the individuals becoming the targets of media exploitation.

Mass Media and "Cultural products"

As a genre, the media has always served as both producer and disseminator of "cultural products"—non-material goods designed for a public audience, typically serving aesthetic or expressive rather than utilitarian functions (Hirsch, 1992). Criticisms of mass-produced culture are not new; Adorno and Horkheimer (Adorno, 1941; Horkheimer & Adorno, 1947/2001) harangued the American media industry[1] in the 1930s for its relentless uniformity and pseudo-individualism and for manipulating society into passivity. The authors viewed the mass media process as stripping cultural products of their uniqueness and critical potential, reducing them to mere commodities. Like capitalism itself, the effect of mass media is totalizing, and designed to replace autonomous and self-determined activities with passive amusements, while inevitably fostering personal discontent (Shippen, 2014). The variety of media content has

[1] The words "industry" and "industrial" as used by Adorno to emphasize the standardization of culture and its existence because of mass production.

now greatly expanded, yet the underlying mechanisms of commodification and profit-driven content production are arguably more pervasive than ever. This suggests that despite new forms and new technologies, the industrial logic that Adorno and Horkheimer critiqued persists.

Advertising has also played a major part in supporting and profiting from the media. Following both social standards and market trends, the advertising sector's representation of bodies in terms of attractiveness, status, and sexual appeal has been predominantly normative or aspirational. For example, keeping to the conventions of the time, advertisements in American women's magazines in the 1950s by and large limited the role placement of women to either wife or mother. The advertising archetype of the "ideal wife" depicted a figure who was enthusiastic, domesticated, and competitive, while the "ideal mother" embodied qualities of pleasantness, nourishment, and thriftiness (Catt, 2014). Despite this portrayal, not all advertisements confined women to domestic roles. There was a growing awareness that women wielded substantial influence over significant purchasing decisions, prompting those with foresight in manufacturing and advertising to capitalize on their spending power and preferences. Recognizing this evolving trend, Goldman et al. (1991) introduced the term "commodity feminism" to describe how feminist discourses were being redirected within mass media and aligned with the logic of commodity relations.

The trend known as "Femvertising" continued to "rehabilitate" feminist ideals such as independence, freedom, and sexual agency in advertising (Varghese & Kumar, 2022). Early initiatives, such as the *Dove Campaign for Real Beauty*, could claim not only to empower women using their products but to cater to women across diverse age groups, skin tones, and body categories. More recent advertisements capitalizing on female empowerment have shifted the focus from excessive thinness to the fit and toned female body, suggesting that the product aligns with the lifestyle of a strong, determined woman combating societal oppression. For example, commercials featuring attractive women "pumping iron" are now relatively commonplace. Many advertisements also position themselves as advocates for mental health and social justice campaigns, including seemingly unrelated entities such as banks, insurance firms and building societies. Simultaneously, the advertising industry closely monitors the demographic trajectories and attitudes of women, with digital profiling significantly expanding the pool of big data available on women's spending behaviors.

It could be said that commodity feminism has changed the way that women look at, and after, their bodies in a positive direction. These new messages of advertising give women permission to express themselves and have fun, potentially lessening the pressure on girls and women to modify and harm their bodies. However, McRobbie (2004, 2011) has argued that the eponymous freedom granted to women in adverts to "be themselves" is simply another form of governmentality which finds its expression through imagery and symbolism, rather than direct political action. It is not, McRobbie says, a question of one step forward and three steps backward, it is rather the creation of a "new form of entrapment made possible through a spurious and superficial sense of equality" (2011, p. 180). No longer aligned with movements of wider social change, feminist culture as it appears in today's media and in corporate messages is largely bound up with neoliberal norms and attributes, such as being endowed with self-confidence and excelling in sports (Fixsen et al., 2022).

While women and their body care—or lack of it—has had a disproportionate amount of media coverage, the contemporary focus on body concerns is less strictly defined by gender. The media of today is particularly keen on "fitspiration" imagery, which has multi-gender appeal (Kiberd, 2015). While seemingly opening its doors to everybody, fitspiration has created a kind of "body fascism," which pushes individuals to go to ever greater lengths to monitor themselves, and to "demonstrate their subjectivity through self-discipline" (Brown, 2021, p. ii). Fitness images on mainstream and digital media emphasize the aesthetics of the physical body at the expense of the processes behind becoming healthy which can be applied to a variety of body types, including those which might not be viewed as conventionally beautiful (Magladry, 2018). This is because the media's ultimate end is to attract a wide range of customers to themselves and other businesses via advertising (Hainneville et al., 2022), and nowadays this means displaying more commitment to equality and diversity. The media can also be a vehicle through which women negotiate their body image in ways which are informed by social and historical experiences. One example cited is singer Beyonce's employment of images of black women in different cultural clothing for the cover of her album

Lemonade. These images honor black women and express their "inner power, beauty, and resilience" (LaVoulle & Lewis Ellison, 2017) yet arguably still represent a type of commodity feminism.

Celebrity bodies have always been admired and emulated, and—where a celebrity is sufficiently famous—the media is likely to be interested in every aspect of their personal life, including their trials and tribulations over body image and/or their "unhealthy" relationship with food. This interest is not gender-specific; male celebrities including Elton John, Ed Sheeran, and Olly Alexander have had their "struggles with body image and an eating disorder" publicly discussed in news media (Parry, 2023). These illness narratives sit side by side with the numerous media features on celebrity workouts, constructing success, bodily perfection, and food consumption as centered around losing fat and building muscle mass and strength (Parasecoli, 2013). Readers are informed of such details as Adele's step-by-step workout routine, and how, coupled with the Sirtfood diet,[2] it enabled the star to lose seven stone. In an article on this topic, journalist Head (2023) adds that Adele's transformation was not for album sales, publicity or to be a role model, but was a personal choice made for herself and her son. These types of statements leave one to ponder their impact on those aspiring to emulate the lives and bodies of role models, without the resources available to elite individuals.

Medicine and the Media

Medical matters are always popular subjects for media representations. Health issues provide not only a rich source of education and entertainment but an opportunity for those in the media to showcase their familiarity with medical topics for validation. While some stories approach medical subjects from an "objective" standpoint, many incorporate sensational and moralistic messages that may resonate with the public in less empathetic ways. Obese and emaciated bodies on screen, suffused with or

[2] The Sirtfood diet was developed by celebrity nutritionists, who advertised the diet as a revolutionary new diet plan that works by turning on the "skinny gene" via *sirtuins*, proteins which have demonstrated some ability to regulate metabolism, inflammation, and lifespan. There is very limited research to back up the specific claims of the diet.

lacking the material qualities of fat, muscle, and bone, have historically been utilized to signify deviance and disorder (Donghi & Wennerholm, 2014). Numerous instances exist in media where storylines featuring individuals with excessive or insufficient weight are accompanied by striking images and cautionary messages from scientists or doctors, aiming to convey seriousness and reliability, but also moral censorship. Sometimes deception is blatant, such as advertisers crafting "news stories" to promote products and services related to weight loss, diet, and surgery—a tactic facilitated by the digitization of media.

An example is a recent article found on a pop-up website, narrating the radical transformation of an "everyday" couple. The story unfolds after navigating through a multitude of advertisements, revealing the unnamed woman's journey through weight loss, cosmetic surgery, and hair treatments, while her husband, driven by insecurity, follows suit by joining a gym and undergoing facial reconstruction surgery. However, as the narrative progresses, the content becomes inundated with advertisements for holidays, life insurance, beauty products, and diet aids. The reader is then bombarded with images of commercial surgeons in blue coats until the page refreshes itself, returning them to the beginning. Despite the overt advertising strategy, the content intersperses moral and emotive messages about self-love, acceptance, and the pursuit of true happiness without the need for change. The contradiction in such posts illustrates how the media hooks into people's desires and anxieties by incessantly generating nonsensical images and text about bodies.

Psychology has been interested in investigating human responses to media and has latterly established its own disciplinary niche on the media stage. In an early study of film, psychologist Hugo Münsterberg (1916) discerned various emotional reactions among audiences watching silent movies, including sympathy for the protagonist and the projection of personal feelings onto the protagonist's emotions. A subsequent study by Arnheim (1944/1969) proposed that identification with characters played a pivotal role in the gratification derived from media consumption, contributing to the success of radio programs. Spurred by the cognitive shift in psychology during the 1960s and 1970s, communication studies increasingly focused on the emotional and psychological processes of media reception, including why certain personalities and age groups appear more susceptible to idealized representations than others (Keery et al., 2004; Mills et al., 2017). Levine and Murnen (2009) identified three key themes in media messages targeted at young audiences: the importance of being sexually attractive, the external sources (primarily media) that shape ideals about beauty and style, and the role of media as enjoyable yet influential sources of information and motivation for achieving attractiveness. They observed that even very young children when exposed to media content rapidly develop socially normative ideas about gender and attractiveness.

In the 1990s, positive psychology gained recognition through figures like Martin Seligman, who popularized now familiar concepts such as "self-esteem" and "resilience" (Seligman & Csikszentmihalyi, 2000). Celebrity psychologists now routinely analyze people's emotions in media, blending entertainment with psychological insights. While arguably fulfilling a public information role, critics argue that the highly ubiquitous "therapy culture" has reshaped our understanding of personhood, pressuring individuals to stay positive and openly discuss vulnerabilities, with failure to do so seen as a flaw (Fineman, 2006; Furedi, 2003). Media has become a major vehicle for this kind of "emotional capitalism"[3]—the harnessing of emotion to the discourses and values of the economic and political spheres (Illouz, 2007, p. 4) where emotions are commodified and scrutinized for hidden meanings, placing the onus of resolving issues on the individual.

The media has particularly sensationalized discussions of emotional upheavals around sexual relations, including where they relate to body appearance and weight. One such example on television is an Oprah Winfrey show aired in 2005. The program features a woman, whose marital difficulties are put down to the fact that the husband did not like her weight gain, and both are placed under the scrutiny of a TV psychologist. The underlying assumption in this scenario is that intimacy is crucial for a healthy relationship. In this context, the woman's weight is perceived as a barrier to intimacy, and her struggle to lose weight is framed as a hindrance to marital bliss. Indeed, the psychologist suggests that the woman

[3] Illouz (2007) points out that the making of capitalism went together with an intensely specialized emotional culture which led to the public performing of the private self.

might have gained weight as a subconscious act of retaliation against her husband. While the woman disputes this notion, she acknowledges that there were unconscious motivations behind her weight gain, asserting that it was a strategy to ward off other men and remain faithful to her husband. The underlying assumption here is that everything contains a concealed, deeper meaning, and purpose, which needs to be uncovered. According to Illouz (2007), it is in this realm where narratives of self-help and suffering intersect. If a person secretly desires misery, the responsibility for alleviating it can be squarely placed on that individual.

Women and the Media Industry

Starting from the premise that representations matter, feminist media studies have sought to understand how images and cultural constructions of bodies are connected to both patterns of inequality and domination and the more hidden pressures of neoliberalism (Gill, 2007, 2017; Rottenberg, 2014). Yet, how women perceive their relationship with media and its impact on their bodies and eating behaviors is less understood. Research often focuses on how viewing idealized images in media influence women's body attitudes, contributing to body dissatisfaction and fat-phobia (Bell & Dittmar, 2011; Levine & Murnen, 2009; Park, 2005; Frost, 2001). Coleman (2008) argues that women's bodies are closely connected to their representations, as they often perceive and experience their bodies through these images. Widdows (2018) adds that media-driven beauty ideals now impose a standard of perfection on all women, with beauty seen as resulting from one's effort and investment, leaving many women dissatisfied with their appearance. The wider the disparity between the culturally constructed ideal body internalized by a woman and her own biological reality, the more likely she is to impose stringent discipline and dietary restrictions on her body to bridge this gap:

> [The] endless pursuit of the perfected screen body can help push the most vulnerable viewers over the razor-thin line that separates what has become the "new normal" of nagging weight worries on the one side from destructive dieting and eating behavior on the other. (Fox-Kales, 2011, p. 4)

The ethics of beauty extend to the film industry which, from its beginnings, was a male-dominated arena. Nowadays, the sexism inherent in media is more hidden (Jones & Pringle, 2015), but in the early years of cinema there was little attempt to hide it. Women on screen often served a decorative purpose or were seen being schooled about how they should present their bodies to remain of sexual interest to men. The 1930s Broadway musical hit, *Keep Young and Beautiful,* is sung by a white actor wearing a black face to a group of peroxide blonde women. The lyrics say it all:

> If your charm still remains
> After you grow old, baby
> You don't have to be a cold baby,
> Keep young and beautiful
> It's your duty to be beautiful
> Keep young and beautiful
> If you want to be loved.
> Don't fail to do your stuff
> With a little powder and a puff
> Keep young and beautiful
> If you want to be loved!

Women acting in early Hollywood were open to sexual abuse and other forms of exploitation. By the 1940s, amphetamine-type stimulants were being commonly prescribed or handed out to female screen actresses, to keep them alert and in shape. A tragic example of this was the actress Judy Garland, who, according to biographic sources, developed both a prescription drug addiction and an eating disorder after being constantly made to diet as a teenage star. Her teenage co-actor, Mickey Rooney, was similarly medicated and fought his addiction for decades (Farren, 2010; Tessier, & Schulman, 2023). Following the *MeToo* movement and famous Hollywood criminal cases, messages about the rights of women working in the film industry to work and progress without fear of being subject to sexual harassment or abuse have been taken more seriously. However, a backlash to this can be seen in the myogenous online media culture, which again places women in the firing line of sexist and hateful comments, as well as body shaming (Dickel & Evolvi, 2023).

During the 1960s, a resurgence of feminism known as the "second wave" emerged, in tandem with left-wing activism and the so-called sexual liberation movement, aligning itself with causes such as civil rights. An early and notable figure in feminist media was the writer Betty Friedan, whose book *The Feminist Mystique* (2010) became something of a best seller. Freidan contended that the myth or mystique lay in the belief that women could derive fulfillment through sexual passivity, male dominance, and maternal love. According to Friedan, urging middle-class American women to withdraw to the home and focus on stereotypically feminine pursuits left them in a state of discontent, melancholy, and despondency (Whitaker, 2017). While Friedan's ideas were not particularly radical, other feminists confronted patriarchal politics more directly, including by establishing their own press outlets. The liberal feminist magazine *Ms* symbolized the internal struggles within the feminist movement and its external conflict with the commercial sector (Farrell, 1998). Its inaugural cover portrayed the goddess Kali performing various tasks with her multiple arms, served as a warning against female exploitation, accompanied by the headline, "The Housewife's Moment of Truth." Applauded by some for its subversiveness (Farrell, 1998), others dismissed *Ms* as feminist consumerism. "The masters tools will never dismantle the masters house," black activist Andre Lorde (2017) declared, emphasizing the need for a more profound transformation. Overall, however, second wave feminism is noted for its alignment with wider movements calling for social equality, including gay and transgender rights and anti-racism policies, and social activism that resulted in clashes with police, and in some cases imprisonment.

Women in media have never spoken with a single voice and "backlashes" against politicized forms of feminism have occurred (Faludi, 2009). A more commercially oriented brand of feminism took root in the early 1990s, marked by its capitalist influences and widespread approval within the media (Fixsen et al., 2022). Third wave or "post-feminism" redefined gender equality within a neoliberal framework, "as an individualistic, entrepreneurial project that can be instilled by the self" (Gill & Orgad, 2015, p. 334). Second-wave feminists contended that "critical social goods" were unevenly distributed within the contemporary gender-structured family (Okin, 1989). The anti-capitalist views of these feminists came to be regarded with contempt by post-feminist writers such as Naomi Wolf, who argued that their "insider mentality" was failing to inspire contemporary women, who were looking instead to the mainstream media discourses for their role models (Wolf, 1994). While second-wave feminism acknowledged systemic gender disparities, this new feminism gave minimal attention to this, emphasizing instead how individual women should focus on self-improvement of mind and body *Facebook* CO, Sheryl Sandberg (2013), in her popular book, *Lean in*, urged women who complain about gender inequalities to first address these issues both within themselves and their immediate workplaces. As a result, industries like the media became intertwined with neoliberal feminism, and its original goals supplanted by objectives that better serve the commercial sector.

More recently, mass media has played a role in amplifying the "gender wars," not only in their binary sense but between those born as or identifying as women. Much has been made of the vitriolic arguments surrounding women like author JK Rowling and academic Kathleen Stock who advocate for biological sex and those standing up for LGBTQ+ rights on social media, on university campuses and more. These arguments have further fractured feminism to the extent that it is no longer possible to speak of feminism as a movement. Rather, feminism is more a term adopted by different groups holding divergent beliefs, often with conflicting goals.

Disordered Eating on Screen

While fashion and advertising focus primarily on normative, beautified bodies, the entertainment business has made considerable capital out of "disordered" bodies, including those with a dietary association. Historical instances include the "living skeletons" and "fat ladies," who were prominent figures in traveling circuses during the eighteenth and nineteenth centuries (Gooldin, 2003). Nowadays, the entertainment industry appears to generate considerable revenue through exhibitions of different body sizes while still focusing on the contrast between fat and thin. A prime example is the TV documentary series "Supersize versus Superskinny," broadcast on Channel 4 from 2008 to 2014. The show brought together individuals with obesity and underweight conditions, instructing them to exchange meals. Close-up shots accentuating the participants' fleshiness or lack of it aimed to evoke awe and potential disgust in the TV audience. The underlying script conveyed psychological messages about the internal issues leading to weight loss or gain, encapsulated in the tagline, "It's not what you're eating, it's what's eating you." The celebrity doctor presenter offered an expert scientific perspective on the proceedings and outcomes. The production heavily relied on shock, humiliation, and blame for entertainment, referencing "dietary crimes" and labeling some participants as "the worst offenders." In one series, obese contestants visited an American cemetery, expressing shame, fear, and remorse about their size and perceived food "addictions." Analyzing the program's narrative structure, Eli and Levis (2014) noted the silencing, distancing, and stylizing of bodies showcased for the viewing pleasure or horror of others, creating an "enfreakment" spectacle reminiscent of but more psychologically perverse than earlier circus performances.

As the topic of eating disorders gained prominence, so mass media realized the public interest value of features about renowned celebrities and their struggles with eating and weight. In the early 1980s, the death of the beloved singer Karen Carpenter (1950–1983) made headlines, serving as the initial exposure to anorexia nervosa for some viewers (Carpenter, 1983). Tales of other female celebrities grappling with eating disorders have since become a prominent avenue through which the viewing public becomes acquainted with various types of eating disorders. "Self-confession" narratives have proved a particularly popular aspect of contemporary media, reaching a point where program presenters are expected to candidly discuss their personal challenges. In some instances, the entire narrative revolves around the broadcaster's personal illness story or that of a friend or family member. A case in point is the documentary "Zara Dermott: Disordered Eating" (BBC, 2023), where the reality TV star and influencer expresses concern about the potential impact of her *Instagram* blog on followers. Zara goes on to visit some of her younger viewers in their homes and eating disorder clinics. During one segment, a group of very young followers suggest that Zara could assist them by sharing more natural images of herself and her life. The program predominantly focuses on the presenter acknowledging her role as a victim of social comparison. While these features shed light on the prevalence of mental health problems and disordered eating, they often fail to address the role played by the burgeoning media industry itself in perpetuating such issues.

TV and big screen films have attempted to dramatize the challenges faced by individuals with eating disorders, which up until recently was usually a white western girl from a middle-class background. One early film of this genre, *Best Little Girl in the World* (1981), tells the story of Casey, a young white American ballerina who struggles with anorexia nervosa. Casey has been encouraged by her ballet teacher to lose some weight if she wants to be successful, while her distracted parents argue over what to do about her troublesome sister. The film explores the themes of body image, perfectionism, and the pressures of the entertainment industry, and does not shy away from portraying the devastating effects of anorexia on a young person's life or its toll on family and friends. The film has some social focus, drawing attention to the considerable pressures on thin body shape facing young women in female-dominated industries such as ballet. At the same time, like other films of this period, it relies on stereotypes and is educational in tone rather than questioning the issues it raises.

Many films about eating disorders turn out to be cautionary tales concerning the poor health outcomes associated with being raised by a flawed family. This fits with commonly held ideas that parents of young people with eating disorders are either highly controlling and perfectionist (Bruch, 1982), or totally neglectful. Life in a dysfunctional, middle-class family was the central storyline of the Hollywood movie, *To the Bone* (2017). The main character, Ellen, struggles with anorexia and reluctantly starts treatment; however, her condition worsens after a disastrous session of family therapy. Her situation further deteriorates until she enters a private eating disorder establishment, where she gets to meet with a wider range of the people with eating disorders. Unusually, the film featured a young white male as ballet dancer with an eating disorder, yet by casting Hollywood actor Keanu Reeves as the gifted male psychiatrist, it falls back on gender stereotypes. Controversially, lead actress Lily Colins was known to be "in recovery" from an eating disorder and lost a lot of weight for the role. Writing in in the *New Statesman,* Leszkiewicz (2017) described the film as "triggering" and noted how quickly the film content had been shared on pro-Ana forums.

Feminists within the film industry have contributed to a more direct commentary on eating disorders as prevalent among women in society. One illustrative example is the Canadian documentary film, "The Famine Within," which delves into the impact of an idealized feminine beauty image on girls and women, exploring the consequences of society's growing fixation on diet and exercise. Critics of the film have raised concerns about its geographic limitations and its emphasis on the psychological makeup of individuals with disordered eating (Archives Publiques de l'Ontario, 2003). Nevertheless, the film stands out as one of the early works addressing these issues partially through a sociocultural lens, departing from the conventional approach of viewing eating disorders as entirely idiosyncratic. It is recognized for its vivid portrayals of the lives of ordinary young American women.

Most of us do not turn to the media for educational purposes alone but for entertainment, and to indulge in the joys and sorrows of others (Eli & Ulijaszek, 2014). Comedy is particularly amenable to these effects, as audiences expect some exaggerated and shocking content, without necessarily breaking the rules of social and political correctness. Fat and thin characters are particularly popular as participants of slapstick in physical comedy, as in the early comedy duos such as Laurel and Hardy. While fun and entertainment was made from weight disparities and out of control behaviors, in earlier cinema this rarely contained any psychological or medical message. In contrast, recent film portrayals are far more moralistic in tone, often emphasizing the neoliberal tropes of meritocracy and authenticity. One such example is the film *Diary of a Wimpy Kid*, which employs the "fat boy" comedy character and explicitly deals with the difficult transition from childhood to adolescence for someone deemed overweight. Based on the best-selling book series by Jeff Kinney, protagonist Greg starts middle school full of dread and desperately tries to fit in, but rapidly learns that normative physicality is decisive in determining social status in this age group. Plotz (2020) points out the ambiguities of the film in terms of its representation of fatness. On the one hand, it confirms and neutralizes the stereotype of the child as fat boy; on the other hand, it ridicules the main character Greg's clumsy, opportunistic way of thinking and his desperate attempts at popularity as counterproductive. The message of the film appears to be about the importance of "being true to oneself," which jars with the narrative that obesity during adolescence necessarily leads to outsider status.

More recently, overweight has been more explicitly framed as consequential to individual failings and to the "wrong kind of eating." Whether or not the topic of eating disorders as actual medical conditions could generate laughs was tested out in 2005, when the situation comedy *Starved* first aired on US television. The program features the lives of four adults with different forms of disordered eating: a male character with ongoing "body-image" and food issues, a black cop with binge eating disorder (BED), a female recovering from anorexia nervosa (AN), and a male character with bulimia nervosa (BN). The audience is entertained (or not) with graphic displays of disordered eating behaviors, including consumption of large amounts of fast foods, self-induced vomiting, and obsessive weighing of the characters' bodies and their food. At times the comedy is brutal, for example, the characters attend a so-called support group called "Belt Tighteners" in which members confess their eating behaviors while the group leader bellows insults to each one, such as "If you were dog, I'd kick you in the face!!" The characters' private struggles are cast in a comedic light, for example, the black cop is seen taking food out of a garbage can, then vomits into what he thinks is a pile of trash, but which turns out to be a homeless man, only to chastise the man for illegally sleeping outside before making a fast exit.

Described by critic Andrew Wallenstein (2005) as "a nasty brutal piece of work [but also] one of the most promising comedies to come along in a while," the comedy failed to win over audiences and ran for little more than a handful of episodes. Possibly, it raised too many contentious issues about the purpose and boundaries of entertainment (Katterman & Klump, 2010). From a sociological perspective, flaws can be seen in the conceptualization of the program's characters. While the program highlights the existence of disordered eating in men and those nearing middle age, it is far from representative of the "normal" distribution of eating disorders across the US population. The camaraderie among the eating disorder group, and the openness with which they act out and discuss their eating disorders in public, is hard to believe. Nevertheless, along with the dark humor are realistic portrayals of the American fast-food industry, the agonies of disordered eating, and the unsubtle nature of the "war against fat" in millennial America.

A more recent feature seeking to turn disordered eating into comedy is the Apple TV miniseries "*Physical*." Presently in its third season, this TV miniseries has showed more staying power than the comic series above, perhaps because this topic is of more relevance to today's medically savvy audience. The story unfolds through retrospection, centering on Sheila, a middle-class West Coast housewife in the 1990s. Unbeknownst to others but revealed to the audience, Sheila engages in episodes of ritualistic binging and purging. Early in the series, several feminist themes are introduced. Sheila, having sacrificed her own academic pursuits to support her misogynistic husband's lectureship in politics, discovers he is on the verge of being fired for misconduct. Set against the backdrop of the West Coast fitness boom, Sheila turns to aerobics to unleash her inner anger and break free from her mundane existence. Sheila embodies two personas: the outward portrayal of the impeccably groomed woman in her prime and the "fucked up," self-critical, and manipulative side, revealed through her frequent internal monologues. Driven and determined, she appropriates a fitness routine from another instructor, using her husband's political campaign fund to produce "her" aerobics video. Sheila's shenanigans are punctuated by covert visits to a drive-through restaurant, where she purchases a large bag of hamburgers, fries, and a shake. She then rents a motel room, strips down to her underwear, gorges the food, then visits the bathroom to throw up and shower. Through all this the viewer hears her inner voice shouting, "You're nothing, you're worse than nothing, you're a ghost; You dumb bitch, stop! Stop right now!! You don't need this anymore!" Then the day after the binge and purge comes the emphatic instruction to herself to behave:

> Today, you will eat clean and healthy foods. You will have a veggie burger. And if you do this list of things, you can have a reasonable serving of cobbler with no ice cream. [Next scene, she's going to the hamburger store, and then buying three cheeseburgers and a chocolate shake]. Tomorrow I will eat clean and healthy. I will not, repeat not.

Throughout the story Sheila fails to find inner peace, until she eventually goes to a private eating disorder clinic, lets out her anger, and "connects" with one of therapy group co-members. Yet Sheila remains dedicated to the neoliberal dream of building a "fitspiration" empire, thus embodying the post-feminist woman on her individual path of discovery and self-revelation. The program poses as a salutary tale of self-hate and low self-esteem, but is ultimately a celebration of western consumerism, punctuated by ambiguous messages about the psychological profiles of those with eating disorders.

The Media and Cultural Stereotypes

Film and TV storylines require actors with different body types and shapes to be used for the various character parts; hence, the industry does not fully fit with the definition of an aesthetic industry. Nevertheless, well-known actors with "attractive" facial looks and body shapes have always made for popular viewing. Even in the eating disorder programs mentioned above, the actors playing the main parts were mostly strikingly attractive and in terms of body weight rarely exceeded what might be considered "comfortable" viewing. Overall, Magladry (2018) argues that the media continues to serve certain kinds of individuals—largely those who occupy white privileged positions in society—rather than benefiting the collective efforts for which feminists of the past have strived. Those who inhabit and work in this celebrity world are seen as the role models for millions of people across the world. To win the broadest audience appeal, big studio films focus not only on the dazzling technical spectacle of action blockbusters but on the bodies of those movie stars recognized for a stylized beauty and glamor, who represent a kind of accepted uniformity of body expectation. After decades working as a clinical psychologist and academic in the States, Fox-Kales (2011) made it her project to study the world of Hollywood and the culture of eating disorders in relation to this celebrity sector. Like others before her, she notes how the women she spoke with shared one implacable theme:

> A troubled relationship to the body's look— its size and shape, sexual attractiveness, its exposure both dressed and undressed—in a consumer culture where the body has become inextricably linked to personal identity and self-worth. Surface has replaced core; internal character virtues such as integrity and courage are subordinated to external manifestations of body control and discipline, while self-concept is synonymous with body image. (Fox-Kales, 2011, p. 2)

Media theorists in the postcolonial context argue that media representations significantly contribute to ethnocentric notions of beauty and health. These western beauty standards are viewed as part of a structural inequality imposed on non-western societies, aligning with the broader project of cultural imperialism (Jha, 2016). Some might say that media output is expressly crafted to neutralize any threat posed by groups who oppose the prevailing governing power structures. Up until recently, women of a non-white ethnicity who did not conform to western beauty standards were largely excluded from media portrayals (Rajan, 2003). Instead, traditional beauty standards have been eroded in favor of westernized body ideals in the media (Basu, 2021; Jha, 2016). In the South Asian film industry, the curvaceous female figure of early Bollywood culture has been replaced by the western silhouette of the slender, female frame. Asian women, in and outside of Asia, grapple with western beauty ideals and whiteness while simultaneously contending with pervasive racial stereotypes in the American film industry. For instance, the typical portrayal of the Asian woman as socially awkward and gauche has often been contrasted with the image of the beautiful, slender, and cool Caucasian woman (Iyer & Haslam, 2006). The various attempts to choreograph feminism and femininity without contradictions have given rise to an ultimately homogenized and depoliticized form of feminism. This has enduring effects on how young women of color, exposed to these images, perceive themselves.

Western screen media has been diversifying in terms of employment of actors for central roles. The industry's efforts to capitalize on gestures toward gender, racial, and body equality and diversity have not, however been without criticism and controversy. An example of this is the 2009 film, *Precious*, which narrates the story of a 16-year-old black girl and her struggles with poverty, family discord, and abuse. The protagonist, Claireece Precious Jones, is an uneducated Black female teenager of sturdy build living on welfare in an abusive Harlem home. Precious has two children by her father and has contracted HIV due to his sexual abuse. The lead actress, Mo'Nique, garnered critical acclaim for her exceptional performance. However, the film itself has been polarizing and extensively discussed by film reviewers and scholars (Mask, 2012). Stoneman (2012) observes that few reviewers failed to comment on the weight and size of the main character: "The 'audacity' of Precious ... consisted in director Lee Daniels' brazen disregard of the fact that his general audience might not be 'ready' for the story of 'an obese Harlem girl' whose family and community unrelentingly terrorize her" (p. 197). The assumption that the representation of fat subjects in visual culture can be neutral in the issue of body size is, Stoneman argues, patently false. In a society ingrained with disgust for the fat body, supported by decades of anti-obesity health policy, obese actors must inevitably encounter challenges.

The making of the film *Precious* raises questions about whether it was a pivotal moment in ending fat stigma and racism, or if the film merely reinforces "noxious stereotypes" of black communities. According to Griffin (2014), the film aligns with the tradition of scrutinizing the black female body through the white gaze. In the film, whiteness is portrayed as a savior; the turning point in Precious' life occurs when a white female school counsellor visits to inform her about an alternative school she can attend after being expelled due to her recent pregnancy. Beyond ideological disputes surrounding the film, disagreements surfaced between Mo'Nique and the film company, which requested her to travel for promotional activities. The actor declined, asserting that it was not part of her contractual obligations. Mo'Nique also made accusations against *Netflix* regarding gender and racial bias, underscoring the intricate and delicate nature of attempts at inclusivity that are not entirely followed through, perpetuating elements of corporate exploitation of socially disadvantaged employees.

Summary

In relation to the construction of eating disorders and disordered eating, representations of bodies in the media clearly matter. Images remain in the public eye and public consciousness, potentially altering the audience member's relationship with their own bodies and that of others. In terms of the fair and dignified treatment of employees in the media such as models and actors, there is still much progress to be made before discrimination and the exploitation of employees' bodies become relics of the past. Those navigating the intersection of factors such as gender, ethnicity, and body size also face the risk of public stigma and prejudice. Nevertheless, societal norms and cultural attitudes are subject to change, and what may have been deemed suitable entertainment material in one era or with one audience can elicit discomfort and dissonance in later generations. Those who produce media inevitably wish to imprint their distinct mark and expression on their creations, aiming to evoke complex emotional responses such as laughter, shock, fear, happiness, safety, and sexual pleasure. While the landscape may seem to have shifted from the era in which Theodore Adorno described the Hollywood "culture industry," breaking through the economic monopoly of global corporations like *Netflix* and *Amazon* is more challenging. These vast platforms inevitably favor work with broad mass appeal. Mainstream media, with some exceptions, traditionally reinforces dominant narratives surrounding socially desirable body shapes and eating behaviors, often in paradoxical and nonsensical ways.

Concerning the impact on eating disorder diagnosis, treatment, and the development of new categories, a host of media mechanisms come into play. Documentaries usually medicalize eating disorders, portraying them as mental disorders rooted in specific psychological profiles. The identification effect occurs as individuals, influenced by the experiences of actors and celebrities with eating disorders, may self-diagnose or seek diagnosis and treatment. Entertainment value is found in emotionally charged or humorous storylines about characters grappling with the indignities of an eating disorder while graphic depictions of behaviors such as binging and purging are largely deemed acceptable. Mainstream media has played a crucial role in drawing the public into the "maelstrom of medical interpretations" (Harbusch, 2022, p. 11). There are many instances where film and television appear to be aimed at educating viewers about the complexities of eating disorders, debunking myths, and reducing stigma. TV portrayals now often include trigger warnings before episodes with sensitive content to alert viewers and provide resources for support. Media are also complicit in reinforcing the need to label eating disorders and to body shame or "out" those known to have, or suspected of having, an "eating problem." Media also contains numerous examples of patient and doctor stereotypes, and plugs for a particular treatment, a cosmetic procedure, or a pharmaceutical drug. Apart from a few exceptions, media treats disordered bodies as cultural products, to be displayed and profited from, while stressing individual and psychological nature over socioeconomic factors.

Following this media theme, Chap. 8, "Disordered Eating in the Virtual World," turns to the role of digital media in the social construction of eating disorders and disordered eating. Topics explored include the ethics of digital surveillance, the pros and cons of online weight-loss programs, the controversies around pro-eating disorder (pro-ED) content online, and the therapeutic and commercial value of "real life" anorexia stories on YouTube.

References

Adorno, T. (1941). On popular music. *Studies in Philosophy and Social Sciences, IX*(1), 17–18.

Archives Publiques de l'Ontario. (2003). *Documenting a province/chronique d'une Province: The Archives of Ontario at 100/Le Centenaire des Archives Publiques L'Ontario*. University of Toronto Press.

Arnheim, R. (1969). *The world of the daytime serial*. Duell, Sloane and Pearce. Original work published 1944.

Basu, P. (2021). The Beauty myth and beyond: Looking at the Bollywood 'Item Number'. In *The Routledge companion to dance in Asia and the Pacific* (pp. 91–102). Routledge India.

Bell, B. T., & Dittmar, H. (2011). Does media type matter? The role of identification in adolescent girls' media consumption and the impact of different thin-ideal media on body image. *Sex Roles, 65*(7), 478–490.

Brechan, I., & Kvalem, I. L. (2015). Relationship between body dissatisfaction and disordered eating: Mediating role of self-esteem and depression. *Eating Behaviors, 17*, 49–45.

Brown, T. (2021). *'App'y Little Dieters: Neoliberalism, post-feminism and genomics in fitness and nutrition apps* (Master's thesis, University of Calgary, Calgary, Canada). Retrieved August 2, 2024, from https://prism.ucalgary.ca. http://hdl.handle.net/1880/113603 Downloaded from PRISM Repository, University of Calgary.

Bruch, H. (1982). Anorexia nervosa: Therapy and theory. *American Journal of Psychiatry, 139*, 1531.

Carpenter, R. (1983, November 21). The Karen Carpenter Story by her brother. *People*. Retrieved August 22 2024, from https://ghostarchive.org/archive/VD93c?url=http://people.com/archive/cover-story-a-brother-remembers-vol-20-no-21/

Catt, C. (2014). *Trapped in the kitchen: How advertising defined women's roles in 1950s America* (Doctoral dissertation). Retrieved August 22, 2024, from https://www.semanticscholar.org/paper/Trapped-in-the-Kitchen%3A-How-Advertising-Defined-in-Catt/183cd91dc5003f414320dc52d6fd9768e3435099

Coleman, R. (2008). The becoming of bodies: Girls, media effects, and body image. *Feminist Media Studies, 8*(2), 163–179.

Dickel, V., & Evolvi, G. (2023). "Victims of feminism": Exploring networked misogyny and# MeToo in the manosphere. *Feminist Media Studies, 23*(4), 1392–1408.

Donghi, P., & Wennerholm, J. (2014). Invisible fat: The aesthetics of food and the body. In K. Eli & S. Ulijaszek (Eds.), *Obesity, eating disorders and the media* (pp. 49–57). Routledge.

Eckersley, R. (2006). Is modern Western culture a health hazard? *International Journal of Epidemiology, 35*, 252–258.

Eli, K., & Levis, A. (2014). From abject eating object being. Media representations of obesity. 'Supersize versus super skinny'. In K. Eli & S. Ulijaszek (Eds.), *Obesity, eating disorders and the Media*. Routledge.

Eli, K., & Ulijaszek, S. (2014). *Obesity, eating disorders and the media*. Taylor & Francis Group.

Faludi, S. (2009). Backlash: The undeclared war against American women. *Psychology of Women Quarterly*.

Farrell, A. E. (1998). *Yours in sisterhood: Ms. magazine and the promise of popular Feminism*. The University of North Carolina Press.

Farren, M. (2010). *Speed-Speed-Speedfreak: A fast history of amphetamine*. Feral House.

Fineman, S. (2006). On being positive: Concerns and counterpoints. *Academy of Management Review, 31*(2), 270–291.

Fixsen, A., Ridge, D., & Porter, A. (2022). Arachne, self-care and 'power-nets' on women's self-development programmes. *Gender and Education, 34*(7), 770–786.

Fox-Kales, E. (2011). *Body shots: Hollywood and the culture of eating disorders*. State University of New York Press.

Freidan, B. (2010). *The feminine mystique*. Penguin Classics. (Original work published 1963).

Frost, L. (2001). *Young women and the body. A feminist sociology*. Palgrave.

Furedi, F. (2003). *Therapy culture: Cultivating vulnerability in an uncertain age*. Psychology Press.

Gill, R. (2007). *Gender and the media*. Polity Press.

Gill, R. (2017). The affective, cultural and psychic life of post feminism. A post-feminist sensibility 10 years on. *European Journal of Cultural Studies, 20*(6), 606–626.

Gill, R., & Orgad, S. (2015). The confidence cult(ure). *Australian Feminist Studies, 30*(86), 324–344.

Goldman, R., Heath, D., & Smith, S. L. (1991). Commodity feminism. *Critical studies in media communication, 8*(3), 333–351.

Gooldin, S. (2003). Fasting women, living skeletons and hunger artists: Spectacles of body and miracles at the turn of a century. *Body & Society, 9*(2), 27–53.

Griffin, R. A. (2014). Pushing into precious: Black women, media representation, and the glare of the White supremacist capitalist patriarchal gaze. *Critical Studies in Media Communication, 31*(3), 182–181.

Hainneville, V., Guèvremont, A., & Robinot, É. (2022). Femvertising or femwashing? Women's perceptions of authenticity. *Journal of Consumer Behaviour, 22*(4), 933–941.

Harbusch, M. (2022). Introduction: Are we all mad here? The normalization of trouble in everyday life. In M. Harbusch (Ed.), *Troubled Persons Industries: The expansion of psychiatric categories beyond psychiatry*. Springer International Publishing.

Head, A. (2023). *18-PT-approved celebrity workouts that promise to make your next sweat session a good one.* Marie Claire. Retrieved August 22, 2024, https://www.marieclaire.co.uk/life/health-fitness/celebrity-workouts-709296

Hirsch, P. M. (1992). Processing fads and fashions: An organization-set analysis of cultural industry systems. *American Journal of Sociology, 77*, 639–659.

Horkheimer, M., & Adorno, T.W. (1947/2001). The culture industry: Enlightenment as mass deception. In G. S. Noerr (Ed.), *Dialectic of enlightenment: Philosophical fragments* (pp. 94–136). Trans. E. Jephcott. Stanford University Press.

Illouz, E. (2007). *Cold intimacies: The making of emotional capitalism.* Polity Press.

Iyer, D. S., & Haslam, N. (2006). Cosmopolitanism: Eating disorders in the context of globalisation. *New Cosmopolitanisms: South Asians in the US*, 138.

Jha, M. (2016). *The global beauty industry. Colorism, racism, and national beauty.* Routledge.

Jones, D., & Pringle, J. K. (2015). Unmanageable inequalities: Sexism in the film industry. *The Sociological Review, 63*(1_suppl), 37–49.

Katterman, S. N., & Klump, K. L. (2010). Stigmatization of eating disorders: A controlled study of the effects of the television show Starved. *Eating Disorders, 18*(2), 153–164.

Keery, H., van den Berg, P., & Thompson, J. K. (2004). An evaluation of the Tripartite Influence Model of body dissatisfaction and eating disturbance with adolescent girls. *Body Image, 1*(3), 237–251.

Kiberd, R. (2015, April 20). *Fitspiration: How strong became the new skinny.* The Guardian. Retrieved August 22, 2024, https://www.theguardian.com/lifeandstyle/2015/apr/20/fitspo-strong-skinny-social-media-food-abs-better-living-body-fascism

LaVoulle, C., & Lewis Ellison, T. (2017). The bad bitch, Barbie Craze and Beyoncé: African American Women's bodies as commodities in Hip-Hop culture, images, and media. *Taboo: The Journal of Culture and Education, 16*(2), 7.

Leszkiewicz, A. (2017, July). *Why Netflix's To the Bone could be triggering*. New Statesman. Retrieved August 22, 2024, https://www.newstatesman.com/culture/2017/07/to-the-bone-netflix-review-glamourises-anorexia-eating-disorders

Levine, M. P., & Murnen, S. K. (2009). 'Everybody knows that mass media are/are not pick one a cause of eating disorders': A critical review of evidence for a causal link between media, negative body image and disordered eating in females. *Journal of Social and Clinical Psychology, 28*(1), 9–42.

Lorde, A. (2017). *The masters tools will never dismantle the masters house*. Penguin Classics.
Magladry, M. (2018). *Fitspiration or fitsploitation? Post feminism, digital media, and authenticity in women's fitness cultures*. PhD thesis, Curtin University. https://espace.curtin.edu.au/handle/20.500.11937/75531
Mask, M. (2012). The precarious politics of Precious: A close reading of a cinematic text. *Black Camera: An International Film Journal (The New Series), 4*(1), 96–116.
McRobbie, A. (2004). Post-feminism and popular culture. *Feminist Media Studies, 4*(3), 255–264.
McRobbie, A. (2011). Beyond post-feminism. *Public Policy Research, 18*(3), 179–184.
Mills, J. S., Shannon, A., & Hogue, J. (2017). Beauty, body image and the media. *Perception of Beauty*, 145–157.
Münsterberg, H. (1916). *The photoplay. A psychological study*. Appleton and Company.
Okin, S. M. (1989). *Justice, gender, and the family*. Basic Books.
Parasecoli, F. (2013). *Routledge International handbook of food studies* (pp. 274–281). Taylor & Francis.
Park, S. Y. (2005). The influence of presumed media influence on women's desire to be thin. *Communication Research, 32*(5), 594–614.
Parry, B. (2023). *Male celebrities who opened up about eating disorders and body image issues: Zyn Malik, Ed Sheeran and more*. Retrieved August 22, 2024, https://www.usmagazine.com/celebrity-body/pictures/male-stars-who-have-talked-eating-disorders-body-image-issues/
Plotz, B. (2020). *Fat on film: Gender, race and body size in contemporary Hollywood cinema*. Bloomsbury Publishing.
Rajan, R. S. (2003). *Real and imagined women: Gender, culture and postcolonialism*. Routledge.
Rottenberg, C. (2014). The rise of neoliberal feminism. *Cultural Studies, 28*(3), 418–437.
Sandberg, S. (2013). *Lean in: Women, work and the will to lead*. Alfred A Kopf.
Seligman, M. E. P., & Csikszentmihalyi, M. (2000). Positive Psychology. *American Psychologist, 55*(1), 5–14.
Shippen, N. (2014). *Decolonizing time: Work, leisure, and freedom*. Springer.
Stoneman, S. (2012). Ending fat stigma: Precious, visual culture, and anti-obesity in the "Fat Moment". *The Review of Education/Pedagogy/Cultural Studies, 34*(3–4), 197–207.

Tessier, B., & Schulman, L. (2023). *Judy Garland–Splendor and Downfall of a Legend*. BearManor Media.
Varghese, N., & Kumar, N. (2022). Feminism in advertising irony or revolution? A critical review of femvertising. *Feminist Media Studies, 22*(2), 441–459.
Wallenstein, A. (2005, November 8). *'Starved': New comedy not hungry for laughs*. npr. Retrieved August 2, 2024, from https://www.npr.org/2005/08/11/4795817/starved-new-comedy-not-hungry-for-laughs
Whitaker, E. (2017). *An analysis of Betty Friedan's The Feminine Mystique*. CRC Press.
Widdows, H. (2018). *Perfect me: Beauty as an ethical ideal*. Princetown.
Wolf, N. (1994). *Fire with fire: The new female power and how to use it*. Fawcett Columbine.

8

Disordered Eating in the Virtual World

As illustrated in the previous chapter, the media industry continues to use an eclectic range of mediums and technologies to disseminate its cultural goods. Increasingly, however, this field is dominated by digital media platforms and their fast-evolving and multipurpose technological applications. Unlike most other forms of media, social media is interactive and user-generated, meaning that it gives the impression of operating as a relatively autonomous, multi-way communication process. Internet technology has been hailed for empowering the "many" to participate actively in the broadcasting process, liberating communication from constraints like time delays and the risk of easy loss of contact. Recent shifts suggest an apparent limitlessness to the online world (Cusumano, 2011). Navigating through social media platforms by swiping and scrolling is as daily activity shared by billions of people.[1] Websites and applications that enable users to create and share content or to participate in social networking have proved especially popular (Kaur & Gurnani, 2022). Using social media, individuals can share images and videos providing glimpses into their activities, opt for voice recordings instead of traditional calls,

[1] According to *Statistica* (May 2023), as of January 2023 there were 5.16 billion Internet users, of which 4.76 billion used social media (59.4 percent of global population).

A. Fixsen, *The Construction of Eating Disorders*, The Politics of Mental Health and Illness, https://doi.org/10.1007/978-3-031-70318-8_8

and update others on real-time locations. But activities on social media are not as user determined as they seem. Social media platforms employ algorithms that tailor content to users' preferences, fostering personalized experiences while also influencing the spread of information and shaping public opinion. Digital media has yet to replicate or control all aspects of human existence, but it has made a good start of doing so. Essentially, digital media operates as a highly effective tool of biopolitics, shaping and sometimes determining how people act upon themselves and interact with one another; the information they receive; the products and services they buy; how they choose to eat, work, love, and spend their leisure; and—centrally to a study of disordered eating—how people seek to shape and modify their real and virtual bodies.

This chapter examines the role of digital media in the construction of eating disorders and disordered eating. Internet platforms and the forums, videos, blogs, and podcasts hosted by them have not only generated new theory around social interaction but have created an archive of information concerning the lived experiences of disordered eating from the perspective of the online generation. Given the vastness of the subject, what follows is a brief synopsis of my own and others' studies concerning the changes wrought by a social life increasingly played out online. After considering the role of sociology in theorizing the functions of social media, the chapter turns to the topic of digital surveillance and "dark" spaces on the Internet. In relation to these covert spaces, the chapter delves into the dynamics of discourses surrounding eating disorders within the context of what have been loosely named pro-eating disorder (pro-ED) forums. The impact of the "selfie society" (Morelock & Narita, 2021) is then discussed, including its shaping of discourses about disordered eating online. Finally, I explain how the illness narratives elucidated in recent online videos have taken a decidedly entrepreneurial turn, with the authors of these videos gaining followings on their subscription channels and diversifying, for example, from their version of a "my anorexia story" to promoting beauty products.

Discourses on disordered eating reflect the complex interplay between personal expression, marketing pressure, community dynamics, and the influence of digital platforms.

New Technology, Old Habits

For decades, sociologists have been keen observers of the social changes wrought by online technologies. The emergence of social media platforms prompted many social scientists and theorists to focus on how these innovations are influencing and transforming social, political, and economic life (Lupton, 2014). Online health support groups have generally been welcomed by health researchers for democratizing health information (Ziebland et al., 2004) and challenging the dominance of expert-driven information systems (Mo & Coulson, 2014). The functions of such member forums to act as places of refuge and to give the "mute" a voice have also been emphasized in the sociological literature (Fixsen & Ridge, 2017; Yeshua-Katz, 2015). At the same time, the misleading and potentially triggering nature of social media content—in terms of increasing users' body dissatisfaction (Boepple & Thompson, 2014) and romanticizing eating disorders (Tragantzopoulou et al., 2024)—has also been highlighted. Social media has also become a key marketing tool. Companies use it to find and engage with customers, drive sales to advertising and promotion, identify fast-moving consumer trends, and collect volumes of personal data. Critical theorists have drawn attention to the governance issues around digital media including the exploitation and manipulation of "Big Data" for commercial ends and the monitoring and controlling of people's inner and outer lives through increasingly sophisticated surveillance tools (Han, 2014; Zuboff, 2015).

Social media may be a novel medium for social interaction, but most of the activities taking place on these platforms embody age-old social and relational processes. The concept of "social facts" has been discussed elsewhere in the book in relation to medical "facts" such as body mass index BMI (see Chap. 6) and can be applied to other collective processes which exist independently of individual manifestations. Social facts, as explained by Durkheim (1892/1982), are external to individuals yet they exert a compelling influence on their behavior, often crystallizing within well-defined social organizations. For example, a relevant social fact concerns the existence of eating disorders as mental illnesses requiring professional treatment. This "social fact" holds true, even if some individuals diagnosed with an eating disorder such as anorexia nervosa

(AN) disagree with their diagnosis and refuse treatment. Social facts can be both material and non-material with only the first kind being directly observed. Non-material facts, such as morality and collective conscience, are inferred from changes in material fact. Deviance is a negative fact which reinforces social norms by setting examples of unacceptable behavior.[2] Once a form of deviance becomes "normalized," it ceases to be an individual concern and becomes a "social fact." Durkheim also introduced the concept of "social currents" to describe phenomena that lack the same objectivity and dominance as social facts over individuals (Casteel, 2011). An example Durkheim provides us with is a public gathering where waves of enthusiasm surpass individual consciousness. These currents, originating externally, can engulf individuals despite their resistance. To quote Durkheim (1982, p. 53):

> Social currents come to each of us from outside and can sweep us along in spite of ourselves. If perhaps I abandon myself to them I may not be conscious of the pressure they are exerting upon me, but that pressure makes its presence felt immediately I attempt to struggle against them … Which leads us to believe we have ourselves produced what has been imposed upon us externally.

What happens on social media has much to do with how we, in contemporary society, approach social facts and social currents. Social media is recognised as a medium through which accepted "truths" can be manipulated or refuted (Cosentino, 2020). It is not uncommon for social posts to challenge or modify social facts, to suit different goals and purposes. Users can become content creators and storytellers, editing photos, videos, and first-hand accounts. Hashtags play a pivotal role in aggregating content around a specific theme or event. They act as amplifiers, for stories to gain visibility beyond individual networks. Through shares, retweets, and viral trends, some stories reach a vast global audience and become "social currents" within a matter of minutes (as in recent posts on the social media platform *X* by Taylor Swift). The social constructionist view of social facts is that they are relative and subject to change, meaning what counts as "disinformation" on social media is also a value judgment on the part of

---

[2] Deviance is used in the sociological sense as nonconformity which needs to be corrected (Scull, 2022).

the receiver. What is undisputable is that hugely profitable social media companies such as *Facebook, Instagram, WhatsApp*, and *Messenger* use power tactics and built in features on their platforms to create or manipulate "social currents," and to entice and ultimately ensnare users—children and young people especially—to compulsively engage, and return again and again, to these spaces, interfering with social life, school, sleep, eating, and other important activities (Richtel, 2023).

Surveillance on the Internet

Digital media now sits uncomfortably at the pinnacle of power. Not only does it represent one of the most significant threats to the principles of governmentality, but it is through digital channels that the present institutions of power seek to exert control over large populations. Several factors contribute to this power. First, there is the massive reach and influence of social media platforms, which allows it to set trends, shape cultural norms, and influence public opinion on a scale previously unimaginable. Second is that social media serves as a primary source of news and information for many people. Platforms can prioritize, amplify, or suppress certain types of content through algorithms, thereby influencing what information is seen and how it is perceived. This control over information flow gives social media companies substantial power over public knowledge and opinion. Third is the enormous economic power of these social media companies, which, coupled with their influence over information and communication, gives them significant leverage over governments, businesses, and individuals. Finally, social media platforms collect vast amounts of data on users, including their preferences, behaviors, and social connections, which can be sold on to government agencies.

Sociologists have conceptualized social media as an inverted Panopticon,[3] since the power relations between individuals and socio-

[3] The Panopticon comes from the Greek word for "all seeing." A panopticon was an institutional building with an inbuilt system of surveillance. The brainchild of reformer and social theorist, Jeremy Bentham, surveillance from a high platform allowed a single correction officer to observe inmates of an institution regardless of whether inmates were aware of being watched. In practice, the full design was never taken up, although it probably influenced the outlay of certain prisons. Michel Foucault later used the idea to explain the operation of modern disciplinary society in his book, *Discipline and Punish* (1975/1991).

technical systems broadly speaking amount to voluntary servitude (Romele et al., 2017).[4] Voluntary servitude, though seemingly paradoxical, encapsulates the simultaneous pursuit of freedom and submission to the system on the part of users. Advancements in media technologies have given rise to an era where individuals inadvertently or willingly contribute vast amounts of personal data through online interactions, social media platforms, and other digital channels. Social media platforms provide a fertile ground from which to gather "digital footprints" to analyze and predict, not just activities but user location, age, gender, level of education, health status, political preferences, and so on. This data can be used for highly targeted advertising and influence campaigns, making social media a powerful tool for marketing, political campaigns, and even social manipulation. Computer algorithms use features to analyze digital traces and levels/time of engagement to establish the strength to which they are associated with attributes and personality traits. Recommendation systems then provide suggestions of media content to be viewed by individual. This extensive data collection has facilitated ongoing social surveillance. Governments, corporations, and various entities leverage digital technologies to observe, analyze, and track individuals' behaviors, preferences, and activities, to inform, advise, or influence (Zuboff, 2015).

The ethical implications for a society subject to so much surveillance are many, and the lack of safeguarding of vulnerable groups is seen by some as alarming. Among the issues of big data collection are privacy invasion, data protection issues, infringement of civil liberties, the potential for abuse of power, and lack of accountability (Zuboff, 2015). In the area of public safety, the replacement of humans with AI content also has an impact on the moderation of content, while automated information spreaders or "bots" are often sources of what counts as disinformation (Hajli et al., 2022). Targeted marketing derived from such information mean that individuals are exposed to adverts that supposedly align with their personal preferences and connect individuals of a similar age and interest with each other. These patterns create the potential for "shadow

[4] *Voluntary servitude* is by no means a modern term but is one that seems applicable to people's relationship to social media. The term was coined in the sixteenth century by Étienne de La Boétie, a young member of the Bordeaux's parliament and a "refined intellectual" (Romele et al., 2017).

profiling" where an individual's undisclosed or private information is revealed or inferred from data which has been accessed to other people in a shared network without their consent (Hinds, 2019).

One of the arguments in favor of greater regulation of social media is the existence of disruptive, illegal, and counter narratives circulating on the Internet, distorting "facts" (Fischer & Klazar, 2020) and leading to personal and social harms (Mörch et al., 2018). It is a rare day when social media is not part of some discussion about expressions of dissidence, misogyny, and antisocial behaviors, including substance abuse, disordered eating, and suicidality. Identifying and countering the culprits who promulgate risky and unscientific (dis)information and encourage antisocial attitudes and behaviors has become a major preoccupation for security forces, politicians, and social and health policymakers across the world (Phelan et al., 2023). Studies suggest that most of the content that becomes popular on social media is posted by just a fraction of users, chiefly made up of self-appointed experts on topics and celebrities (Zafar et al., 2016; Welles & González-Bailón, 2018). Social media algorithms play a role in shaping the visibility of stories. As well as enhancing the global reach of certain narratives, they contribute to the formation of "echo chambers," where users are exposed to information aligned with their existing beliefs. If social media is the new God, he is a god who speaks with a forked tongue.

However, not all forms and functions of social media are met with disapproval by the authorities. One example relating to disordered eating has been the emergence of digital platforms which "educate" users about weight-loss surgery and other such interventions (Ferry & Richards, 2015). These sites have met with support from health organizations, including the World Health Organisation (WHO) (Jane et al., 2018). As with mental health policy, the thinking has been that delivering weight-loss interventions via social media could be highly effective in terms of reducing costs, time saving, and delivering materials to hard-to-reach populations on a much larger scale. Some researchers interested in these forums emphasize the positive functions of such sites for those undergoing or considering bariatric surgery (surgical procedures which are aimed to help with weight loss), including managing people's expectations, decision-making, and signposting; providing social and emotional support;

helping others with access to healthcare professionals; and managing blame (Jane et al., 2018; Robinson et al., 2020).

Yet even sponsored programs are bound to vary in type and quality. While some evidence exists to support the efficacy of specific programs, it has proved difficult to determine or compare the combined impact and utility of different weight-loss platforms for public health, due to variations in levels of health literacy among different populations and to the mixture of professionally led support and peer support programs (Chang et al., 2021). One systematic review of social media weight-loss interventions among teenagers and young adults (mostly on Facebook) looked at the extent to which younger audiences engage in these platforms and their messages about exercise and healthier eating choices, and the ability of studies to identify effective tools for weight-loss management (Lozano-Chacon et al., 2021). The principal advantage of weight-loss platforms was the more accurate monitoring of weight loss, leading to improvements in the data collection and surveillance processes of the target population. However, the effectiveness of these platforms in terms of weight loss was tied in with factors including socioeconomic status and social and family support. The authors argue that greater homogeneity in the methodology of studies and application of interventions is needed before any conclusions can be drawn about these sites (Lozano-Chacon et al., 2021).

Discourses on disordered eating reflect the complex interplay between personal expression, marketing pressure, community dynamics, and the influence of digital platforms. There are also ethical and conflict of interest issues which weight-loss forums raise. Features sponsored by advertisers are likely to downplay the side effects of such things as bariatric surgery, including loss of appetite, and to emphasize the necessity of surgical procedures. The "before and after" stories and images on these sites can be viewed as a form of "cultural fraud" (Eckersley, 2005), in that they promote images and ideals of the good life which serve the economy, but which may fail to reflect personal and social realities. In a society that disapproves of obesity, overweight is portrayed as a miserable burden, but the message that increased weight necessarily leads to unhappiness or a lower quality of life may be flawed (Thommasen et al., 2005).

Public health statements and professionally run programs now compete with social media channels communicating their own narratives about bodies and health, often projecting public health advice as "out of sync" with the needs and desires of certain groups and consumers. While lay generated content on social media may be accompanied by a greater sense of connection and trust (Chang et al., 2021), following the messages on these sites can result in unsound life and health choices, potentially with dire effects on individual and community health outcomes (Greškovičová et al., 2022). Digitalization also means that official forms of knowledge can be easily repurposed or by-passed by messages designed to connect more directly with the inclinations of the digital audience. How messages around thinness and disordered eating play out on the Internet will be explored in depth in the following sections.

Online Narratives of Disordered Eating

As individuals increasingly turn to the Internet and other forms of digital media to share their experiences, seek support, or contribute to the perpetuation of certain beliefs and behaviors, personal narratives about disordered eating have become a significant aspect of the digital landscape, and also a popular research topic. One abiding question for health scientists and statisticians is whether viewing social media should be described as a *risk factor* or a *causation* of eating disorders. Various studies have set out to establish the relationship between time spent viewing certain forms of media and other factors, including low body satisfaction (Mills et al., 2017), as well as female gender and pre-existing mental health problems (Anderson & Jiang, 2018). The portrayal of idealized body types on social media platforms, often characterized by unrealistic beauty standards, has been identified as a key factor influencing individuals' perceptions of their own bodies. Studies have found a strong correlation between exposure to idealized images on platforms such as *Instagram* and increased body dissatisfaction (Perloff, 2014). The rise of "thinspiration" and "fitspiration"[5] content on platforms like *Pinterest* and *Tumblr* is thought

[5] *Fitspiration* broadly aims to inspire individuals to exercise and keep healthy. *Thinspiration* idealizes depictions of excessively thin and lean bodies. On social media sites fitspiration and thinspiration can converge in their portrayal of the ideal, fat-free body.

to have further contributed to the normalization of extreme dieting and exercise behaviors (Boepple & Thompson, 2016; Tiggemann & Slater, 2013). The anonymity provided by social media is also considered to have created an environment in which cyberbullying—the use of electronic communication to intimidate, harass, or humiliate others—can thrive (Cheng et al., 2023; Day et al., 2022).

As well has general content concerning idealised body images, dedicated platforms exist on which participants share stories and content about ultra-thin bodies and restrictive eating regimes. It seems likely that what came to be known as the pro-eating disorder (Pro-ED) "movement" (Hammond, 2014) first emerged among affected individuals, seeking to share their personal stories with like-minded others online. Pro-ED social media chat forums have been present since the early 1990s, a time when eating disorder therapy was still scarce. The anonymity offered by these online spaces allowed individuals to candidly discuss their experiences and exchange "tips and tricks" that might be difficult in face-to-face interactions. So-called Pro-Ana (promoting Anorexia) and Pro-Mia (promoting Bulimia) websites seemingly rejected the idea of passive, isolated suffering, but rather support members in their efforts to further restrict their diets and lose weight. Typically organized and managed by lay individuals, these forums provided platforms for those engaged in self-starvation and purging, or those directed by algorithms from meta platforms, to engage in conversations, share images, and exchange ideas and experiences online (Day & Keys, 2008). Most of the recent sites feature blogs, dieting tips and tricks, BMI calculators, and photo/video galleries that offer "thinspiration" for extreme weight loss (Boepple & Thompson, 2014, 2016; Stapleton et al., 2019). The desire "to be part of" draws people into a secretive social world that may become increasingly hard to resist. Girls identifying themselves with pro-Ana sometimes wear a red bracelet resembling a thin string on their right wrist as a badge (Hoffmann, 2018). Those who wish to create a "buzz" on these sites often do so through stories about more "outrageous" diets and behaviors, encouraging others to gravitate toward such extremes. A regular "vlogger" and self-proclaimed veteran of the pro-Ana movement describes in one online *YouTube* video the craziness, hyper-competitiveness, and sisterhood which characterized pro-Ana early forums:

> What actually goes on in forums I think is shrouded in mystery enough, let alone what goes on when you actually bring together a whole bunch of these teenagers and all of their many dysfunctions and let them run riot around London, particularly in the early 2000s when meeting up with people from the Internet was not something you did.

The "Vlogger" explains how in the early hours she would be able to talk with others about their attempts to be skinniest or engagement in binges and purges:

> It sounds dark and sick to say this, [but] it was a lot of fun and there was a lot of crazy stuff that went on then, I mean I remember one girl posting a load of pictures … on her forum [with her] username written in puke on the toilet seat! This was the kind of antics that we got up to.

People who voice disapproval are, according to the vlogger, always the ones with no first-hand experience, such that it seems a form of bigotry: "I swear to God every single time [that] those the people who get offended are the people who have never had eating disorders or addictions themselves; they just get offended on general principle." In this way, Pro-Ana forums became an opportunity for these youngsters to share experiences and create a sense of camaraderie. In the same video, the vlogger also mentions the sad cases of members who subsequently died from their condition, underscoring the fragile nature of these relationships.

As these types of forums mushroomed, so they began to evoke moral panic and garnered widespread criticism among many in the medical, media, and public sector. The information on these sites is considered by many to be inaccurate, risky, or subversive, or to pose a threat to public safety (Boepple & Thompson, 2014; Christodoulou, 2012; Rouleau & von Ranson, 2011). On so-called pro-eating disorder websites, obtaining a thin body is portrayed as desirable and stringent weight control practices are promoted (Holland & Tiggemann, 2016; Au & Cosh, 2022). The search terms "pro-ana" (for anorexia nervosa) and "pro-mia" (for bulimia nervosa) (Borzekowski et al., 2010) have made these sites relatively quick and easy for browsers to locate. Operating outside of any official clinical or medical model, they have been viewed, by medics and those in child protection, as part of a "dark net," whose countercultural narratives pose a serious threat to child safety (Christodoulou, 2012; Fairplay, 2022).

A specific area of concern is that the main audience for social media is drawn from younger age groups, who are considered more vulnerable to extreme messages. A recent report highlighted how *Instagram* has been profiting from the growing number of pro-eating disorder "bubbles" appearing on its platform, largely directed at very young audience members (O'Sullivan et al., 2021). According to Fairplay (2022), the "pro-eating disorder bubble" on *Instagram* alone had two million unique followers, some as young as nine years of age. On these sites, visitors are exposed to extreme ideas about food, diet, appearance-related content, and also bullying, humiliation, and grooming activities (Da Rocha & Long, 2008; Tragantzopoulou et al., 2024). Media stories speak of shocking things such as the sadistic practices employed by online coaches and the sexual exploitation of young people on platforms such as *Tumblr* (Sukenesan, 2021). Pro-Ana material on social media is believed to trigger social comparison, creating a "vicious" feedback loop, whereby young people feeling bad about themselves go on to social media to self-soothe, then end up viewing the types of post which led to their anxieties in the first place (Heilweil, 2021). As individuals seeking help may inadvertently stumble upon these harmful platforms, the potential for misinformation and reinforcement of destructive behaviors can derail efforts to promote healthier dialogues and support networks on mainstream social media. The effects of these unofficial sites on shaping alternative discourses around "self-care" might also perpetuate the idea that "clean" forms of eating (such as a raw food diet) represent an elevated form of self-care, while traditional or standard eating norms are viewed as inferior and even disgusting.

Those who escape predators on social media are still victims of data mining. With the use of algorithms, psychological profiling, and advertising on media platforms such as *Facebook,* digital industries can make tidy profits from disordered eating. This is not small fry in economic terms, platforms such as *Instagram* and *Tiktok* earn millions of dollars by using algorithms on these sites to deliver content related to topics or themes, with the aim of maximizing the time users spend on a platform (Fairplay, 2022). Following the UK Online Safety Act (UK Parliament,

2024), Internet platforms have a legal duty to minimize harmful content and a duty to protect children from accessing harmful age-inappropriate content, including that relating to eating disorder content. Nevertheless, the organization BEAT (2024) suggests that more must be done to ensure that all viewers are protected from harmful content while it remains unclear how eating disorder content will be defined. The Act also fails to consider the impact of diet and fitness content and role of algorithms in targeted online advertising. In a recent BEAT (2024) survey, 91 percent of people with lived experiences of an eating disorder had encountered content that was harmful in the context of their disorder, while many described being bombarded with triggering content and imagery in adverts.

From the beginning, researchers in the feminist community have grappled with how to describe pro-ED websites (Cobb, 2017; Day & Keys, 2008). It has long been suspected that those with eating disorders perceive their illness very differently to the way professionals understand it; hence, a reductive approach to these sites would appear to be unhelpful. Qualitative researchers have found a notable discrepancy between professional accounts and how people conceptualize their eating disorder as less of an illness and more of a life choice, with benefits that only those who share this world view can understand (Da Rocha & Long, 2008; Dias, 2003; Tragantzopoulou et al., 2024; Yeshua-katz, 2015). Dias (2003) noted how little heed was paid to the words and perceptions of individuals with eating disorders during normal clinical practice, which contrasts with the empathic tone of some of the moderators on these pro-ED forums. While efforts have been made to make ED consultations more patient-centered, the idea that something as precarious as AN might be conceived of as desirable remains almost inexplicable to many outside these communities. In contrast, these points of view are frequently discussed on Pro-Ana websites by users, articulating the pro-Ana collective perspective.

Members of the pro-Ana movement challenge established biomedical and paternalistic ideas surrounding the treatment of AN based on the "normalization" of body shape and weight; however, their messages appear to go further than just resisting established body norms. In a grounded theory study by Norris et al. (2006), religious metaphors, lifestyle descriptions, and "thinspiration" (inspirational photo galleries and quotes that aim to serve as motivators for weight loss) were frequently present on pro-Ana sites. Ward (2007) argues that the pro-Ana group offers a model of "being" and "knowing" and facilitates the emergence of a coherent anorexic subjectivity, which is sustained by the development of an "ana-language" and the legitimacy and validation of ana rituals and behavior patterns on these forums. Yeshua-Katz and Martins (2013) suggest that these sites operate as places of stigma resistance. Those visiting these pro-Ana sites appear to be seeking some stability through the advice and companionship of people who know what it feels like to live with ana (Ward, 2007; Stapleton et al., 2019). The fervor and ritualistic attitudes and behaviors legitimated on these sites, with "Ana" sometimes spoken of as "god" (Stapleton et al., 2019; Tragantzopoulou et al., 2024), suggest distinct parallels between the "holy anorexia" reported on by mediaeval chroniclers and the devotional acts of starvation described on pro-Ana sites.

One of the insights gained from investigations of pro-Ana forums and materials concerns how their messages and potential membership have changed over time. As suggested in the earlier vlogger interview, more established members may employ social equality arguments to expose what they see as the fallacy of portraying "Ana" purely as a mental illness rather than a chosen lifestyle (Hoffmann, 2018). However, as the pro-Ana audience gets younger, its tone has changed accordingly. Cobb's (2017) thesis on pro-Ana online spaces takes the long view of these sites, noting how the association between third-wave feminism and AN had diminished in the last decade. On line spaces continue to provide a space for expression beyond the medical gaze (Ging & Harvey, 2018). Their political potential has been stymied by and replaced with something more individualistic and populist. In her study of posts concerning the film, *Frozen* on pro-Ana sites Holmes (2015) offers a functional view of these videos and interprets them as places where these young women can find validation and support for views and behaviors that mainstream society has labelled as dangerous. Nevertheless, she points out how, because of pro-Ana users' individualism, they have "no clear affinity with the feminist approaches which persistently foreground the culture-bound nature of eating disorders" (p. 116).

A Study of Powerplays on Pro-ED Sites

The arguments above suggest that the apparently countercultural discourses on pro-ED forums and platforms are seductive because they appear to offer opportunities and solutions unavailable in conventional society. They also create a kind of moral fervor which centers on the disciplining and modification of the body. For some individuals, membership to these sites might instill a sense of purpose and significance as they embark on a project, with forum members ready to provide guidance and criticism. The study that will be described in this section utilized critical discourse analysis, following Fairclough's methodology (2001), to scrutinize the language, messages, and powerplays on pro-eating disorder (pro-ED) sites, and to compare them with healthy eating (HE) websites (Tragantzopoulou et al., 2024). Study data was collected exclusively from publicly available websites using keywords and terms over a four-month period in 2021. Multiple texts were examined for recurring language, and phrases were identified across various posts and threads. Codes were organized based on similarities, leading to the creation of a thematic framework. The themes encompassed expertise in diet and restriction, health and food-related anxieties, critiques of bodies and motherhood, reward and punishment, and discipline and devotion.

In contrast to the authors on HE sites, who were eager to showcase their professional credentials in nutrition, contributors on pro-eating disorder (pro-ED) sites seemed to have taken on the roles of "experts" and "coaches" based on their knowledge of specific techniques for achieving and maintaining a low BMI. Many of these self-proclaimed "authorities" had adhered to restrictive diets for extended periods, conveying the idea that pro-Ana could be a lifestyle choice. Both HE and pro-ED site authors drew connections between fasting, restrictive diets, and notable improvements in physical conditions such as clearer skin. However, the primary focus on pro-ED sites was not on achieving optimal health but rather on avoiding weight gain associated with calorie-rich foods. Consequently, discussions on these sites predominantly centered around sharing lists of so-called impure or weight-inducing foods, with food fears playing a significant role in the conversations.

Another theme concerned the conceptualization of the "female body" and "motherhood" on websites. Several HE websites referenced motherhood, featuring both positive and negative representations of mothers. In contrast, pro-ED sites did not associate motherhood with eating, possibly due to the younger demographic of the pro-ED community or a deliberate avoidance of topics linked to female development and pregnancy. Another distinction between HE and pro-ED forums was evident in the attitudes toward discipline and devotion expressed on the sites. While both encouraged a sense of community and loyalty, pro-ED sites placed greater emphasis on guilt and punishment, often featuring self-deprecating and sadistic language. Some coaches even made promises like "I will make your ED worse" or "I will traumatize you," seemingly targeting those willing to sacrifice self-worth for weight-loss tutorials.

Studying user-generated content on ED platforms can help us to understand how those controlling the narrative online may come to assume power over people's lives and why they are such a popular way in which to broadcast one's own story about an eating disorder. Our study indicates that real and perceived power inequalities operate online, which are reinforced, not only through status effects but by use of disciplinary language. However, characterizing the relationships between coaches and visitors on these sites as mere coercion and bullying would be to oversimplify their dynamics. Members appear to view these methods as legitimate pathways toward self-realization and fulfillment, involving reshaping both the mind and body. This suggests that people do find meaning and purpose through pro-ED sites, even if these goals appear unwholesome or harmful from a psychological and clinical perspective. In summary, disciplining the female body on both type of site aligns with a broader concept of power and identity associated with neoliberalism, emphasizing self-entrepreneurial activity and self-striving. In the context of pro-Ana, the pursuit of thinness, while appearing as an act of rebellion, may represent a form of self-imposed servitude which in terms of individual satisfaction is ultimately counterproductive.

Online ED "selfie culture"

We have already noted, as in other literature, how individualism and emotional capitalism have created a societal pressure on individuals facing mental health issues to "open up" as a means of safeguarding their mental well-being and showcasing authenticity (Cohen, 2016; Harbusch, 2022). This type of thinking is not a recent development. As Foucault elucidated, the act of confession or "truth telling" originated in the classical world between a master and an acolyte, evolving into "one of the West's most highly valued techniques for producing truth" (Foucault, 1989, p. 59). Foucault would no doubt have had much to say about the abundance of "confessional" content on current social media, viewing it as a technology of power.[6] However, a new dimension concerning truth has emerged for social media users, as it is increasingly difficult to discern between the real and the virtual online. Nor are the relationships established on social media necessarily mirrored in the real world. For instance, it is recognized that, overall, people who are connected on social media may spend less time face-to-face with friends and family, and more time sharing digital images and information with a faceless audience (Morelock & Narita, 2021). Self-promotion has long been a feature of human relationships, while self-mediated portraits and stories about oneself and one's achievements are nothing new. However, in the digital age, the selfie symbolizes a more complex social reality, since speaking out about one's vulnerabilities can be both a sign of personal strength and an entrepreneurial opportunity. Neoliberalism applauds the ability of people to create personal capital out of just about anything; hence, self-care and self-entrepreneurism are now regarded as bedfellows, rather than being somehow at odds with one another.

In our so-called selfie society (Morelock & Narita, 2021), eating disorder identities and discourses can manifest themselves, not just on anonymous chat forums but on more open, image-based platforms such as *Instagram*. On these platforms, posters can use emotive and evocative language to describe their damaged bodies and identities, as in "written

[6] By *technologies of power* is meant those forms of discourses and actions, which determine the conduct of individuals and submit them to certain ends or domination.

in the scars of the stories, I can't explain" (Ging & Garvey, 2018). Countless self-made videos of anorexia have now been posted by "vloggers" on *Facebook, Tiktok, Instagram, YouTube*, and blogs. The study by Ging and Harvey (2018) found thousands of pro-Ana images being shared on *Instagram* daily. The authors concluded that the proliferation of pro-Ana hashtags, along with multiple tagging, meant that the images could be easily searched and found by the pro-Ana audience, and by other users whose interests span a range of topics from dieting and fitness to self-harm, suicide, and depression. It is this overlap between the selfie culture, depression- and self-harm-related content, and pro-recovery material which, for the authors, challenged stereotypes of the pro-anorexic who desires to hide themselves away and wishes to communicate only with others with the same problem and world view. Rather, those posting on online platforms appear to be seeking a likeminded, empathic audience to share their embodied pain, in ways that professionals are unwilling or unable to do (Fixsen & Ridge, 2017).

Drawing on Gidden's (1991) theory of the body as project, Holmes (2015, 2017) set out to explain how girls use popular culture as a resource for identity construction; how they navigate issues of reception, representation, and production; and the questions this raises about "mediated subjectivities, self-representation, and gendered forms of corporeal production in teenage girls" (Holmes, 2017, p. 5). In data searches of "my anorexic stories" on YouTube, Holmes detected common stylistic features among videos which positions them within the wider genre of digital illness narratives and teenage "suffering" narratives. Similar conclusions were reached in the study by Loewen (2021) who focused on "performing anorexia" on YouTube and how it assumes three functional forms—confessionals, food videos, and life stories. Confessional videos may enable YouTubers to repair their self-narratives, become active witnesses, and use their bodies to communicate their stories. Food videos seem uniquely suited to assist those with anorexia work through their paradoxical fascination and fear around food. Finally, life story videos may increase feelings of empowerment, embodiment, and selfhood. The comments from viewers following these videos may also generate affective ties which affirm the YouTubers' decision to share their stories and to increase the visibility of anorexia as an illness.

The online platform *YouTube* was launched in 2005 as a user-friendly site to upload, store, and share videos. In 2006 it was bought by Google for $1.65 billion and became a primary site for the marketing of music, movies, and television. As both a top-down and bottom-up platform, *YouTube* has retained much of its original identity but has increasingly become a site for self-promotion and the creation of the "self-brand" (Banet-Weiser, 2011). One of the factors that has led to *YouTube's* popularity is its community-oriented format, where users videoblog on a single common platform accessible to everyone, although individually hosted blogs are viewed mostly by people within the blogger's circle. YouTube is a virtual public sphere where the marketplace of ideas is both vast and disorderly. As Banet-Weiser et al. (2020) explain, broadcasting and branding on *YouTube* have become one and the same, as the ways in which individuals communicate their personal values, ideas, and beliefs, and employ strategies and logic from brand culture, are increasingly applauded in the present economic environment. These videos are often part of a series from which the host vlogger or organization can acquire further followers and generate income. This behavior is reinforced by the influencer culture, where personal narratives, including those related to mental health, can become a commodity. There are economic advantages of choosing social media as a form of promotion, since compared to mainstream media, posting online is usually a low-cost medium. Nevertheless, there are also drawbacks and risks to posting videos on social media. A certain amount of courage is required to stream videos with highly personal content, and the consequences of doing so are often outside of the vlogger's control. Popular or sensational videos can "go viral," for better or worse. Heated conversations can take place in the comment sections on people's social media accounts. If people post comments about pictures and videos, they are then publicly available unless action is taken to delete them.

"Anorexia and me"

In 2021, we (myself and students at our university) conducted online research on video stories addressing AN that were freely available on *YouTube*. We utilized search terms such as "eating disorder" or "anorexia," in conjunction with phrases like "my story," "my survival," "my recovery," and "my journey," focusing on videos which had been viewed by at least several thousand people. Sixteen of these videos were then selected, reviewed, and transcriptions were subjected to a secondary analysis. This comprehensive analysis not only delved into the shared messages of the videos but examined their style, content, and the various hooks and devices employed by vloggers to engage their audiences. Common characteristics among these vloggers included identifying as female, communicating in English, and residing in countries where English was the primary language. The videos explored recurring themes, such as depicting anorexia as another entity in one's life; grappling with body insecurity and the fear of rejection; ongoing concerns about food and weight; the impact of their illness on family and friends; navigating the challenges of in-patient treatment; and reclaiming one's life.

We noted how all the videos recorded in the first person had adopted the conventional style of narrative by including a beginning, middle, and outcome to the story. The illness narratives often commenced with a reflection on how, despite engaging in disturbing actions, the speaker initially failed to recognize any behavioral changes. A prevalent theme among participants revolved around the genesis of anorexia nervosa, often rooted in a perceived sense of control. This aligns with research suggesting that anorexia represents not just a means of gaining mastery over one's weight but control over one's life. Another rationale cited for adopting anorexic behaviors was the perceived connection between weight loss and a healthier lifestyle. Authors spoke about their belief that shedding pounds would enhance their lives and protect them from negative comments, e.g., "*I correlated getting skinny with getting to be like an incredible girl*"; "*I felt like my friends wouldn't have liked me if I was big as I was before, I felt scared of the idea of gaining weight.*" Anorexia nervosa came to symbolize a "safe haven" for participants, in which they could establish their own rules. However, at some point, anorexia turned into a malign presence and/or a voice that was constantly judging one's mirror image, leading to the marking of evermore foodstuffs as "out of bounds" and dangerous to one's integrity. The terrible impact on people's family lives was only really understood in retrospect:

> They say anorexia is a disease that affects the entire family, and personally, I couldn't agree more. I can only imagine what it must have been like for my family and for my friends seeing me disintegrate into a black, shadowy shell of myself and distance myself from everyone.

In all these videos, participants spoke of a slow and bumpy treatment journey, usually involving several episodes as in-patients and sometimes a near-death experience. Years of people's lives were impacted, with opportunities in education, work, and leisure lost along the way. Nevertheless, most videos ended on a positive note, with hopes expressed for a better future and gratitude for those who had patiently stood by them, e.g., "I can't describe it in words really. I'm just really grateful to be here today … My teenage years they weren't great, but we can sort of move on from that."

As explained above, the chosen videos were also analyzed for their style, content, and the techniques and strategies utilized by vloggers to captivate their audiences. Some, but not all, videos included shock-provoking photographs of vloggers at different stages of severe weight loss. Most videos included pictures of the vloggers alongside family, friends, and pets, emphasizing the shrinking proportions of their own bodies. Also widely photographed were pictures of food; indeed, one video contained multiple shots of different meals which were rejected. Music was frequently added to create an emotional ambience. Selfies were often shot in soft focus lending an air of romance to these stories.

In one emotive video produced by a young American girl in her 20s, the speaker explains in much detail about her years of mirror watching, calorie counting, purging, and excessively exercising due to what she describes as her "disease" and "body dysmorphia." Apart from a few selfie images of the speaker at her lowest weight, the video is a long-spoken monograph. The soft and repetitive background music, reminiscent of a yoga relaxation tape, adds a rather spiritual dimension. The juxtaposition between the sweet and delicate appearance and voice of the young woman, her pristine environment, and the brutal tale of self-castigation and purging creates a compelling but shocking effect. The speaker begins with a trigger warning, then goes into detail how her low body weight was achieved. These "tips," along with her pleasant appearance, create an allure which some might see as encouraging rather than leading interested listeners away from this path.

Overall, these representations of anorexia nervosa fit with much of what is conventionally known about this disorder, to the extent that there was a certain textbook approach to the downslide and "recovery" narratives. Most of these first-person videos had a subscription option, and in some cases, viewers were directed by "vloggers" to other videos and blogs, where products like make-up and fashion advice were available for purchase. This is not to doubt the sincerity of the person producing the video in wishing to help others, and to make the tribulations of anorexia nervosa for themselves and their families more widely known. Rather, it is to point out the extent to which posting illness and recovery videos has become a commercial opportunity, which is bound to impact both their look, content, and likability. Moreover, studies suggest that Internet users who post about anorexic experiences largely identity as female, upper-middle-class, western, and white (LaMarre & Rice, 2016). Broadly speaking, the most widely viewed English language videos in our sample also fitted this demographic. However, in her study of self-representations of Russian-speaking women with anorexia on YouTube, Mikhaylova (2022) found similar findings and draws conclusions akin to ours in that the content and scope of narratives produced by vloggers largely mirrored mainstream explanatory models of anorexia.

Social media platforms have normalized the sharing of personal experiences, including personal struggles and challenges about eating disorders. These videos represent and conspire in the "illness entrepreneurism" that has found a home on social media. Individuals may feel compelled to disclose their eating disorder experiences in the same way people share other aspects of their lives. The blurred boundary between public and private spheres online can contribute to this trend. The idea of the entrepreneurial illness blogger or vlogger is not novel. Stage's (2014) definition of entrepreneurial illness blogging is "the explicit intertwinement of individual, often very intimate, stories of physical suffering and large projects of political and social change" (p. 168). Stage draws on the concept of the "wounded storyteller" (Frank, 2013/1995) to depict the blogger as preoccupied with personal transformation but also as socially and politically motivated, intent on raising public awareness or fund-raising on behalf of a charity. Yet, trends change swiftly on social media, and we have entered the period of the social media influencer. These entrepreneurial illness role models, while paying lip service to social change, are openly engaged in promoting themselves and establishing their online business. Like other social media influences, they are likely to use sponsored content and covert marketing tactics (Hudders et al., 2021).

While some may use their platforms to challenge body and gender stereotypes, our study suggests that conventionally modelled discourses on these sites are more typical. With superstars like Taylor Swift speaking out on media about overcoming an eating disorder (Willman, 2020), it is likely that those on social media, including the less famous influencers, look to these highly successful people as role models. However, it should be emphasized that individuals' motivations for sharing their experiences with eating disorders on social media are diverse and may vary widely. Rather than judging the content of social media in terms of its alignment with medical knowledge and ethics, a comprehensive and compassionate approach is required to appreciate and understand the cultural, social, and economic dynamics at play in this complex landscape.

Conclusions

Early studies of digital media marveled at the potential of online spaces to democratize health information and to provide a vast and easy to access source of information. This position has changed, with the hard-to-regulate and sometimes impenetrable realm of social media seemingly blamed for most of society's ills. However, digital media never functions in isolation from the wider structures of power and governance. Digital media operates as a form of biopower and as an avenue for "psychopolitics" (Cohen, 2016). Much of what happens on social media sites, including those which focus on body image and disordered eating, mirrors, edits and amplifies messages and information which emerge from the commercial and biopolitical economy. Therefore, any measures designed to reduce harmful activities on social media sites need to factor in overarching pressures on people of all backgrounds and ages to rise to the demands of the digital economy. They must also be viewed as an aspect and outcome of our surveillance society, in which confession obtained by force has been replaced by the torturous, compulsive pull of the smart phone (Jeffries, 2017).

As illustrated by studies presented in this chapter, the construction of eating disorders and disordered eating is rapidly evolving. Digital technology has been linked to not just the proliferation of thinspiration images and narratives but the development of new mental pathologies based on modern obsessions, including orthorexia nervosa, the "unhealthy" fixation with eating only "natural," healthy foods. Chapter 9, "Orthorexia Nervosa: Eating Disorder for a Pro-health Era," explores the debates concerning the pros and cons of healthy eating including the politicization of "healthism" and the efforts to measure levels of orthorexia nervosa in different populations and to see it included as a distinct mental disorder in the DSM. Finally, the chapter summarizes findings from a series of qualitative studies, which sought to capture and compare the perceptions and experiences of different stakeholders with an investment in managing or pursuing more extreme healthy eating practices.

References

Anderson, M., & Jiang, J. (2018). *Teens, social media & technology*. Pew Research Center. Retrieved August 22, 2024, from https://www.pewresearch.org/internet/2018a/05/31/teens-social-media-technology-2018/

Au, E. S., & Cosh, S. M. (2022). Social media and eating disorder recovery: An exploration of Instagram recovery community users and their reasons for engagement. *Eating Behaviors, 46*, 101651.

Banet-Weiser, S. (2011). Branding the post-feminist self: Girls' video production and YouTube. In M. Kearney (Ed.), *Mediated girlhoods: New explorations of girls' media culture* (pp. 277–294). Peter Lang Publishers.

Banet-Weiser, S., Gill, R., & Rottenberg, C. (2020). Post-feminism, popular feminism and neoliberal feminism? Sarah Banet-Weiser, Rosalind Gill and Catherine Rottenberg in conversation. *Feminist Theory, 21*(1), 3–24.

BEAT. (2024, April 8). *How many people have an eating disorder in the UK?* https://www.beateatingdisorders.org.uk/get-information-and-support/about-eating-disorders/how-many-people-eating-disorder-uk/

Boepple, L., & Thompson, J. K. (2014). A content analysis of healthy living blogs: Evidence of content thematically consistent with dysfunctional eating attitudes and behaviors. *International Journal of Eating Disorders, 47*(4), 362–367.

Boepple, L., & Thompson, J. K. (2016). A content analytic comparison of fitspiration and thinspiration websites. *International Journal of Eating Disorders, 49*(1), 98–101.

Borzekowski, D. L., Schenk, S., Wilson, J. L., & Peebles, R. (2010). e-Ana and e-Mia: A content analysis of pro–eating disorder web sites. *American Journal of Public Health, 100*(8), 1526–1534.

Casteel, P. D. (2011). Durkheim & social facts. In *Early theorists & the science of society* (pp. 35–47). Salem Press.

Chang, L., Chattopadhyay, K., Li, J., Xu, M., & Li, L. (2021). Interplay of support, comparison, and surveillance in social media weight management interventions: Qualitative study. *JMIR mHealth and uHealth, 9*(3), e19239.

Cheng, C. M., Chu, J., Ganson, K. T., Trompeter, N., Testa, A., Jackson, D. B., et al. (2023). Cyberbullying and eating disorder symptoms in US early adolescents. *International Journal of Eating Disorders, 56*(12), 2336–2342.

Christodoulou, M. (2012). Pro-anorexia websites pose public health challenge. *The Lancet*. https://doi.org/10.1016/s0140-6736(12)60048-8

Cobb, G. R. (2017). *Critiquing the thin ideal in pro-anorexia online spaces* (Doctoral dissertation, University of Sussex). Retrieved August 22, 2024, from https://sussex.figshare.com/articles/thesis/Critiquing_the_thin_ideal_in_pro-anorexia_online_spaces/23445089

Cohen, B. M. Z. (2016). *Psychiatric hegemony: A Marxist theory on mental illness*. Palgrave Macmillan.

Cosentino, G. (2020). *Social media and the post-truth world order*. Palgrave Pivot.

Cusumano, M. A. (2011). Platform wars come to social media. *Communications of the ACM, 54*(4), 31–33.

Da Rocha, L. N. C., & Long, C. (2008). *Alternative portrayals of anorexia nervosa and its symptoms on pro-anorexic websites: A thematic analysis of website contents* (Doctoral dissertation, University of the Witwatersrand). Retrieved August 22, 2024 from https://wiredspace.wits.ac.za/items/041d1bd9-242e-42ca-8c42-35adc6784cf9

Day, K., & Keys, T. (2008). Starving in cyberspace: A discourse analysis of pro-eating-disorder websites. *Journal of Gender Studies, 17*(1), 1–15.

Day, S., Bussey, K., Trompeter, N., & Mitchison, D. (2022). The impact of teasing and bullying victimization on disordered eating and body image disturbance among adolescents: A systematic review. *Trauma, Violence, & Abuse, 23*(3), 985–1006.

Dias, K. (2003). The ana sanctuary: Women's pro-anorexia narratives in cyberspace. *Journal of International Women's Studies, 4*(2), 31–45.

Durkheim, E. (1982). *The rules of sociological method.* Free Press. First published 1892.

Eckersley, R. (2005). 'Cultural fraud': The role of culture in drug abuse. *Drug Alcohol Review, 24*, 157–163.

Fairclough, N. (2001). Critical discourse analysis as a method in social scientific research. *Methods of critical discourse analysis, 5*(11), 121–138.

Fairplay. (2022). *Designing for disorder: Instagram's pro-eating disorder bubble.* Fairplay. Retrieved August 22, 2024, from https://fairplayforkids.org/wp-content/uploads/2022/04/designing_for_disorder.pd

Ferry, M. D., & Richards, C. (2015). Biopedagogy digitalized: 'Educational' relations among participants on an online weight loss surgery forum. *Critical Public Health, 25*(1), 63–77.

Fischer, R., & Klazar, E. (2020). Facts, truth, and post-truth. *The International Journal of Information, Diversity, & Inclusion, 4*(3/4), 5–19.

Fixsen, A. M., & Ridge, D. (2017). Stories of hell and healing: Internet users' construction of benzodiazepine distress and withdrawal. *Qualitative Health Research, 27*(13), 2030–2041.

Foucault, M. (1975/1991). *Discipline and punish. The Birth of the Prison.* Trans. A. Sheridan. Penguin Books.

Foucault, M. (1989). Technologies of self. In L. H. Martin, H. Gutman, & P. H. Hutton (Eds.), *Technologies of the self: A seminar with Michel Foucault* (pp. 16–50).

Frank, A. W. (2013/1995). *The wounded storyteller.* University of Chicago Press.

Giddens, A. (1991). *Modernity and self identity* (p. 256). Polity Press.

Ging, D., & Garvey, S. (2018). 'Written in these scars are the stories I can't explain': A content analysis of pro-ana and thinspiration image sharing on Instagram. *New Media & Society, 20*(3), 1181–1200.

Greškovičová, K., Masaryk, R., Synak, N., & Čavojová, V. (2022). Superlatives, clickbaits, appeals to authority, poor grammar, or boldface: Is editorial style related to the credibility of online health messages? *Frontiers in Psychology, 13*, 940903.

Hajli, N., Saeed, U., Tajvidi, M., & Shirazi, F. (2022). Social bots and the spread of disinformation in social media: The challenges of artificial intelligence. *British Journal of Management, 33*(3), 1238–1253.

Hammond, M. D. (2014). *The pro-eating disorder movement: A qualitative study* (Doctoral dissertation, Wheaton College).

Han, B.-C. (2014). *Psychopolitics: Neoliberalism and new technologies of power*. Verso.

Harbusch, M. (Ed.). (2022). *Troubled Persons Industries: The expansion of psychiatric categories beyond psychiatry*. Springer International Publishing.

Heilweil, R (2021, May). *YouTube's Kids App Has a Rabbit Hole Problem,* Vox. Retrieved August 22, 2024, from https://www.vox.com/recode/22412232/youtube-kids-autoplay.

Hinds, J. (2019). *Behaviour prediction: The challenges and opportunities of big data*. Centre for Research and Evidence on Security Threats (CREST). https://crestresearch.ac.uk/comment/hinds-behaviour-prediction/

Hoffmann, B. (2018). Pro ana (1): Eating disorder or a lifestyle. *Trakia Journal of Sciences, 16*(2), 106–113.

Holland, G., & Tiggemann, M. (2016). A systematic review of the impact of the use of social networking sites on body image and disordered eating outcomes. *Body image, 17,* 100–110.

Holmes, S. (2015). 'That perfect girl is gone': Pro-ana, anorexia and Frozen (2013) as an 'eating disorder' film. *Participations, 12*(2), 98–120.

Holmes, S. (2017). 'My anorexia story': Girls constructing narratives of identity on YouTube. *Cultural Studies, 31*(1), 1–23.

Hudders, L., De Jans, S., & De Veirman, M. (2021). The commercialization of social media stars: A literature review and conceptual framework on the strategic use of social media influencers. *International Journal of Advertising, 40*(3), 327–375.

Jane, M., Foster, J., Hagger, M., Ho, S., Kane, R., & Pal, S. (2018). Psychological effects of belonging to a Facebook weight management group in overweight and obese adults: Results of a randomised controlled trial. *Health & Social Care in the Community, 26*(5), 714–724.

Jeffries, S. (2017, December 30). *Psychopolitics: New technologies of Power by Bynug-Chun Han—Review*. Retrieved August 21, 2024, from https://www.theguardian.com/books/2017/dec/30/psychopolitics-neolberalism-new-technologies-byung-chul-han-review

Kaur, K., & Gurnani, B. (2022). Commentary: Impact of social media applications like Instagram, Facebook, Twitter, and YouTube on ophthalmological education. *Indian Journal of Ophthalmology, 70*(9), 3253–3254.

LaMarre, A., & Rice, C. (2016, March). Embodying critical and corporeal methodology: Digital storytelling with young women in eating disorder recovery. In Forum Qualitative Sozialforschung/Forum: Qualitative Social Research (17, No. 2).

Loewen, R. (2021). *Performing Anorexia on YouTube: The Aesthetics, Narratives, and Functions of Video Testimonials* (Doctoral dissertation, Carleton University). Retrieved August 22, 2024, from https://repository.library.carleton.ca/concern/etds/5m60qs89t

Lozano-Chacon, B., Suarez-Lledo, V., & Alvarez-Galvez, J. (2021). Use and effectiveness of social-media-delivered weight loss interventions among teenagers and young adults: A systematic review. *International Journal of Environmental Research and Public Health, 18*(16), 8493.

Lupton, D. (2014). *Digital sociology*. Routledge.

Mikhaylova, O. (2022). Self-representations of the experience of anorexia on YouTube: The joint influence of the explanatory model and the web platform. *New Media & Society*. https://doi.org/10.1177/14614448221099172

Mills, J. S., Shannon, A., & Hogue, J. (2017). Beauty, body image, and the media. In M. P. Levine (Ed.), *Perception of beauty* (pp. 145–157). Intech.

Mo, P. K. H., & Coulson, N. S. (2014). Are online support groups always beneficial? A qualitative exploration of the empowering and disempowering processes of participation within HIV/AIDS-related online support groups. *International Journal of Nursing Studies, 51*(7), 983–993.

Mörch, C. M., Cote, L. P., Corthesy-Blondin, L., Plourde-Léveillé, L., Dargis, L., & Mishara, B. L. (2018). The Darknet and suicide. *Journal of Affective Disorders, 241*, 127–132.

Morelock, J., & Narita, F. Z. (2021). *The society of the selfie: Social media and the crisis of liberal democracy*. University of Westminster Press.

Norris, M. L., Boydell, K. M., Pinhas, L., & Katzman, D. K. (2006). Ana and the Internet: A review of pro-anorexia websites. *International Journal of Eating Disorders*. https://doi.org/10.1002/eat.20305

O'Sullivan, D., Duffy, C., & Jorgensen, S. (2021). Instagram promoted pages glorifying eating disorders in teen accounts. *CNN Business*. Retrieved August 22, 2024, from https://edition.cnn.com/2021/10/04/tech/instagram-facebook-eating-disorders/index.html

Perloff, R. M. (2014). Social media effects on young women's body image concerns: Theoretical perspectives and an agenda for research. *Sex Roles, 71*(11–12), 363–377.

Phelan, A., White J., Wallner, C., & Patterson, J. (2023). Introductory guide to understanding misogyny and the far right. Centre for Research and Evidence on Security Threats (CREST). Retrieved August 22, 2024, https://crest-research.ac.uk/resources/introductory-guide-to-understanding-misogyny-and-the-far-right/

Richtel, M. (2023, October 25). *Is social media addictive? Here's what science says.* The New York Times. Retrieved August 22, 2024, from https://www.nytimes.com/2023/10/25/health/social-media-addiction.html

Robinson, A., Husband, A. K., Slight, R. D., & Slight, S. P. (2020). Digital support for patients undergoing bariatric surgery: Narrative review of the roles and challenges of online forums. *JMIR Perioperative Medicine, 3*(2), e17230.

Romele, A., et al. (2017). Panopticism is not enough: Social media as technologies of voluntary servitude. *Surveillance & society, 15*(2), 204–221.

Rouleau, C. R., & von Ranson, K. M. (2011). Potential risks of pro-eating disorder websites. *Clinical psychology review, 31*(4), 525–553.

Scull, A. (2022). *Desperate Remedies: Psychiatry and the mysteries of mental illness.* Penguin Books.

Stage, C. (2014). 10 The entrepreneurial illness blogger. *Enterprising Initiatives in the Experience Economy: Transforming Social Worlds*, 168–187.

Stapleton, K., Evans, S. L., & Rhys, C. S. (2019). Ana as god: Religion, interdiscursivity and identity on pro-ana websites. *Discourse & Communication, 13*(3), 320–341.

Statistica. (2023). *Number of internet and social media users worldwide as of January 2023.* Retrieved August 22, 2024, from https://www.statista.com/statistics/617136/digital-population-worldwide

Sukenesan, S. (2021). 'Anorexia coach': Sexual predators online are targeting teens wanting to lose weight. Platforms are looking the other way. *The Conversation.* Retrieved August 22, 2024, from https://theconversation.com/anorexia-coach-sexual-predators-online-are-targeting-teens-wanting-to-lose-weight-platforms-are-looking-the-other-way-162938

Thommasen, H. V., Self, B., Grigg, A., Zhang, W., & Birmingham, C. L. (2005). The relationship between self-rated health, stress, health care, overall quality of life and weight in a rural population. *Eating and Weight Disorders-Studies on Anorexia, Bulimia and Obesity, 10*, e66–e69.

Tiggemann, M., & Slater, A. (2013). NetGirls: The Internet, Facebook, and body image concern in adolescent girls. *International Journal of Eating Disorders, 46*(6), 630–633.

Tragantzopoulou, P., Fixsen, A., Ridge, D., & Cheshire, A. (2024). 'You are not alone, we've got you': Power plays, devotion, and punishment on Healthy Eating and Pro-Eating Disorder websites. *Qualitative Health Research.* https://doi.org/10.1177/10497323241238628

UK Parliament. (2024, August 14). *Preparedness for online safety regulation.* Retrieved August 22, 2024, from https://publications.parliament.uk/pa/cm5804/cmselect/cmpubacc/73/report.html

Ward, K. J. (2007). 'I love you to the bones': Constructing the anorexic body in 'pro-ana' message boards. *Sociological Research Online, 12*(2), 122–135.

Welles, B. F., & González-Bailón, S. (2018). *The Oxford handbook of networked communication* (B. F. Welles & S. González-Bailón, Eds.). Oxford University Press.

Willman, C. (2020, January 23). *Taylor Swift opens up about overcoming struggle with eating disorder (EXCLUSIVE).* Variety. Retrieved August 22, 2024, from https://variety.com/2020/music/news/taylor-swift-eating-disorder-netflix-documentary-miss-americana-1203478047/

Yeshua-Katz, D. (2015). Online stigma resistance in the pro-Ana community. *Qualitative Health Research, 25*(10), 1347–1358.

Yeshua-Katz, D., & Martins, N. (2013). Communicating stigma: The pro-ana paradox. *Health communication, 28*(5), 499–508.

Zafar, M. B., Bhattacharya, P., Ganguly, N., Ghosh, S., & Gummadi, K. P. (2016). On the wisdom of experts vs. crowds: Discovering trustworthy topical news in microblogs. In *Proceedings of the ACM Conference on Computer Supported Cooperative Work and Social Computing (CSCW)* (pp. 438–451).

Ziebland, S., Chapple, A., Dumelow, C., Evans, J., Prinjha, S., & Rozmovits, L. (2004). How the internet affects patients' experience of cancer: A qualitative study. *BMJ, 328*(7439), 564.

Zuboff, S. (2015). Big other: Surveillance capitalism and the prospects of an information civilization. *Journal of Information Technology, 30*, 75–89.

9

Orthorexia Nervosa: Eating Disorder for a Pro-health Era

The rhetoric of healthy eating seems to be everywhere. Messages about which specific components of foods to eat or avoid (such as fats and salt) now appear in government documents, commercials, food packaging, celebrity blogs, advice from friends, on our smart phone apps, and much more. Traditional nutrition models now face competition from emerging perspectives, such as the association between dairy products and cancer (Wang et al., 2020). Long-established food items have been rebranded as "superfoods," (Singh et al., 2022; Jagdale et al., 2021) celebrity endorsements, such as in the word "kale" appearing on clothing worn by super-star Beyoncé (Luckhurst, 2015). Simultaneously, traditional farming lobbies have continued to defend staples like meat and dairy to protect their livelihoods (Thorning et al., 2016). Courtesy of social media, arguments around food have become more polarized, contributing to what some describe as a "post-truth food culture"[1] (Overbend, 2020). The medicalization of food has not been limited to its effects on physical health. As the food and nutrition debates rage on, so the epistemologies of psychiatry have also been gaining traction including in

[1] The term "post truth culture" describes a state of society where information based on emotions and personal beliefs outweigh scientific data.

A. Fixsen, *The Construction of Eating Disorders*, The Politics of Mental Health and Illness, https://doi.org/10.1007/978-3-031-70318-8_9

areas association with daily life choices and often outside of the discipline itself. Increasingly, non-psychiatric actors have displayed an interest in categorizing new mental states along psychiatric lines, including those involving unhealthy or excessive lifestyle options (Krug et al., 2022; Mosley, 2009), in some cases linking them with "celebrity diets" (Micallef, 2023). One candidate for this emerging taxonomy is orthorexia nervosa (ON)—an eating disorder (ED) based on an over-preoccupation with heathy eating—which, for over two decades has been garnering a lot of scientific and media attention (Arguedas, 2020; Costa et al., 2022; Håman et al., 2015, 2016; Valente et al., 2022). Despite its absence from DSM-V (APA, 2013), a vast number of Internet searches related to orthorexia nervosa and its associated terms have been performed, while ON is recognized as an eating disorder on prominent websites such as healthline.com and NEDA (National Eating Disorders Association). So concerned are some experts with the problem of extreme healthy eating , that they have lobbied for its inclusion in the next DSM (Bratman et al., 2017). From a sociological perspective, the emergence of ON as a diagnostic category reflects the "shifting engines of medicalization" (Conrad, 2005), highlighting the involvement of multiple stakeholders in the formation of new psychiatric labels.

This chapter explores the origins and recognition of ON, its uncertain clinical parameters and overlaps with other EDs and mental disorders. Also discussed are philosophical and sociological explanations for society's seeming obsession with food provenance, including radical changes to food ecologies and institutional structures, neoliberal capitalism's emphasis on self-cultivation, and the promotion of healthism as a means of diverting attention from social and economic ills. Obsessive healthy eating practices are reported as having significant and multifaceted effects on people's lives, including mental and physical health, social life, daily routine, body image, and financial state (Bratman & Knight, 1997; Cheshire et al., 2020). The final part of this chapter looks at empirical data taken from studies that examined the views of professional and lay participants concerning excessive healthy eating (Cheshire et al., 2020; Fixsen et al., 2020; Fixsen & Cheshire, 2022; Tragantzopoulou et al., 2024). Findings suggest that while there are multiple explanations given for why people might take to extreme forms of eating, including as a means of disguising efforts to lose weight, ultimately ON emerges as an aspect of psychiatric expansionism, and the continued use of reductionist explanations for complex social, economic, and political trends.

The Birth of ON

Since mental illnesses are not inherently biological phenomena, their existence is contingent upon their construction within a social context where they are recognized as real, and their treatment by medical experts is seen as imperative. Examining the unconventional origins of orthorexia nervosa (ON) may thus shed light not only on the popularity of ON but also why, despite its increasing usage in media and clinical settings, psychiatry has yet to include it in its official taxonomy. Coined by Dr Steven Bratman in the late 1990s, ON (derived from the Latin "ortho" meaning "proper" and "orexias" meaning "appetite") refers to an eating disorder characterized by an extreme fixation on the quality and purity of one's diet, accompanied by an intense preoccupation with avoiding foods perceived as unhealthy or impure (Bratman & Knight, 1997; Cheshire et al., 2020; Zickgraf, 2020). Bratman (2017) describes ON as a "disease disguised as a virtue" because unless significant weight loss occurs, this unhealthy fixation on food may go unnoticed by health professionals. In his first book on the topic, Bratman (2017) recounts his personal experiences as a "health food junkie," before coming to recognize this extreme behavior as pathological. ON, he explains, usually begins innocuously, often stemming from a desire to combat chronic illness, shed excess weight, or rectify perceived shortcomings in the American diet. Motivated by warnings about the dangers of certain foods, the person comes to restrict their dietary choices to an unreasonable extent. Bratman delineates the personal traits exhibited by individuals with ON: "Iron willpower and self-discipline" are requisite for avoiding foods deemed impure, resulting in "a somber sense of self-righteousness that overwhelms all other sources of joy and meaning." The life of the "orthorexic" becomes increasingly narrow with time consumed by meal planning, food procurement, preparation, and eating, leaving little opportunity for other pursuits. Social gatherings are eschewed due to concerns and guilt regarding dietary transgressions, leading to physical and emotional seclusion. Bratman's story "hit a nerve with the popular public" (Hanganu-Bresch, 2019, p. 312), and by early 2010s his concept had gained traction, with popular reports claiming the existence of orthorexia nervosa (ON) in print and online media.

While the fundamental characteristics of ON appear relatively straightforward, determining its clinical parameters and prevalence has proven to be challenging. Its perceived overlap with other mental disorders, such as obsessive-compulsive disorder (OCD) (Brytek-Matera, 2012; Dell'Osso et al., 2016; Pontillo et al., 2022) and anorexia nervosa (AN) (Bhattacharya et al., 2022; Musolino et al., 2015), has raised concerns about its potential misinterpretation in clinical contexts (Brytek-Matera, 2021). The physiological implications of ON symptoms remain unclear, besides it being distinguished from other restrictive disorders by its high emphasis on food quality and lack of emphasis on weight loss (Bratman, 2017; Bratman & Knight, 1997; Koven & Abry, 2015). Statistical studies have reported widely varying prevalence rates for ON, ranging from as low as 1 percent (Dunn et al., 2017) to over 90 percent (Turner & Lefevre, 2017). Contradictory findings also exist regarding the biometrics of ON (Dell'Osso et al., 2016; Fidan et al., 2010), while no clear gender link has been established (Noebel et al., 2023). However, a significant relationship has been proposed between ON and "alternative" or "clean" eating practices (Allen et al., 2018) with vegetarianism, veganism, raw food diets, and macrobiotics all mentioned in different research studies (Brytek-Matera, 2021; Çiçekoğlu & Tunçay, 2018; Segura-Garcia et al., 2014). While not a feature of the early ON literature, the link between ON and excessive exercise has been increasingly highlighted (Meyer et al., 2011), with sports persons and bodybuilders considered to be high risk groups (Bo et al., 2014; Håman et al., 2017; Parisi et al., 2021; Selvi & Bozo, 2020). One of the markers of a psychiatric diagnosis is its specificity (Horwitz & Grob, 2016). Yet, even among those who accept the necessity for some type of clinical diagnosis, no consensus has been found as to exactly *which* factors to include in ON scales (Cheshire et al., 2020). Lacking a present official diagnosis, clinical "presentations" of ON are likely to be placed in a generic eating disorder (ARFID[2] or OSFED[3]) category. It also remains unclear whether the contradictory findings over ON suggest its non-existence or indicate the poor quality of measuring tools, which have been unable to distinguish between healthy eating and ON (Bratman, 2017; Douma et al., 2021).

Explanations for ON

With the "science" underpinning ON remaining in doubt, scholars have turned their attention to establishing the driving forces behind the growing trend in healthy or "clean" eating[4] (Staudacher & Harer 2018). Writing about the widespread nature of alimentary fears today, Nicolosi (2006) proposed the idea of the "orthorexic society" and noted various influences contributing to this phenomenon, including the waning impact of traditional institutions like religion, ethnicity, and community on dietary behaviors. In likelihood, Nicolosi writes, the "primitive" body functioned within a collective framework, with communal dining serving as a social platform for expressing cultural dietary traditions. In contrast, the modern consumer often eats alone and lacks the traditional structure and eating norms prevalent in tightly knit communities. A further contributing factor Nicolosi (2006) notes is the widespread skepticism toward biotechnologies, stemming from the growing detachment between food producers and consumers. The argument goes that today's average consumer is largely disconnected from the sources, locations, and processes involved in food production, leading to a knowledge gap that fuels concerns about food origin, safety, and integrity (Diemling, 2015). Alongside this are the now familiar studies appearing to corroborate the link between poor quality food, chronic disease, and early mortality (Pagliai et al., 2021). So concerned are some about the poor quality of

[2] Avoidant restrictive food intake disorder.

[3] Other specified eating and feeding disorder.

[4] The term "clean eating" broadly refers to foods which are seen as being as close to their natural state as possible, with minimal use of fertilizers, chemical additives, and preservatives. The food may also be organic, plant-based, sugar-free, or gluten-free.

modern cuisine, and the loss of tradition, that they have called for return to the dietary practices of our grand parents (Pollan, 2008).

Other scholars have highlighted the inherent contradictions between neoliberal ideals of bodily citizenship and consumption patterns promoted by market-driven food systems (Pirie, 2016; Strahler & Stark, 2020). Since self-interest is central to neoliberalism, its claims to moral virtue vis-a-vis notions of public good, fairness, and justice can be called into question. Neoliberalism considers itself to be a bastion of emotional freedom; however, one needs to pay close attention to the set of emotions and self-cultivation practices that are being promoted or marginalized, and how these factors lead to a sense of social disconnection, competition, and aloneness (Becker et al., 2021). As Foucault asserts, neoliberalism produces a kind of freedom, but "this very act entails the establishment of limitations, controls, forms of coercion and obligations relying on threats" (Foucault et al., 2008, p. 64). In this case the implicit threat is that of being perceived as a "bad consumer." These moral judgements typically fall on women, who are expected to make "healthy" food choices for their families. One study on food choices among Canadian women shed light on the pressures of healthism experienced by concerned female consumers. The perpetual quest for reliable information within a complex and conflicting food landscape, coupled with fluctuating expert advice, contributed to feelings of anxiety regarding food choices and a sense of helplessness in navigating available information among participants (Rangel et al., 2012). The authors concluded that the pivotal factor in food selection today, more than other societal factors, was the constant exposure participants had to discourses around food risks.

From a governance perspective, practicing healthy eating has emerged as a primary method through which individuals in neoliberal societies engage with various "technologies of the self" (Foucault, 1988). While the stated aim of self care is to "improve" one's body, thoughts, and behaviors, contemporary citizens can also acquire status and capital by engaging in pro-health activities, even when performed alone—since these behaviors are often reported to doctor, friends and colleagues. Workplaces also increasingly monitor and demand their employees' engagement in pro-health activities (Fixsen et al., 2017). Why we have become so obsessed with health also has to do with the way in which we have come to view our bodies as mouldable projects. With a diminishing focus on collective entities like family or religious communities, this cultivation of personal identity through projects of bodily management and self-care has become increasingly prominent (Martínez et al., 2021; Shilling, 2016). Although, ultimately, illness and mortality lie beyond the individual's control, modern consumers are encouraged to view their bodies and lifespans as dependent on the degree of effort and capital they put in to improving their health. Writing on this topic decades earlier, Crawford (1980) characterized the ideology of "healthism" as politically driven and emerging from a desire to curtail healthcare expenses by portraying health as largely attainable through self-discipline and moral behavior. Healthism has since evolved into a major marketing strategy and a pervasive "super-value" symbolizing the ideals of a good life (Kristensen et al., 2016). This individualistic trend has not been always welcomed by the medical profession, who must face the demands of middle-class, articulate, health-conscious patients and parents who, under healthism's influence, flout "anti-scientific" opinions (Greenhalgh & Wessely, 2004). In the following journal piece, a general practitioner echoes this sentiment in relation to clean eating:

> Food should be our pleasurable fuel, not our quest and destination. We're all going to die, regardless of how much quinoa we eat. If we've "had enough of experts," as one UK politician recently claimed, this sort of thing can only proliferate. (McCartney, 2016)

However, the notion of healthism as some radicalized, middle-class trend is contradicted by the evidence. The principles of healthism fit well with the ethics of capitalism and have thus been widely embraced by authorities, as a means of expanding health markets and reducing public healthcare expenses. Government-led food campaigns have been utilized for decades to heighten public consciousness regarding health and dietary practices (Diemling, 2015), employing media-generated messaging to emphasize the distinction between "healthy" and "unhealthy" food choices (Goodman et al., 2017). In educational establishments, these food policies and pedagogies operate as imperatives or calls for obedience, even while mediated by economic, cultural, and familial relations

(Fernández et al., 2021; Leahy, 2014). The arena of food politics has become fiercely competitive, aiming to stimulate economic growth and influence consumer purchasing behaviors (Nestle, 2013). Furthermore, the free market makes selecting options and conforming to normative behaviors increasingly challenging, compelling individuals to seek out the latest products claiming to cater to our health-driven capitalist society. Societal pressure now exists to elevate one's food choices based on quality, while social esteem can be garnered through purchasing foods which are labeled as "organic," "fair trade," "sustainably sourced," or other advertising terms that fit in the category of "greenwashing" (de Freitas et al., 2020). Scholars also note how societal health ideals have become more aggressive due to the commercialization of the fitness culture, with personal training one of the fastest growing career options in western culture (Håman et al., 2017). Within the setting, strict diets and high volumes of exercise constitute the prevailing norms of the gym.

Back in mid-1990s, Lupton (1995) noted the growing influence of technology in the rise of healthism. Since then, the Internet has enabled unprecedented efforts to promote and commodify healthy eating, both independently and alongside other fitness regimes. Healthy eating (HE) sites—interactive platforms where users share and access health-related content—have become a widespread feature of digital media (Tragantzopoulou et al., 2024). These sites—which disseminate nutritional information, share recipes, and guide healthier lifestyle choices—seem to support public health policy objectives (Mete et al., 2019). However, the largely unregulated nature of the Internet means that anyone can create a website and claim nutritional expertise. While some platforms are managed by non-profits and charities, such as the American Heart Association and NHS Eatwell, many are operated by private companies or individuals sponsored by food and supplement manufacturers with commercial interests. From a medical perspective, there are concerns that these sites may exacerbate food and body anxieties, promoting extreme diets to attract customers and drive sales (Cesiri, 2016). The authoritative, often messianic language used on these sites may contribute to the growing obsession with the perfect diet, potentially culminating in orthorexia nervosa (Boepple & Thompson, 2014; Hanganu-Bresch, 2019; Tragantzopoulou et al., 2024).

Lay and Professional Perspectives

Despite the widespread interest in ON, the ways in which different actors interpret and appraise their own or others pro-health food regimes have not been widely studied. Over the past few years I have been part of a team investigating professional and lay people's perspectives of healthy eating behaviors and ON through a social constructionist lens (Cheshire et al., 2020; Fixsen et al., 2020; Tragantzopoulou et al., 2024). Our aim has been to understand the meanings which different cohorts with an interest in healthy eating ascribe to their own and others' diets and its effects on their lifestyle or work practices. The data described in the following section was taken from six studies and comprises: 25 interviews with people who self-identify as "extremely preoccupied with healthy eating" (HEs); 10 interviews with health professionals who specialized in eating disorders and were familiar with ON (HPs); 10 fitness instructors (FIs); 9 bodybuilders (BBs); and people posting anonymous messages on open access eating disorder support forums (Posters). All parts of the study were approved by the same University Research Ethics Committee. Any identifying data was removed before analysis. Secondary inductive thematic analysis, focusing on patterns, themes, and categories of analysis that emerged out of the data, was combined with a modified constant comparison approach[5] to achieve rigor (Glaser, 1965). As themes emerged, they were organized first separately and then across the entire data. All names used in the following accounts are pseudonyms.

Food Marketing

In contrast to an individualistic approach to unhealthy and disordered eating behaviors, accounts from our participants underscored the problematic and contradictory nature of food marketing, and its variable

[5] Glaser (1965) suggests four stages for constant comparison: (1) comparing incidents applicable to each category; (2) integrated categories and their properties; (3) delimiting the theory; (4) writing the theory. A modified constant comparison approach may diverge from these stages but remains true to the idea of constantly referring to the source material and comparing sections of text with each other.

impact on contemporary consumers. Healthy eaters (HEs) were especially critical of the pervasive marketing of convenience foods, which for many had been part of their childhood diets. Specifically, they criticized the overconsumption of high-calorie, sugary, and processed foods, as well as the deceptive use of "greenwashing" tactics, such as labeling products as "Mediterranean" to imply healthiness. HE Tina noted that many people deluded themselves into believing they were eating healthily, despite doing things like loading their plates with five tablespoons of mayonnaise. In the UK, processed and high-calorie foods were frequently served at family meals, as illustrated by one participant's recollection of their grandmother's meals made with corned beef, which they considered very poor cuisine. In contrast, some HEs from Greece spoke positively about the traditional Mediterranean diet served by families but also noted the emotional significance of feeding others in Greek culture. Food restriction and deprivation were historically associated with rural poverty, while the absence of widespread adoption of public health messages, such as "Eat your 5 a day," in Greece was attributed by HE Anya to the historical experiences of hunger among the Greek population:

> Greek kids always used to be chubby … that's seen as a sign of health, and it goes back to the days of poverty when you were skinny because you didn't have enough to eat so … you know it is not that many decades [ago].

Health professionals (HPs) and fitness instructors (FIs) were in agreement with lay participants concerning the pervasive influence of modern advertising and social media on food choices. However, the emphasis of HPs was more on the excessive marketing of health foods, leading to "idiosyncratic irrational ideas about the power of food to influence health and well-being." One HP who worked in Los Angeles spoke about the pervasive billboard and advertising campaigns all around the city, amounting to the virtual demonization of fats and carbohydrates. The proliferation of dietary advice on social media was also a growing problem, especially as unqualified people were giving nutritional guidance online, along with fake imagery, a lot of which was "airbrushed."

In contrast to professional opinions, lay participants thought that at least some of the information on social media about health and diet could be helpful and even life changing. Pointing out the popularity of platforms like *TikTok* within the South Asian community, HE Shivali shared how his exploration of various body transformation videos led him to discover one channel that had altered the way he has thought about himself and his body, "So, it went from, you know, making me feel bad about myself to making me feel good, it helped me." Social media content provided powerful imagery and shocking statistics about such things as factory farming and use of growth hormones. At least some of the HEs in the study had adopted healthy (plant based) eating for environmental reasons, and this sort of content was influential in these decisions. For example, Jane explained how, after watching the documentary "Cowspiracy," she had finally stopped eating animal products: "It's about how the meat and dairy industry is bad for the environment- and it encouraged me to go vegan."

Health Professionals and ON

Health professionals (HPs) in the study were recruited based on their familiarity with eating disorders and the term orthorexia. Consequently, they had much to say on the topic and described the types of clients who adopted extreme healthy eating at length. For some time, registered dietitian Raquel had noted a "very interesting trend" in Southern California where an entire family could develop "extreme core beliefs" around health and food: "I've seen both cases where it's the mother running it, and then also the father running it." Clinical psychologist Sheila, who also worked on the West Coast of America, thought that this type of extreme healthism was becoming increasingly prevalent in the Latin American community. The "trendiness" of healthy eating compounded the difficulties for health practitioners in trying to modify or change their clients' beliefs and behaviors. Sue, a clinical psychologist with decades of experience, described clients obsessed with healthy eating as "murder to treat" because of their absolute disgust for "normal" eaters, which she suspected included herself. This perspective, that orthorexia represents a search for a superior way of eating, was echoed by sports therapist Catherine, who distinguished it from the drive for weight loss seen in anorexia:

> They [people with ON] are looking for a pathway to eat in a particular way that they believe is evangelist, is superior to everybody else, and it makes them feel better about themselves, at least to start with anyway.

This gradual restriction of "unhealthy" foods was seen as dangerous in child and adolescent clients, who used it as another method of cutting calories: "First, they cut out sugar, and then they cut out everything." In family therapist Jane's opinion, lack of shared family mealtimes contributed to the problem; hence, her first treatment action was to insist that regular family meals be instigated. US dietician Ann, whose private client base was perhaps a little older, sometimes called out her health-obsessed clients by taking them for a shared ice cream, to disrupt their inflexible eating patterns. Dietitian Liz, on the other hand, thought that not all food fears were irrational; she had seen many clients who developed healthy eating obsessions alongside gastric illnesses such as ulcerative colitis, celiac disease, or Crohn's disease where "the stomach pain almost feeds the orthorexic cycle."

While agreeing that extreme views on healthy eating were a real problem, health professionals were divided over whether orthorexia nervosa should be a separate category in the DSM. Clinical psychologist and sports therapist Catherine advocated the creation of ON as an official psychiatric category and had been actively promoting this on a working group. Clinical psychologist Sue, on the other hand, argued that psychiatric labels were misleading; "The label is dangerous because it may blind us to what is going on underneath." Clinical psychologist Jenny also expressed concern about pathologizing "picky eaters," which could then potentially include her teenage son with Asperger's syndrome.

Diet and Fitness: Professional Views

Studies suggest that the highly competitive environment of the fitness industry can leave professionals and enthusiasts feeling under considerable pressure to achieve personal body and fitness goals. This in turn placed the onus on fitness instructors and personal trainers to be on the lookout for signs of disordered eating behaviors in clients (Andreasson &

Johansson, 2016; Wojtowicz et al., 2015). However, the identification of EDs for those employed in the fitness industry remains something of a grey area. For a start, instructors themselves may also pursue rigorous diets, confounding their ability to recognize disordered eating in others. This conundrum was born out in our interviews with fitness instructors (FIs), who expressed considerable uncertainty about what constituted an "eating disorder." Fitness instructor (FI) Dave thought that for a behavior to be called an eating disorder it needed to be "triggered mentally" and to exceed "what is classified as normal"—but then added, "what is normal to be honest, anyway?" FI Lee believed the issue was not about eating healthily but about not eating enough: "I've seen some people do extremely, extremely strict diets but … as long as they're not going crazy – so long as they not make themselves ill and sick … I think that's to me quite acceptable." While conceding that certain colleagues and clients appeared to fit the ON description, trainers were reluctant to challenge what were regarded as normative behaviors in the industry. "Loads of people" were consuming smoothies and raw salads; hence, this was more indicative of a health fad than an eating disorder. Some FIs conceded that working out at the gym might conceal an individual's disordered eating, but distinguishing between orthorexia and healthy restrictive eating was challenging. As one instructor noted, "If you can't visibly see that they've got an eating disorder, they could be eating healthily and maintaining their weight – I would just assume they were on the slim side." Similar findings emerged in Håman et al.'s (2017) study, where personal trainers (PTs) feared falsely accusing clients of being "pathological" and saw extreme behaviors as legitimized by an aggressive exercise trend in society.

Lay Perspectives: Disciplining the Body

For those in the study who reported adopting extreme healthy eating habits—HEs and body builders (BBs)—changing or adhering to a healthy diet required self-discipline to avoid relapsing and falling back into "unhealthy" eating patterns. Forward planning and monitoring were needed to maintain a stricter dietary regime; "The main challenge is not to be lazy. To get the right food that I need instead of ordering take outs, or just eating whatever without thinking about it." These lay participants explained in detail, not just their everyday dietary practices and food regimens, but their perceived importance for immediate and future health and well-being. For the more mature HEs, eating "good quality" food was viewed as a form of medicine; "It's a preventative measure to eat well and to eat good produce now, rather than loads of herbicides, pesticides, all that kind of stuff." HE Luke believed that refraining from low-quality foods could go a long way toward preventing future illness: "Now that I'm getting older you have to start worrying about things like cancer, Parkinson's, Alzheimer's, all that type of stuff." HE Chrissie was convinced that her "clean" diet had saved her from going down the pharmaceutical medical route: "I'm 61 years old, I'm almost 62, my last check-up was great. I feel good, I don't have to take a lot of medications and ultimately, the proof's in the pudding."

Younger participants, on the other hand, focused more on using diet to achieve a desired body shape, e.g., "My appearance … I literally wanted to change myself." A subset of lay female participants had, at least initially, been motivated by weight loss, and some had spent years trying out different diets. Several participants had faced criticism about their weight during young adulthood or voiced concerns about avoiding obesity which affected other family members. While women were often interested in losing weight, the younger male participants tailored their diets toward increasing muscle mass. This was especially the case for body builders (BBs), since a very low-carb, high-protein diet was seen as necessary for achieving the required muscle bulk and the "sculpted" body shape for competitions. For example, BB Conner explained his typical meal in training as "like fifteen egg whites just scrambled up together, and then put in some salad".

There were other perceived advantages to changing one's shape: one male participant admitted that he had initially taken up body building and changed his diet to make him more sexually attractive to women and had experienced more success in that area. Before competitions the BBs would follow stringent regimes, which could be "boring," but was considered a better option than using anabolic steroids. Female romantic partners were generally portrayed as playing a supportive role, both in encouraging more variation in diet and, as in Leon's case, cooking him tasty meals which still aligned with his goals as a bodybuilder:

> She's quite good at understanding what I need and how I need it, and that benefits me a lot more than how I used to live, where it was literally just plain chicken, plain rice and "perinaise" (a spicy sauce) drizzled on top … and [her food] would taste nicer, so I'll eat more of it.

Posting Online About ON

On eating disorder threads concerning orthorexia or "ortho," there was more debate around the desirability of obsessing over healthy foods. Most of the posters had been diagnosed with one or other form of eating disorder (typically anorexia or bulimia) and on balance, being obsessed with healthy eating was seen as a move in the right direction, e.g., "I honestly believe being orthorexic isn't that bad … I'm eating whole plant foods and not eating donuts, pizza and crap." The low-calorie content of many healthy foods was also a big appeal. One Poster described feeling, "kinda safe when I binge on fruits and vegetables even if it's high calorie, because there's a limit with them where I stop naturally." Clean eating was seen as a good thing, but as one poster admitted, it was also "a mixture of how much I eat (the quantity) and what I eat (the quality)."

Anxiety and guilt at deviating from one's diet is regarded in the literature as an indicator of eating pathology (Blythin et al., 2020). While most of the lay participants admitted to a certain amount of disappointment and guilt when they deviated from their dietary guidelines, the obsession and remorse described by posters on ED forums was of a different magnitude. On one thread entitled, "what are some of the things you obsess over?", members prioritized activities such as calorie counting, weight loss, and maintaining a specific image, with one individual remarking, "I only eat healthy foods since you can't get fat from them." Those posting online spoke of having "so many food rules and fears" and "making them stricter and stricter." Some combined their "clean eating" with binging and purging, as they worried about eating too little or too many calories. Even when Posters were eating a plant-based diet, the anxiety about gaining extra weight for some remained: "Yesterday.... I deffo binged on fruit and veg- and ended up with 2350 calories!".

Healthy Eating: Trendy Setting or Antisocial?

A common assertion about disordered eating practices concern their solitary and even secretive nature (Diane Barth, 2008; Musolino et al., 2015). This finding was partly borne out in our study of posters, some of whom expressed deep frustrations and even anger with social gatherings, where they felt compelled to consume "unhealthy" foods against their preferences, e.g., "I'm tired of being upset about all the nasty food my mom makes me sit down and eat against my will." Conversely, anonymous online forums were perceived as safe spaces to openly express fears and emotions. For some posters, sharing their struggles and concerns was a source of immense relief, as indicated by the sentiment, "Realizing that I'm not alone. That it isn't just a failure on my part but a biological response."

In contrast, HEs we interviewed spoke of feeling much more comfortable about social eating now that veganism and clean eating were more socially acceptable and even desirable. Some HEs had partners, family members, and friends who had followed on and adopted similar healthy eating practices. For BBs the situation remained more difficult since their perceived need to eat frequently, including at work, could result in complaints from managers. Running one's own business was seen as advantageous in this respect and had motivated some to train as online fitness instructors or personal trainers. At this point, some people were able to earn a living from advising others about the diet. The aesthetic and entrepreneurial advantages of having a body which is perceived as fit and healthy were especially noted by those for whom looking good was an essential part of their online business promotion:

> I think a lot of people in the bodybuilding world are more … they're very concerned with their appearance. More so like the people on *Instagram* and that is like, what other people think about their appearance. (Ben, BB)

Discussion

Deeply rooted in sociocultural factors, ON, arguably more than any other form of so-called "disordered eating," reflects broader societal, political, and economic shifts and struggles. While perceptions of what constitutes a "healthy" or "pure" diet vary, it may be the first time in history that concerns about food quality and provenance are transcending age, ethnicity, and socioeconomic divides (Fernández et al., 2021). The pressures on people today to seek out ways to "clean up" their diets and become "healthy eaters" are mounting and seem to come in every direction. The medical profession warns of the dangers of unhealthy diet in terms of long-term disease and costs to the health service, while those in ecological camp remind us of the ethical and environmental issues relating to animal husbandry. At the same time, those who take to healthy eating in ways or to degrees which, from a clinical perspective, are considered excessive may well find themselves labeled with a mental disorder. By comparing the stories of individuals with different viewpoints and positions, insights into the cultural and medical conflicts surrounding diet could be gained, and the difficulties of judging and categorizing health-conscious individuals in ways which make sense to professionals and lay persons alike further explored.

Health professionals (HPs) in our study, including some with a personal stake in promoting healthy eating, strongly criticized society's fixation with healthy foods and the extreme attitudes of some of the parents of their clients. Their responsibility was to identify and alter these obsessive behaviors before they caused any significant psychological or physical harm. HPs were divided on the necessity of assigning a specific diagnosis to complex patient issues, with some expressing reservations about the future inclusion of orthorexia nervosa in the DSM. However, this did not prevent them from challenging clients about their healthy eating or considering these behaviors to be problematic. Conversely, fitness instructors (FIs) in this study worked in an industry where restricted, health-oriented diet is normative, and the likelihood of encountering individuals who could be clinically categorized as "orthorexic" is considered high (Bo et al., 2014; Håman et al., 2017; Parisi et al., 2021; Selvi & Bozo, 2020).

Yet as a group the FIs felt unqualified or uncomfortable about approaching a client or colleague about their eating habits. This conundrum was compounded by the fact that some criteria for an eating disorder could fit with their own preoccupations. Hence, for most of the FIs in our study, only rapid weight loss was considered a valid enough reason to approach a client about their "disordered eating."

Lay participants in this study were broadly of the opinion that their healthy eating practices were beneficial to their well-being and sometimes to society and the environment. As in other studies (Valente et al., 2020), these views were supported by a host of justifications, ranging from a desire to allay future illness, protecting animals and the environment (Li, 2017) to achieving a fitter and more socially desirable body shape. One rationale for pathologizing healthy eating is that an excessive anxiety about "unhealthy" foods can result in greater body dissatisfaction and social isolation (Dunn & Bratman, 2016). Among the lay participants we interviewed there was little evidence of this; while some had suffered from poor body image in childhood and adolescence, most reported a general satisfaction with their present body shape, while male participants thought that it gave them a sexual advantage. Those posting online expressed greater upset about their present lives and bodies, but still welcomed the ability of healthy eating to lift them "above the food chaos" (Cinquegrani & Brown, 2018).

Findings from this study confirm that those who would want to see ON included on the DSM must also contend with the high normativity of extreme healthy eating, its strong appeal to certain groups and particular sectors of society and the many different justifications which support this behavior. Aside from the matter of illness and disease management, environmental concerns and ethical beliefs, this study draws attention to the status effects of having a visibly fitter and healthier body. In our identity obsessed times, those with the fittest and most attractive bodies are more likely to succeed in the biosocial and economic sense. Since capitalism denigrates poor health as costly and socially burdensome, those who follow pro-health behaviors, including those who earn a living from them, can be seen as practicing "moral citizenship" (Kristensen et al., 2016). Social media has contributed to this trend though excessive claims about specific dietary and fitness regimes, encouraging people to seek status or income from these activities (Brown & Tiggemann, 2016). Rather than labeling them as psychopathological, those who follow careful, even stringent diets may, from this perspective, be regarded as efficient users of health and cultural capital, and in alignment with "the new spirit of capitalism" (Boltanski & Chiapello, 2005). However, as Boltanski and Chiapello (2005) attest, the new "freedoms" of capitalism, in the sense of the emphasis on individual achievement, come at the cost of material and psychological security. The vision might be utopian, but the reliance on personal capital means the average person needs to be concerned about their individual security and, with diminishing state help, must ensure their own health, social, and employment status.

What has been said so far relates to the growing fixation with a healthy diet under neoliberalism, but it does not fully explain how or why such a diet has come to be widely considered as potentially pathological, and for this we must look to how medical taxonomies evolve. According to Brossard (2019), a "medical taxonomy" vector includes two facets. The first is internal to medicine, as in: where in the psychiatric categorization does the illness fit? The second is external, as in: what are the competing categorizations outside psychiatry where the illness could possibly fit? Besides the general expansion of ED labels as a form of psychiatric hegemony (Cohen, 2016), our study findings confirm that the concept of orthorexia nervosa (ON) holds value for some clinicians and the public. The continuing popularity of ON as a topic in media and in academic circles attests to its potential to capture public and scholarly interest, and to cater for an emerging trend within the new cultural landscape. However, a dilemma for ED clinicians is that in contrast to some diagnoses like bulimia nervosa (BN) and binge eating disorder (BED), which have more dubious moral and physical implications, among those struggling with restricted eating the appropriation of the ON label has virtuous and attractive connotations. Posters online saw being "ortho" as something to be applauded. Hence, it may well be that many clinical cases that *appear* to fit the ON label are culturally novel presentations of restrictive eating patterns resembling anorexia nervosa, a view that has been expressed by others researching in this area (Bhattacharya et al., 2022).

In summary, our own and other studies of psychiatric expansionism highlight the dangers of narrowing the perimeters of normality such that *not* having some mental health or eating disorder becomes the exception. The temptation within the research community has been to categorize more and more people as medically and socially "deviant," even while others are seeking to understand and interpret eating choices and behaviors in less reductionist ways (Fixsen et al., 2023; Mitrofanova, et al., 2021). Whether or not one believes that the categorizing of mental disorders is expanding to reflect emerging social realities or is resulting in a diagnosis for all of life's misfortunes (Paris, 2020) remains a matter of perspective. Some have argued that psychiatry can only survive by being more conscious of cultural variations and changes and expanding its criteria to accommodate them (Claudino et al., 2019). Others believe that the only ones who really profit from this expansion are the pharmaceutical companies (Frances, 2013). Whatever one's perspective, the growth of mental health categories leaves society with a very practical problem; by skewing the resources available for treatment, it results in further backlogs in public health systems, potentially leaving highly vulnerable individuals at risk for longer periods.

Finally, we can reflect on the irony that ON—which emerged from the "hippie" culture—has become one of the psychiatric labels catering for the "casualties" of new capitalism—in the sense of persons who take their own neoliberal self-cultivation to greater extremes. Just as capitalism has compounded our psychological problems, so it seeks to sell us the apparatus to rescue ourselves. According to Brossard and Chandler (2022) there remain some "not yet-labelled-troubles"; however, zealous healthy eating, along with fitness pursuits, have been swept into realms of psychiatry and clinical psychology, with their teleological ways of demonstrating the construction of social and personal ills.

The final part of this book, "Chapter 10: Conclusions: Cultural and Technological Transformations," brings together and expands upon its central themes—the politics of bodies; the costs of dietary freedom; the economics of obesity; our diagnostic culture; psychiatry and ethics; the crisis in mental health services; and finally, the dubious claims that neuroscience, genetics, and advanced technologies will fix all our eating problems.

References

Arguedas, A. A. R. (2020). "Can naughty be healthy?": Healthism and its discontents in news coverage of orthorexia nervosa. *Social Science & Medicine, 246*, 112784.

Allen, M., Dickinson, K. M., & Prichard, I. (2018). The dirt on clean eating: A cross sectional analysis of dietary intake, restrained eating and opinions about clean eating among women. *Nutrients, 10*(9), pii: E1266.

American Psychiatric Association. (2013). *Diagnostic and statistical manual of mental disorders (DSM-V)*. American Psychiatric Association Publishing.

Andreasson, J., & Johansson, T. (2016). 'Doing for group exercise what McDonald's did for hamburgers': Les Mills, and the fitness professional as global traveller. *Sport, Education and Society, 21*(2), 148–165.

Becker, J. C., Hartwich, L., & Haslam, S. A. (2021). Neoliberalism can reduce well-being by promoting a sense of social disconnection, competition, and loneliness. *British Journal of Social Psychology, 60*(3), 947–965.

Bhattacharya, A., Cooper, M., McAdams, C., Peebles, R., & Timko, C. A. (2022). Cultural shifts in the symptoms of Anorexia Nervosa: The case of Orthorexia Nervosa. *Appetite, 170*, 105869.

Blythin, S. P., Nicholson, H. L., Macintyre, V. G., Dickson, J. M., Fox, J. R., & Taylor, P. J. (2020). Experiences of shame and guilt in anorexia and bulimia nervosa: A systematic review. *Psychology and Psychotherapy: Theory, Research and Practice, 93*(1), 134–159.

Bo, S., Zoccali, R., Ponzo, V., Soldati, L., De Carli, L., Benso, A., Fea, E., Rainoldi, A., Durazzo, M., Fassino, S., & Abbate-Daga, G. (2014). University courses, eating problems and muscle dysmorphia: Are there any associations? *Journal of Translational Medicine, 12*, 1–8.

Boepple, L., & Thompson, J. K. (2014). A content analysis of healthy living blogs: Evidence of content thematically consistent with dysfunctional eating attitudes and behaviors. *International Journal of Eating Disorders, 47*(4), 362–367.

Boltanski, L., & Chiapello, E. (2005). The new spirit of capitalism. *International Journal of Politics, Culture, and Society, 18*(3/4), 161–188.

Bratman, S. (2017). Orthorexia vs. theories of healthy eating. *Eating and Weight Disorders, 22*(3), 381–385.

Bratman, S., & Knight, D. (1997). *Health food junkies: Orthorexia nervosa: Overcoming the obsession with healthful eating*. Random House.

Bratman, S., Cuzzolaro, M., Depa, J., Dunn, T., Missbach, B., Setnick, J., Varga, M., Cena, H., García, C. S., & Donini, L. M. (2017). The Orthorexia Nervosa Task Force (ON-TF): Objectives and key strategies. *Eating and Weight Disorders, 22*, 563–598.

Brossard, B. (2019). Why mental disorders flourish and wither: Extending the theory of ecological niches. *Social Science & Medicine, 237*, 112445.

Brossard, B., & Chandler, A. (2022). *explaining mental illness*. Bristol University Press.

Brown, Z., & Tiggemann, M. (2016). Attractive celebrity and peer images on Instagram: Effect on women's mood and Body Image. *Body Image, 19*, 37–43.

Brytek-Matera, A. (2012). Orthorexia nervosa—An eating disorder, obsessive-compulsive disorder or disturbed eating habit? *Archives of Psychiatry and Psychotherapy, 14*(1), 55–60.

Brytek-Matera, A. (2021). Vegetarian diet and orthorexia nervosa: A review of the literature. *Eating and Weight Disorders-Studies on Anorexia, Bulimia and Obesity, 26*, 1–11.

Cesiri, D. (2016). The blog is served: Crossing the 'expert/non-expert 'border in a corpus of food blogs. In *COLLOQUIUM* (Vol. 1, No. 1, pp. 47–62).

Cheshire, A., Berry, M., & Fixsen, A. (2020). What are the key features of orthorexia nervosa and influences on its development? A qualitative investigation. *Appetite, 155*, 104798.

Claudino, A. M., Pike, K. M., Hay, P., Keeley, J. W., Evans, S. C., Rebello, T. J., et al. (2019). The classification of feeding and eating disorders in the ICD-11: Results of a field study comparing proposed ICD-11 guidelines with existing ICD-10 guidelines. *BMC Medicine, 17*, 1–17.

Çiçekoğlu, P., & Tunçay, G. Y. (2018). A comparison of eating attitudes between vegans/vegetarians and nonvegans/nonvegetarians in terms of orthorexia nervosa. *Archives of Psychiatric Nursing, 32*(2), 200–205.

Cinquegrani, C., & Brown, D. H. (2018). 'Wellness' lifts us above the Food Chaos': A narrative exploration of the experiences and conceptualisations of Orthorexia Nervosa through online social media forums. *Qualitative Research in Sport, Exercise and Health, 10*(5), 585–603.

Cohen, B. M. (2016). *Psychiatric hegemony: A Marxist theory of mental illness*. Springer.

Conrad, P. (2005). The shifting engines of medicalization. *Journal of Health and Social Behavior, 46*(1), 3–14.

Costa, M. F., Prado, S. D., & Carvalho, M. C. D. V. S. (2022). Orthorexia in social media: Reflections between health and disease. *Saúde E Sociedade, 31*(2), e210760en-e210760en.

Crawford, R. (1980). Healthism and the medicalization of everyday life. *International Journal of Health Services, 10*(3), 365–388.

de Freitas Netto, S. V., Sobral, M. F. F., Ribeiro, A. R. B., & Soares, G. R. D. L. (2020). Concepts and forms of greenwashing: A systematic review. *Environmental Sciences Europe, 32*, 1–12.

Dell'Osso, L., Abelli, M., Carpita, B., Pini, S., Castellini, G., Carmassi, C., & Ricca, V. (2016). Historical evolution of the concept of anorexia nervosa and relationships with orthorexia nervosa, autism, and obsessive-compulsive spectrum. *Neuropsychiatric Disease and Treatment, 12*, 1651–1660.

Diane Barth, F. (2008). Hidden eating disorders: Attachment and affect regulation in the therapeutic relationship. *Clinical Social Work Journal, 36*(4), 355–365.

Diemling, M. (2015). The politics of food: Kashrut, food choices and social justice (tikkun olam). *Jewish Culture and History, 16*(2), 178–119.

Douma, E. R., Valente, M., & Syurina, E. V. (2021). Developmental pathway of orthorexia nervosa: Factors contributing to progression from healthy eating to excessive preoccupation with healthy eating. Experiences of Dutch health professionals. *Appetite, 158*, 105008.

Dunn, T. M., & Bratman, S. (2016). On orthorexia nervosa: A review of the literature and proposed diagnostic criteria. *Eating Behaviors, 21*, 11–17.

Dunn, T. M., Gibbs, J., Gibbs, J., Whitney, N., Whitney, N., Starosta, A., & Starosta, A. (2017). Prevalence of orthorexia nervosa is less than 1 %: Data from a US sample. *Eating and Weight Disorders, 22*(1), 185–192.

Fernández, E., Kitching, K., & Horgan, D. (2021). Young girls' experiences of 'good' food imperatives in a working-class school community: Rethinking food desire? *Cambridge Journal of Education, 51*(5), 543–561.

Fidan, T., Ertekin, V., Işikay, S., & Kırpınar, I. (2010). Prevalence of orthorexia among medical students in Erzurum, Turkey. *Comprehensive Psychiatry, 51*(1), 49–54.

Fixsen, A., Cheshire, A., & Berry, M. (2020). The social construction of a concept—Orthorexia Nervosa: Morality narratives and psycho-politics. *Qualitative Health Research, 30*(7), 1101–1113.

Fixsen, A., & Cheshire, A. (2022). Orthorexia Nervosa: The medicalization of extreme healthy eating practices. In M. Harbusch (Ed.), *Troubled persons industries: The expansion of psychiatric categories beyond psychiatry* (pp. 147–170).

Fixsen, A., Cranfield, S. & Ridge, D. (2017). Self-care and entrepreneurism: An ethnography of soft Skills development for Higher Education staff. *Studies in Continuing Education, 40*(2), 181–197.

Fixsen, A., Ridge, D., Ponsford, O., Holder, M., & Saran, G. (2023). Battles over 'unruly bodies': Practitioners' interpretations of eating disorders and the utility of psychiatric labelling. *Sociology of Health & Illness, 45*(3), 560–579.

Foucault, M. (1988). Technologies of the self. In *Technologies of the self: A seminar with Michel Foucault* (Vol. 18, p. 170).

Foucault, M., Davidson, A. I., & Burchell, G. (2008). *The birth of biopolitics: Lectures at the Collège de France, 1978–1979*. Springer.

Frances, A. (2013). Saving normal: An insider's revolt against out-of-control psychiatric diagnosis, DSM-V, big pharma and the medicalization of ordinary life. *Psychotherapy in Australia, 19*(3), 14–18.

Glaser, B. G. (1965). The constant comparative method of qualitative analysis. *Social problems, 12*(4), 436–445.

Greenhalgh, T., & Wessely, S. (2004). 'Health for me': A sociocultural analysis of healthism in the middle classes. *British Medical Bulletin, 69*, 197–213.

Goodman, M. K., Johnston, J., & Cairns, K. (2017). Food, media and space: The mediated biopolitics of eating. *Geoforum, 84*, 161–168.

Hanganu-Bresch, C. (2019). Orthorexia: Eating right in the context of healthism. *Medical Humanities, 46*(3), 311–322.

Håman, L., Barker-Ruchti, N., Patriksson, G., & Lindgren, E. C. (2015). Orthorexia nervosa: An integrative literature review of a lifestyle syndrome. *International Journal of Qualitative Studies on Health and Well-Being, 10*.

Håman, L., Barker-Ruchti, N., Patriksson, G., & Lindgren, E. C. (2016). The framing of orthorexia nervosa in Swedish daily newspapers: A longitudinal qualitative content analysis. *Scandinavian Sport Studies Fórum, 7*.

Håman, L., Lindgren, E. C., & Prell, H. (2017). "If it's not Iron it's Iron f* cking biggest Ironman": Personal trainers' views on health norms, orthorexia and deviant behaviours. *International Journal of Qualitative Studies on Health and Well-being, 12*(sup2), 1364602.

Horwitz, A. V., & Grob, G. N. (2016). The troubled history of psychiatry's quest for specificity. *Journal of Health Politics, Policy and Law, 41*(4), 521–539.

Jagdale, Y. D., Mahale, S. V., Zohra, B., Nayik, G. A., Dar, A. H., Khan, K. A., et al. (2021). Nutritional profile and potential health benefits of super foods: A review. *Sustainability, 13*(16), 9240.

Koven, N. S., & Abry, A. W. (2015). The clinical basis of orthorexia nervosa: Emerging perspectives. *Neuropsychiatric Disease and Treatment*, 385–394.

Kristensen, D. B., Lim, M., & Askegaard, S. (2016). Healthism in Denmark. *Health, 20*(5), 485–504.

Krug, I., Fuller-Tyszkiewicz, M., Hughes, E. K., & Roncero, M. (2022). What do we know about Other Specified Feeding or Eating Disorders, Unspecified Feeding and Eating Disorder and the Other EXIAs (eg, Orthorexia, Bigorexia, Drunkorexia, Pregorexia etc.)? *Frontiers in Psychology, 13*, 953402.

Leahy, D. (2014). Assembling a health [y] subject: Risky and shameful pedagogies in health education. *Critical Public Health, 24*(2), 171–181.

Li, A. M. (2017). Ecological determinants of health: Food and environment on human health. *Environmental Science and Pollution Research International, 24*(10), 9002–9015.

Luckhurst, P. (2015, February 23). *The holy kale. Beyoncé wants London to full crazy in love with her new nutrition plan.* The Standard. Retrieved August 22 2024, from https://www.standard.co.uk/going-out/foodanddrink/the-holy-kale-beyonce-wants-london-to-fall-crazy-in-love-with-her-new-nutrition-plan-10064170.html

Lupton, D. (1995). The imperative of health: Public health and the regulated body. *The Imperative of Health*, 1–192.

Martínez, N., Connelly, C. D., Pérez, A., & Calero, P. (2021). Self-care: A concept analysis. *International Journal of Nursing Sciences, 8*(4), 418–425.

McCartney, M. (2016). Clean eating and the cult of healthism. *BMJ (Online)*. https://doi.org/10.1136/bmj.i4095

Mete, R., Curlewis, J., Shield, A., Murray, K., Bacon, R., & Kellett, J. (2019). Reframing healthy food choices: A content analysis of Australian healthy eating blogs. *BMC Public Health, 19*, 1–9.

Meyer, C., Taranis, L., Goodwin, H., & Haycraft, E. (2011). Compulsive exercise and eating disorders. *European Eating Disorders Review, 19*(3), 174–189.

Micallef, R. (2023, April 5). *An eating disorder specialist reacts to Gwyneth Paltrow's diet. What is orthorexia nervosa?* YouTube. Retrieved August 22, 2024, from https://www.youtube.com/watch?v=LFZdIAZSvf0

Mitrofanova, E., Pummell, E. K., Mulrooney, H. M., & Petróczi, A. (2021). Using behavioural reasoning theory to explore reasons for dietary restriction: A qualitative study of orthorexic behavioural tendencies in the UK. *Frontiers in Psychology, 12*, 685545.

Mosley, P. E. (2009). Bigorexia: Bodybuilding and muscle dysmorphia. *European Eating Disorders Review: The Professional Journal of the Eating Disorders Association, 17*(3), 191–198.

Musolino, C., Warin, M., Wade, T., & Gilchrist, P. (2015). 'Healthy anorexia': The complexity of care in disordered eating. *Social Science and Medicine, 139*, 18–25.

Nestle, M. (2013). *Food politics* (10th ed.). University of California Press. https://doi.org/10.1525/j.ctt7zw29z

Nicolosi, G. (2006). Biotechnologies, alimentary fears and the orthorexic society. *Tailoring Biotechnologies, 2*(3), 37–56.

Noebel, N. A., Vela, R. B., Arreguin, D. H., & Oberle, C. D. (2023). Orthorexia nervosa symptomatology in the LGBTQ community: Gender and sexual orientation differences. *Eating Behaviors: An International Journal, 50*, 101771–101771.

Overbend, A. (2020). *Shifting Food Facts: Dietary discourse in a post-truth culture.* Routledge.

Pagliai, G., Dinu, M., Madarena, M. P., Bonaccio, M., Iacoviello, L., & Sofi, F. (2021). Consumption of ultra-processed foods and health status: A systematic review and meta-analysis. *British Journal of Nutrition, 125*(3), 308–318.

Paris, J. (2020). *Overdiagnosis in psychiatry: How modern psychiatry lost its way while creating a diagnosis for almost all of life's misfortunes*. Oxford University Press.

Parisi, L., La Grutta, S., Lo Baido, R., Epifanio, M., Carotenuto, M., Operto, F., et al. (2021). Bigorexia and orthorexia: An indissoluble relationship? *Minerva Psychiatry, 62*(4), 203–208.

Pirie, I. (2016). Disordered eating and the contradictions of neoliberal governance. *Sociology of Health & Illness, 38*(6), 839–853.

Pollan, M. (2008). *In defence of food: The myth of nutrition and the pleasures of eating*. Penguin UK.

Pontillo, M., Zanna, V., Demaria, F., Averna, R., Di Vincenzo, C., De Biase, M., et al. (2022). Orthorexia nervosa, eating disorders, and obsessive-compulsive disorder: A selective review of the last seven years. *Journal of Clinical Medicine, 11*(20), 6134.

Rangel, C., Dukeshire, S., & MacDonald, L. (2012). Diet and anxiety. An exploration into the Orthorexic Society. *Appetite, 58*(10), 124–132.

Segura-Garcia, C., Ramacciotti, C., Rania, M., Aloi, M., Caroleo, M., Bruni, A., Gazzarrini, D., Sinopoli, F., & De Fazio, P. (2014). The prevalence of orthorexia nervosa among eating disorder patients after treatment. *Eating and Weight Disorders, 20*(2), 161–166.

Selvi, K., & Bozo, Ö. (2020). The dark side of bodybuilding: The role of bodybuilding activities in compensation of frustrated basic psychological needs. *Motivation and Emotion, 44*(2), 190–208.

Shilling, C. (2016). *The Body: A very short introduction*. Oxford University Press.

Singh, M. P., Soni, K., Bhamra, R., & Mittal, R. K. (2022). Superfood: Value and need. *Current Nutrition & Food Science, 18*(1), 65–68.

Strahler, J., & Stark, R. (2020). Perspective: Classifying orthorexia nervosa as a new mental illness—Much discussion, little evidence. *Advances in Nutrition, 11*(4), 784–789.

Staudacher, H. M., & Harer, K. N. (2018). When clean eating goes dirty. *The Lancet Gastroenterology & Hepatology, 3*(10), 668.

Thorning, T. K., Raben, A., Tholstrup, T., Soedamah-Muthu, S. S., Givens, I., & Astrup, A. (2016). Milk and dairy products: Good or bad for human health? An assessment of the totality of scientific evidence. *Food & Nutrition Research, 60*(1), 32527.

Tragantzopoulou, P., Fixsen, A., Ridge, D., & Cheshire, A. (2024). 'You Are Not Alone, We've Got You': Power plays, devotion, and punishment on healthy eating and pro-eating disorder websites. *Qualitative Health Research*. https://doi.org/10.1177/10497323241238628

Turner, P. G., & Lefevre, C. E. (2017). Instagram use is linked to increased symptoms of orthorexia nervosa. *Eating and Weight Disorders, 22*(2), 277–284.

Valente, M., Syurina, E. V., Muftugil-Yalcin, S., & Cesuroglu, T. (2020). "Keep yourself alive": From healthy eating to progression to orthorexia nervosa A mixed methods study among young women in The Netherlands. *Ecology of Food and Nutrition, 59*(6), 578–597.

Valente, M., Cesuroglu, T., Labrie, N., & Syurina, E. V. (2022). "When are we going to hold orthorexia to the same standard as anorexia and bulimia?" Exploring the medicalization process of orthorexia nervosa on Twitter. *Health Communication, 37*(7), 872–879.

Young, G. (2013). Breaking bad: DSM-V description, criticisms, and recommendations. *Psychological Injury and Law, 6*, 345–348.

Wang, X. J., Jiang, C. Q., Zhang, W. S., Zhu, F., Jin, Y. L., Woo, J., et al. (2020). Milk consumption and risk of mortality from all-cause, cardiovascular disease and cancer in older people. *Clinical Nutrition, 39*(11), 3442–3451.

Wojtowicz, A. E., Alberga, A. S., Parsons, C. G., & von Ranson, K. M. (2015). Perspectives of Canadian fitness professionals on exercise and possible anorexia nervosa. *Journal of Eating Disorders, 3*, 1–10.

Zickgraf, H. F. (2020). Chapter 2—Treatment of pathologic healthy eating (orthorexia nervosa). In *Advanced Casebook of Obsessive-Compulsive and Related Disorders Conceptualizations and Treatment* (pp. 21–40). Academic Press. https://www.sciencedirect.com/science/article/

10

Cultural and Technological Transformations

DiNicola (1990) posed a critical question: if our lives are shaped by forces beyond our control, who or what governs these forces? This book has examined this question in the context of disordered eating and eating disorders. The debates over the distinction between "external forces" and what is considered "essential" within an individual are ongoing. The book argues that, capitalism, colonialism, western medical ideology, food conglomerates, and the media have all influenced the construction—and sometimes deconstruction—of disordered eating. The definition of an eating disorder (ED), both medically and sociologically, has been shaped by the interests of biomedical, legal, pharmaceutical, media, marketing, and consumer groups, whether they collaborate or compete. The evolving food landscape, the medicalization of food, the rise of individualism, and ongoing psychiatric classifications all contribute to the construction of EDs and disordered eating. In matters of mental health, western cultural and industrial imperialism have worked for centuries to marginalize alternative perspectives. Not only have other explanations for mental distress been dismissed as inferior to psychiatric ones, but political, social, and economic factors influencing food choices and behaviors have also been obscured, in favor of commodified, psychological solutions.

A. Fixsen, *The Construction of Eating Disorders*, The Politics of Mental Health and Illness, https://doi.org/10.1007/978-3-031-70318-8_10

However, psychiatry's far-reaching influence is not the result of maintaining exclusivity. While the discipline itself has evolved only modestly, its classifications and concepts have permeated society. Psychiatric ideas have spread globally, transforming everyday emotions into symptoms and dietary preferences into eating disorders. The process of medicalization has shifted from a top-down approach to one involving various stakeholders across different sectors. While some may favor psychiatry's expansion, critics argue that this aspect of western medicalization has led to the decontextualization of social problems (Harbusch, 2022) and the spread of western concepts of mental illness to contexts where they were previously unfamiliar, potentially reinforcing the very ethnic stereotypes they aim to challenge (Nuckolls, 2022). In this final chapter, I revisit and further debate the book's central themes—the politics of bodies, the costs of dietary freedom, the economics of obesity, our diagnostic culture, psychiatry and ethics, the mental health crisis, and the rise of advanced technologies—to offer my concluding reflections.

The Biopolitics of Bodies

A key idea explored in this book is the relationship between contemporary bodies as objects of radical transformation and the development of eating disorders. Not so long ago, most people spent a lot of time engaged in the pursuit of physical labor; working bodies were used to fix or make things, whereas now the bulk of people's work is performed through keyboards, gadgets, and other devices (Orbach, 2019). Aesthetics of bodies have always mattered; however, it seems unlikely that bodies have ever before been the objects of self-beautification (in the flesh and in images) to the extent that they are today. In this sense the body in our time has become the subject of its own work; it is seen as a flexible, malleable project which can be shaped according to the subjective desires of the individual. "We have become responsible for the design of our own bodies," Giddens wrote (1991, p. 102). This concept, that individuals can be trained, or can train themselves, to perceive their bodies differently, underpins most self-development programs, including those aimed at the prevention of eating disorders, which use cognitive and psychological techniques to address body dissatisfaction (Stice et al., 2013). These ideas align with the idea of the person as the natural locus of belief and desire and essentially responsible for their own well-being. What Rose (1998) calls the "regime of the self" includes the prospect of self-invention such that we are led to believe that our bodies can be anything we choose, so long as we can pay for this.

Most of us in western societies are no longer the subjects of feudalism; however (as described in Chap. 2), from a governance perspective, the contemporary body remains more acted upon than autonomous (Turner, 2008). A more liberal stance in matters such as sexual preference, manner of dress, and so on, may exist, yet the human body is now the subject and object of social and technological control in unprecedented ways. The body is central to economic growth—not only in the traditional areas of medicine, culture, fashion, sports, fitness, and entertainment, but as a key subject of the emerging biotechnological and genetic industries. This technological revolution, which some argue is ushering in a "post-human future" (Fukuyama, 2003), promises not just plastic bodies but ones capable of withstanding nature's challenges, potentially leading to a utopian existence where our bodies no longer struggle, experience pain, produce unwanted flesh or parts, or engage in many of the processes traditionally associated with being alive and human.

The impact of capitalism and consumerism on body image and their role in the genesis of eating disorders is a subject that has occupied feminists and other scholars for decades. One theory concerning the increase in diagnosis since the 1960s of anorexia nervosa (as covered in Chap. 3) is that it is an unfortunate outcome of pressures on women to be slim as they entered the office workplace in greater numbers (Bruch, 1979; Orbach, 1978, 1986; Tyler & Wilkinson, 2007). This proposal still has traction, however as women have sought greater social and economic equality, so the norms and expectations around their bodies have changed. Emerging in the 1990's, "Girl power" was a youth-oriented feminist trend which sought to change the way that women viewed their bodies and appearance as their own source of power. Women (and girls) were seen as right to use their bodies to further their personal and professional aspirations, so long as this was done of their own free will. Whatever its original intentions, the "girl power" slogan was rapidly adopted as a marketing tool to sell music, film, clothing, accessories, magazines and more. Inevitably, this neoliberal version of feminism has come at a price, both in terms of the additional consumer pressures it places on girls and young women to purchase the latest products and services and to display the qualities associated with it, and the effects it has on their emotional and psychic life (Gill, 2017). Another trend, body positivity, saw its origins in the alternative social and political movements of the 1960s and fat activism (Cooper, 2021). Although the body positivity movement has encouraged greater inclusivity regarding body look and size, this too has been manipulated by capitalism as corporations have used body diversity to sell their brands. Moreover, it has yet to eliminate structural forms of fat phobia in society, while with the promoting of slimming drugs such as *Ozempic,* some of the arguments around weight as a personal choice may lose their power.

The contemporary body improvement infrastructure is not solely aimed at females. Alongside the commercial pressures on women, the neoliberal health and beauty market has expanded to include a wide range of cultural products and services tailored for use on men's bodies and those of trans people, many of them billed as "essential" (Soulliard et al., 2022; Wooldridge & Lytle, 2012). This is not just about pampering, contemporary bodies are also subjected to new types of violence, not only in the form of sexual exploitation but by way of sometimes punishing, self-inflicted regimes to move, shape, and decorate bodies in extreme ways. In the health and fitness world, the cultural and medical emphases on a more muscular and athletic physique have proved highly profitable, since maintaining such a body requires significant and ongoing investment in personal fitness routines and dietary programs. The fitness and body building industry has boomed, with personal training one of the fastest growing business sectors (Chekhovska, 2017). Corporate advertising, social media, and government health messages collectively promote a vast array of products and devices aimed at keeping bodies of all ages in optimal shape and "fit for purpose." Celebrities and well-known influencers promote these campaigns, pushing their healthy diets and beauty regimes beyond mere self-care, to suggest that an ultra-fit body can be also a marker of social and professional success (Berardi, 2019). Many enthusiasts are led to believe that they can build a career around their physical fitness, though the market is crowded, and not everyone succeeds.

The pursuit of fitness is not the only way that people go about changing the appearance and anatomy of their bodies. Tattooing and body piercing, once fringe activities, have become an important aspect of the aesthetic and biopolitical economy. The international market for cosmetic surgery has soared and among some social groups is almost a required form of self-improvement (Sarwer, 2019). Of the 17.5 million cosmetic surgical treatments performed between 2016 and 2017 in the US, as recorded by the American Society of Plastic Surgeons (2018), the majority were minor procedures, such as Botox injections; however, some were more invasive, including those linked to weight concerns such as liposuction[1] and abdominoplasty[2]. Heyes (2007) points out that cosmetic surgery is not always an attempt to achieve a perfect beauty; nevertheless, it is closely linked to the cult of identity and the process of normalization inherent in biopower. The more that cosmetic surgery becomes normalized, the greater the social pressure to seek ways to externally express one's authentic identity and to regard body modification and augmentation as an essential aspect of self-care.

As discussed in Chap. 7, in areas of entertainment, cultural representations of bodies often emphasize and moralize extremes, deliberately linking overweight or emaciated bodies with social deviance or poverty. Bordo (1996) describes television's "freak shows," where audiences were either shocked by emaciated bodies or given detailed accounts of binge eating. Nearly 30 years later, not much has changed; the media continues to caste moral and aesthetic judgment on body shapes and eating behaviors that deviate from the norm. In advertising, a common strategy involves contrasting "perfect" body parts like smooth, toned arms and bellies with ones that are flabby or "flawed." These images are designed to drive up sales of dietary, cosmetic, and surgical products by raising consumer hopes or exploiting their anxieties. Images and videos of bodies also feature prominently on popular social media platforms (discussed in

[1] A technique in cosmetic surgery for moving excess fat from under the skin by suction.

[2] Removal of excess skin, fat and stretch marks, and tightening the abdominal muscles.

Chap. 8) such as *Tiktok, Reddit,* and *Facebook,* with some of this content glorifying thinness and promoting excessive weight loss (Blackburn & Hogg, 2024; Tragantzopoulou et al., 2024). Member only "pro-Ana" forums have also gained much traction and according to figures are now viewed by very young audiences (Fairplay, 2022). Much of this can be put down to algorithmic weighting used by social media, which governments have consistently failed to reign. While a target to increase the protection of children online has been set by the UK government, they acknowledge that measures adopted by the Online Safety Act will take years to implement (UK Parliament, 2024). In the meantime, it remains the case that any child or young person can be directed to pro-ED content in the space of a few clicks.

Social media has normalized the sharing of personal experiences, including the physical and emotional struggles associated with eating disorders. Online communities can provide a sense of belonging and understanding that might be missing in offline lives. Often, individuals aim to raise awareness about eating disorders, their complexities, and their impact on lives. There is also a growing trend of monetizing illness and recovery stories, with people sharing their experiences to build a following or personal brand. As their audience grows, vloggers may be seen as influencers, especially within communities focused on mental health and disordered eating. Additional revenue streams include sponsorships and partnerships with brands, promotion of products and services, advertising revenue, affiliate marketing, crowdfunding, and donations. In essence, social platforms have not only democratized discussions around eating disorders but have also given rise to "illness entrepreneurship." The intersection of self-disclosure and entrepreneurship is epitomized in the self-revelatory ED story. While most of these narratives are solitary, their tendency is to perpetuate the idea that disordered eating is disconnected from broader social forces, some romanticizing the notion of having an eating disorder though emotive music and photographs. Overall, content related to eating disorders on social media tends to be individualistic and psychologized, reflecting neoliberal society's fixation on self-identity.

The Illusion of Dietary Freedom

As neoliberal consumers, we are led to believe that we enjoy unprecedented freedom to plan our diets, and that it is our own foremost responsibility to protect our health. As I have argued in this book, this freedom of choice is partly illusory, and it comes at cost. As argued in Chap. 5, the vast range of products available in "rich world" food outlets command prices too high for many living in the countries in which they are produced. The modern food industry is increasingly dominated by a handful of powerful corporations whose primary focus is maximizing profit (FFCC, 2024), often at the expense of quality, environmental sustainability, public health, and social equity. The intersection of food production and corporate greed has led to numerous challenges that threaten both the planet and its people. Monoculture farming, where large tracts of land are devoted to a single crop, is a prime example. This practice depletes soil nutrients, increases vulnerability to pests, and drives the overuse of chemical fertilizers and pesticides. Many of these chemicals not only harm local ecosystems but also contribute to water pollution and the decline of biodiversity. Furthermore, large-scale industrial farming is a significant contributor to greenhouse gas emissions, particularly methane from livestock and carbon dioxide from deforestation for agricultural expansion. Many agricultural workers have poor working conditions and low wages, and are exposed to hard physical labor and/or harmful chemicals. Despite these known impacts, many corporations continue to push for intensive farming methods that maximize yields and profits, ignoring the long-term consequences for the environment.

The push for healthy eating, while celebrated for encouraging nutritious diets, has exposed a complex and often contradictory dietary landscape. The global rise in demand for "superfoods" like quinoa and avocados has led to significant environmental and social impacts, including over-farming and ecological degradation in regions where these crops are staples (Magrach & Sanz, 2020). This surge can disrupt local economies and ecosystems, revealing that the effects of dietary trends extend well beyond individual health. Healthism—an individualistic trend whereby personal health has become a super value (Crawford, 1980;

Kristensen et al., 2016)—is (as described in Chap. 9) closely tied to neoliberal capitalism. Neoliberalism's focus on personal branding has turned the body into a vehicle for a multitude of psychosocial symbols, demanding an endless array of consumable products. Empire-builders and their food conglomerates have led to an expectation that any type of food and diet is available at a price. With media now the new empire-builder, many dietary items and disciplines are now promulgated virtually. Vast fortunes are made not only by multinational food companies but also by celebrity entrepreneurs like Gwyneth Paltrow and Beyoncé, who leverage mainstream media and e-commerce to promote their branded nutrition programs and products, often promising a "spiritual and physical cleanse" (Luckhurst, 2015). These business moguls follow in the footsteps of earlier figures like Sylvester Graham and John Harvey Kellogg, acting as "moral entrepreneurs" (Cohen, 1972) and linking their wholesome products to a sense of spiritual superiority (Tompkins, 2009). Attempting to emulate these modern Titans are numerous social media influencers, endorsing various health and fitness brands.

For those who can afford to buy based on "quality," food has become less about such things as satiation and companionship, and more about status and achieving a particular lifestyle. Consumers who try to follow these eating trends will notice that foods labeled "organic," "local," and "superfoods" come with premium prices. Nothing in the food cupboard is safe from gentrification, or "yassification" (slang for "makeover"), including dressed up staples like canned fish, cooking oil, salt and vinegar. Food snobbery is nothing new, however as health and fitness standards become increasingly stringent and widely applied, those who fail to meet them may be viewed as morally deficient or deviant, both by themselves and others (Jönsson, 2009). Yet, vast contradictions exist between the types of consumption promoted by governments and market-based food systems and the social and economic realities many people face. Studies indicate that health inequalities, including numbers of adolescents classed as overweight and obese, have been increasing in wealthy countries (Kestens & Daniel, 2010). Healthy food consumption is closely linked not only to income but to higher cultural and social capital. Supportive measures at school, including nutritional school meals, have been identified as crucial for reducing social inequality and improving health outcomes according to a large-scale international study by de Clercq et al. (2017). These types of measures require government funding to put them into place, whereas many private markets appear to be more interested in profits than people.

For around half a century a powerful "anti-obesity" campaign (as discussed in Chap. 6) has been raging that hinges on the neoliberal assertion that everyone is responsible and accountable for their own health, with fatness being viewed as a personal choice. Measures to cut fat in the diet mark out certain bodies as disordered and influence the stereotypes of who is at risk of developing restrictive or binge-purge–type eating disorders and obesity. Those from middle and upper classes are often assumed to "know better" than to engage in behaviors assumed to result in fatness (McPhail, 2013). Others from lower socioeconomic classes and minority ethnic groups may be considered more prone to ignorance and unruliness, while social circumstances and beliefs are not considered. In the realm of food marketing, corporate influence over food production has led to the proliferation of highly processed foods that are inexpensive to produce but low in nutritional value. "Big Food" (mass market, processed foods), is, according the Food, Farming and Countryside Commission (FFCC, 2024), costing UK society £268 billion in terms of chronic disease, with the greatest burden falling on those with lower incomes.

These ultra processed products, which are flooding food markets, are typically packed with artificial additives and preservatives, added sugars, unhealthy fats, and excessive salt, contributing to rising rates of obesity, diabetes, and other diet-related diseases. The aggressive marketing of such products, particularly in low-income areas and to children, has significantly exacerbated the problem. In contrast, wealthy individuals in affluent countries are statistically less obese due to their consumption of a lower-calorie, high-quality diet, whereas those with lower economic status in the same economy can only afford or choose a higher-calorie diet (Mathieu-Bolh & Wendner, 2020). As the cost of obesity to the public purse increases, so various biopolitical strategies have been employed to manage it. Suggested measures to tackle those forces feeding into the"obesogenic environment" include the promotion of physical activity, the regulation of food advertising (especially to children), the enforcement of penalties of fast food companies and the implementing of taxes on sugary drinks. However, some of these policies also economically penalize the poor, since fresh and nutritious foods are often more expensive and are sold in more affluent areas, making them less accessible to lower-income populations. This creates a paradox where malnutrition and obesity coexist, even within the same communities. Making it a right for every citizen to have access to sufficient, affordable healthy food from childhood (FFCC, 2024) is not yet on the horizon.

Social injustice associated with food and eating has historic roots, no more so than in the story of sugar (touched upon in Chap. 6). The cruel exploitation of black slaves on sugar plantations has now been brought to light; however, the "sugar ecologies" (a complex network of economic, political, scientific, and ideological practices) remain intertwined with racism and even slavery. Hatch et al. (2019) highlight how the harmful effects of sugar are amplified by contemporary forces that direct sugar into black bodies, leading to extraordinary levels of toxicity and chronic metabolic disease among black people in the US (p. 595). The authors argue that binge eating is encouraged by food manufacturers as it is essential for corporate growth. Meanwhile, the exploitation of individuals from low socioeconomic backgrounds continues; modern sugar plantations are known to rely on coercive labor practices, including threats of violence, wage withholding, forced indebtedness, withholding of identity documents, child labor, and outright slavery (Hatch et al., 2019; Verité, 2012). While obesity is not classified as an eating disorder, there are clear overlaps between these concepts, in terms of diagnosis (McCuen-Wurst et al., 2018), associations with socioeconomic status, and implications for mental well-being. In one large-scale study of community surveys by Kessler et al. (2013), most respondents with lifetime binge eating disorder also met the criteria for one or more DSM disorder.

Fat stigma has deeply penetrated a society marked by social and economic disparities. Obesity is now viewed as a global economic burden (Santomauro et al., 2021), but this also means that discrimination against the obese begins in childhood and perpetuates the cycle of socioeconomic disadvantage (Children's Commissioner, 2024). When people of lower socioeconomic status (SES) seek services, they may face longer waiting times and receive lower levels of care and attention from providers (Huryk et al., 2021). Binge eating disorder (BED) has been specifically identified as a social justice issue due to its association with lower SES (Bray et al., 2022; Mitchison et al., 2014). From an intersectional perspective, race, ethnicity, and gender can influence stigmatized beliefs about eating disorders, further impairing mental health literacy, treatment-seeking, and recovery (Ali et al., 2017).

A Diagnostic Culture

While "unhealthy" eating is more broadly understood as socially and economically constructed, eating disorders remain widely accepted as individual phenomena. As a product of western medicine, the concept of an eating disorder rests on the belief that a set of western psychiatric templates can generate a universally valid knowledge base, above and beyond any specific society and culture (Summerfield, 2012). In line with this thinking, the definition of an eating disorder by the World Health Organization (WHO) embraced the International Classification of Disease Related Health Problems (now ICD-11 (WHO, 2019)), which typifies the way in which eating disorders as mental illnesses are rendered classifiable and diagnosable. This assumption, that western health expertise can be exported from the global north across the world in the form of a neutral relocation of knowledge and practice, has been contested (Cox & Webb, 2015). The World Health Organization's Mental Health Action Plan 2013–2020 outlines steps for all member states to reduce the global burden of mental illness, emphasizing the need for mental healthcare to be provided in a "culturally appropriate" way. Cox and Webb (2015) contend that this requirement is problematic, primarily because these directives are still influenced by the normative assumptions of western medical and psychological practices, along with their associated ethical, legal, and institutional perspectives. The authors point out several important issues concerning the exploitation of mental health expertise from the global north to the global south, including that of presumptive methodologies based on western notions of selfhood, exclusion of indigenous traditions and practices, and other ethical considerations.

Beside the broad criticisms around the imposition of inappropriate and potentially inaccurate western bio-psychiatric definitions on non-western populations, there is the issue of a prescribed western disease model of health being used globally to expand its own power, along with global capitalist ethics and pharmaceutical products through which medical authorities maintain their power (Wildeman, 2013). Both DSM and ICD systems of classifying symptoms reinforce the notion that mental distress relates to diagnosable illness; however, these classifications are more convenient than scientific and, as has been argued, are certainly not culturally grounded (Summerfield, 2008). They are, according to Summerfield (2012), part of a medical imperialism which transfers western concepts of normal and abnormal to mental distress in different cultural environments. The training of evermore individuals (professionals and other stakeholders) in the language and methodologies of western psychiatry appears to have become a primary goal of the American Psychiatric Association and its publicity arm. This is not just a one-way process, in answer to criticisms, psychologists were far more involved in the decision-making process for the *Diagnostic and Statistical Manual of Mental Disorders, Fifth Edition, Text Revision* (DSM-V-TR). Published in 2022, the revised manual is advertised online as "the most comprehensive, current, and critical resource for clinical practice available to today's mental health clinicians and researchers." This version, which has made efforts to employ more culturally and inclusive language, describes itself as a "valuable resource for other physicians and health professionals, including psychologists, counselors, nurses, and occupational and rehabilitation therapists, as well as social workers and forensic and legal specialists" (APA Publishing, 2022). Welcoming other professionals into the psychiatric fold may seem democratic; however, the strategy also functions as a "conversion" process, with an ever-widening constellation of stakeholders potentially feeling inclined to employ the reductionist language of the DSM in their professional lives, "systematically serving the interests of the powerful" (Cohen, 2016, p. 8). As discussed in Chap. 4, even if they disagree with psychiatric labels from an ideological standpoint or are not directly involved in diagnostic decision-making, professionals and others working in mental health are likely to regard the use of psychiatric diagnostic labeling as a necessary part of their job (Fixsen et al., 2023).

Western psychiatry can pride itself on having catalogued, revised, expanded, and sold on its large taxonomy of mental disorders, by asserting that these criteria are, by way of recent revisions, applicable to *all* individuals, irrespective of place and background. However, a prevailing criticism concerning the mental categories of the DSM or ICD is that these symptom clusters remain assembled by people, in this case, members of a committee, and not by nature. The argument that normal anxieties of life are being labeled as illness is now many decades old. Some of the strongest critics have come from within psychiatry itself, beginning with the architects of the "anti-psychiatry" movement such as Thomas Szasz (1920–2012) and R.D. Lang (1927–1987). Psychiatrist Derek Summerfield (cited above) is best known for his criticism of the "invention" of post-traumatic stress disorder (PTSD), which he regards as a political construct designed to subsume trauma into the everyday descriptions of life's vicissitudes (Summerfield, 2001). Arguing along similar lines, psychiatrist Joel Paris bemoans psychiatrists' propensity to pathologize all manner of reactions to ordinary life (Paris, 2020). Both authors agree that psychiatry has lost its soul on the way; however, for Paris, the problem lies not so much in the categories themselves, but the selective way in which certain more "fashionable" labels are liberally used by practitioners. Summerfield (2001), on the other hand, seems especially concerned about the victim culture which, due to the labeling of emotional problems as post-traumatic stress disorder (PTSD), has become commonplace.

This does not mean that western psychiatry has remained wholly untouched by other cultural influences. Some changes to the DSM and ICD have been influenced by findings involving non-western populations (Lee, 2001), along with wider criticisms of the DSM and ICD concerning their lack of cultural and ethnic sensitivity (Claudino et al., 2019; Thomas et al., 2013). Furthermore, other versions of psychiatric manuals exist, including the *Chinese Classification of Mental Disorders* (CCMD). However, the CCMD is still written along similar lines to the DCM and ICD, in that it is primarily concerned with signs and symptoms of mental disorders rather than the underlying causes. It still relies on the same operational definitions and concepts, such that "mental disorders" like depression and anorexia are defined by specific measurable criteria based on observable behavior and specific timelines. It does not diminish the potential harm of labels and the invitation of social stigma and discrimination attached to them. The threat of mental health stigma was borne out in a qualitative study of professionals employed in the treatment of eating disorders on mainland China, conducted by Zhao (2022). Professionals interviewed for the study, who were trained in western medicine, spoke of how it was still commonplace to regard the diagnosis of a mental disorder as bringing shame and dishonor to the subject's family. As a result, parents and some practitioners were inclined to attribute major weight loss in a child or young adult to physiological factors such as a stomach disease or menstrual problem.

ED diagnoses have largely been spared the criticisms afforded other forms of psychiatric labeling, but they too exist as part of the western culture of diagnosis. EDs are founded on the belief that disordered eating must be psychiatric in origin and that they cannot be remedied without being categorized. As with other psychiatric labels, ED labels hold the potential for social stigma and discrimination, change of status based on diagnosis, and a potential impact on social relationships. Fundamentally, labels oversimplify complex human experiences, reducing a person to a diagnosis and ignoring the individuality of their experiences within the broader context of their life. Some individuals may feel that the diagnosis comes to define them. Being awarded a diagnosis may remove a person's control and autonomy and pressurize them to conform to the expectations associated with the label. The eating disorder taxonomy is also subject to frequent additions and revisions. Along with the body dysmorphic conditions, eating behaviors linked with the contemporary emphasis on health and diet as a lifestyle, such as orthorexia nervosa—an "unhealthy" preoccupation with "healthy" eating—have been seeking to establish their place in the official psychiatric taxonomy (Fixsen et al., 2020a). A new type of lifestyle- oriented psychiatry has come to pass, with labels such as "bigorexia" (fixation on building body mass) and "orthorexia" entering popular and clinical vocabulary (Krug et al., 2022).

The Question of Harm

One of the arguments against the excessive use of psychiatric diagnoses concerns the potential, and sometimes inevitable distress and harm afforded those who are detained and treated against their will. Psychiatry is frequently used in the development of policies related to mental health and criminal justice, including laws on involuntary commitment, sentencing for mentally ill offenders, and the provision of mental health services in prisons. In countries such as the UK, the reach of mental capacity law is immense. Under UK law, a person with a mental disorder may be formally detained in hospital (or "sectioned") in the interest of their own safety or for the protection of other people. These numbers have been steadily rising, with 53,337 new detentions recorded under the 2021–22 Mental Health Act, with overall national totals expected to be higher (NHS England Digital, 2022). Eating disorders are generally considered harmless to others; nevertheless, they can lead to incarceration in a similar manner to a criminal act. Compulsory inpatient treatment is enforceable in the UK under the Mental Capacity Act 2005, the Mental Health Act 2007, and 2021–22 as well as the Children's Act 1989 (NICE, 2021). In cases of anorexia nervosa (AN) involuntary admission, detention, and nasogastric tube feeding have been widely described in the literature (Clausen, 2020). In one register-based study in Demark, all possible involuntary measures had been used with patients with AN, including enforced medication and mechanical or physical restraint (Clausen et al., 2018). Clearly, the issues around enforcing potentially life-sustaining treatment on a person are complex and ethically fraught. The idea of allowing a person, especially a minor, to place themselves at risk of harm and death may seem unbearable and often overrides appeals to the principle of respect for a patient's autonomy. Added to this are the potential risks of refeeding syndrome to consider which, while relatively rare, can be fatal (Mehanna et al., 2008).

Ultimately psychiatry functions as a system of power. As Lyons and O'Malley (2002) argue, there is ample potential for the present system of psychiatric diagnosis to be used as a weapon of exploitation and for psychiatry's taxonomy to reinforce not just social norms but political interests. The employment of psychiatry for punitive purposes may seem alien to life in a western democracy; however, we should not forget the overarching power and paternalism associated with medical intervention. That the vast majority of those who receive treatment for an ED, both voluntary and involuntary, are intelligent females, has troubled generations of female writers (Bordo, 1994; Hepworth & Griffen, 1995;

Holmes et al., 2021; Umezulike, 2020). Loss of autonomy, erosion of trust of family and professionals, social stigma, and isolation are just some of the potential drawbacks of compulsory detainment. From the human rights perspective, Umezulike (2020) points out that involuntary treatment entails not just uncomfortable, painful, and risky methods of feeding, but the constant surveillance of day-to-day activities of patients while institutionalized. In studies of patients being treated for AN, the perception of being placed under a high degree of coercion was overwhelming (Guarda et al., 2007). Even where patients retrospectively acknowledge a treatment as lifesaving, they continued to regard this as a form of punishment, which should be short-lived (Clausen, 2020; Seed et al., 2016). Giordano (2005) points out that many believe that respect for individual autonomy should be suspended in psychiatry, since mental illness compromises a person's ability to make decisions and care for themselves. The author goes on to strongly argue that beliefs connecting AN with a lack of competence are false. Lack of engagement with the subjective meaning of self-starvation, a "doctor knows best attitude" and denial of the patient voice are significant obstacles to creating the conditions for recovery—as is the use of punitive behavior and patients being required to earn trust in ways that they experience as dehumanizing and demotivating (Holmes et al., 2021; Umezulike, 2020).

As McBride (2022) reminds us, state sponsorship of psychiatry has bestowed on it cultural legitimacy and institutional authority, as well as political power, offering governments an ethical basis and practical means to manage its most troubling citizens. Studies suggest that thousands of political prisoners have found themselves confined and abused in psychiatric hospitals, in China,[3] Eastern Europe, and Russia (van Voren, 2010, 2016). In addition to obvious human rights infringements, there is the potential for food refusal to be employed in political protests and for authorities to act forcefully against it. Prisoners, suffragettes, and others have employed hunger strike where they felt there were no other means

[3] The Chinese government's campaign against the popular movement of Falun Gong (a discipline with roots in Buddhism and Taoism) has led to the incarceration of thousands in mental hospitals, despite their families refuting the presence of mental illnesses in their relatives. These measures have been reinforced by forensic psychiatry and the workings of the judicial system in China (Lyons & Malley, 2002).

of protest, and many have been subjected to forced feeding and punishment for doing so (Miller, 2016; Scanlan et al., 2008). It is easy to shake our heads at these blatant examples of violence and abuse, yet one thing remains unchanged; declaring a person as mentally ill claims authority over the body and mind of the person so diagnosed. While there is some acknowledgment of the historical contingent nature of current psychiatric classification, modern psychiatry continues to grapple with, not just its racist legacy (Thomas & Casper, 2019) but its present discriminatory practices. A deep distrust toward "white medicine" among certain socially oppressed and medically abused communities persists, rooted in a history of mistreatment and exploitation by the healthcare system. Notable instances such as the highly unethical Tuskegee syphilis study[4] serve as enduring reminders of this troubling past. Although—as Keene (2024) points out—at any time, anyone of us could find ourselves (deemed) incapable of caring for our own health, welfare, and finances, some groups are more represented in this respect than others.

These statistics emerging from established institutions point to the precarious and potentially discriminatory foundations upon which the psychiatric diagnostic classification system is built. Furthermore, factors such as lack of cultural competence among healthcare providers, limited access to healthcare services, and disparities in insurance coverage contribute to the disenchantment felt by individuals from black communities toward the healthcare system. Within this context, psychiatric categories often serve more as tools for detainment rather than avenues for treatment, particularly for people of color. For instance, in the UK in 2023, black or black British people were 3.6 times more likely to be

[4] In 1932, the US Public Health Service (USPHS) began an experiment in Macon County, Alabama, to observe the progression of untreated, latent syphilis in African American males. The study involved 400 impoverished African American men with syphilis and 200 uninfected men who served as controls. The men were promised free medical treatment. Despite the widespread availability of penicillin as the preferred treatment for syphilis starting in the 1950s, none of the infected participants were provided with penicillin. There were instances where the USPHS actively discouraged treatment for syphilis. It was not until 1972, when reports of the study surfaced in the national media, that the Department of Health, Education and Welfare halted the experiment. It is estimated that more than 100 participants died directly due to advanced syphilitic lesions (Brandt, 1978). The study, which was clearly an abuse of human rights, is believed to have led to a deep distrust of white public health systems, including that some drug treatments are man-made weapons of racial warfare.

involuntarily detained under the Mental Health Act (Royal College of Psychiatrists, 2024). Psychiatric detention rates are also clearly linked with social deprivation; rates of detention in the most deprived areas of the UK are more than three and a half times higher than the rate of detention in the least deprived areas (NHS England Digital, 2022). Yet, increasingly the public and especially ethnic minorities are being urged not to delay seeking help for a mental health problem, with eating disorders especially highlighted as requiring rapid treatment (BEAT, 2023). While many believe that western psychiatry can help people deal with the hurt and trauma left by colonization, psychiatry and medicine clearly needs to eliminate not only the racist elements of the health system but psychiatry's interpretation of mental health as separable from people's history.

The Mental Health Crisis

A supporting argument for psychiatric diagnosis is that, while the existing taxonomy and accompanying legislation have their flaws, formal assessment tools and measures are essential for a smoothly functioning mental health system and for a safe society. Diagnostic labels can both aid communication and collaboration between practitioners, patients, and their families, and guide subjects down appropriate treatment pathways to avoid long term harm. The importance of early detection and treatment is backed up by statistical studies suggesting that, as a global society, the number of people with mental disorders is increasing. Around a quarter of the population in western countries are now considered to be suffering from a mental health problem, with young people reporting the highest levels. In the UK, the number of individual prescriptions for antidepressants rose by 2 percent from 2022 to 2023 to 86 million, while prescriptions for central nervous stimulants and drugs for ADHD increased by 33 percent in adults over 18, and 12 percent in children under 17 in the same period (NHS Business Services Authority, 2023). The role of pharmaceutical drugs in the treatment of different eating disorders is less clear; however, since most diagnosed eating disorders are considered co-morbid with at least one other mental disorder (Hay,

2020), we can assume that many ED patients will be prescribed a psychotropic medication. Statistics generated during and following the Covid pandemic bear out the widespread but unequal impact of poor living conditions, social and economic disadvantage, and difficulty accessing medical and social care on people's quality of life and health outcomes, including those associated with disordered eating (Gao et al., 2022).

Most worrying is the apparent decline in the mental health of children and young people. A rise in depression, anxiety, suicidality, and eating disorder diagnoses have been reported among children, adolescents, and young adults in the US since Covid-19 (Office of the Surgeon General, 2021). In the UK, NHS figures also show a large increase in the number of hospital admissions for eating disorders between 2015 and 2021, with almost half those admitted being under the age of 25 (NHS England, Digital 2021). Despite calls for early detection, the period between and ED diagnosis and start of treatment has considerably lengthened. Not only has the number of children starting treatment more than doubled since 2016 to 2017, in the last quarter of 2022 to 2023, 45 percent of urgent cases were waiting more than 12 weeks to start treatment (Children's Commissioner, 2024). Most of these hospitalized cases pertain to restrictive eating disorders (NHS England, 2021). Over a similar timeframe there has been a notable increase in childhood obesity cases, placing the UK among the countries with the highest rates of childhood obesity in Europe. The link between social deprivation and obesity is particularly evident in this age group, with children from the most deprived areas being more than twice as likely to be obese compared to those from the least deprived areas (Children's Commissioner, 2024).

As with most problems related to mental health, much of what would be described as "disordered eating" remains hidden within the same social structures which serve to maintain inequalities. For example, the number of men and women with eating disorders in prisons has largely gone unrecorded but is believed to be substantial (Farber, 2013; Tyler et al., 2019). People in prisons have significant mental health problems, yet typically their health needs are underserved (Tyler et al., 2019). Writing on this topic, Waldman (2014) notes that prisoners may under-report their symptoms of inducing vomiting and possession of diet pills, laxatives, and diuretics because it would subject them to disciplinary action.

Prison environments can also be highly stigmatizing, leading to an increased focus on weight. Many people in prisons will have experienced trauma and a good number will have moved back and forth from psychiatric hospitals to prisons. With little to do when confined to cells and spurred on by media, some prisoners may spend excessive amounts of time in the gym, resulting in more extreme dietary behaviors. Poor prison food may also exacerbate eating problems. Yet very few scholars have explored these aspects of extreme or disordered eating, while prison numbers continue to rise.

As with other areas of mental health, cultural and racial stigma surrounding eating disorders continue to contribute to the uneven distribution of treatment (Moreno et al., 2023). Eating disorders are now recognized as being linked to ethnic and intersectional disparities. Historically, discussions about eating disorders have largely excluded Black, Indigenous, and other People of Color (BIPOC) due to inherent biases in western medical systems and culture. This systematic neglect and exclusion have resulted in a lack of diversity within the medical system itself. A recent study of eating disorder providers in the US revealed that 73 percent of the workforce in this field is comprised of white individuals (Jennings et al., 2020). Respondents to the study highlighted unrecognized biases and prejudices among current gatekeepers, Eurocentric perspectives, and clinical and educational elitism. The absence of cultural diversity also means that few providers have first-hand experience or understanding of the chronic stresses associated with systemic racism, repeated microaggressions, discrimination, intergenerational racial trauma, marginalization, and their various direct and indirect impacts. These experiences significantly affect the well-being and overall health of individuals from BIPOC communities.

Paradoxically, the shift away from psychiatric labeling may stem from political motives rather than one grounded in neuroscience or social justice. With a mental health disorder now ranking as the most prevalent condition among economically inactive individuals due to health reasons (IPPR, 2022), there has been a growing political backlash against those who are signed off work with a mental health disorder. Recent headlines in the UK press highlighted the remarks from the then Work and Pensions Secretary Mel Stride, who suggested that the discourse surrounding mental health had become excessively open (Gutteridge, 2024). Similarly, Conservative Deputy Chair Rachel MacLean voiced alarm about the lack of acceptance that life is hard and stated that "is it normal to feel happy all the time?" (Tapsfield, 2024). It must be emphasized that critiquing the present psychiatric diagnostic system as flawed does not equate to accusing individuals of exaggerating or fabricating their experiences of mental distress to avoid work, as insinuated by some right-wing politicians. A survey conducted by the UK charity Mind (2013) revealed that work is the most significant source of stress for people, surpassing concerns about debt, financial difficulties, or health issues. Notably, stress and burnout rates are particularly high in "people" professions, with teaching being identified as the most stressful sector of employment (Glass, 2024).

Advanced Technology: Brave New World?

While much has been written supporting and critiquing the DSM/ICD classification system, the role of biotechnology in the treatment of disordered eating has yet to be fully explored from the social constructionist perspective. This is an omission, because in terms of social and biological engineering, AI and other advancements have significant implications for us all. In contrast to the sociological studies cited in this chapter, work published in the neuroscience and biotechnology field paints a more optimistic picture of our future minds. Enthusiasm with these new sciences has been expressed by sociologists including Shilling (2016), who points out how developments within the "new" biology associated with the Human Genome Project[5] and other initiatives which highlight the body can reveal important information about the operation of not just individual bodies but societies. Similarly, Rose and Abi-Rached (2013) urge sociologists and neuroscientists to work toward a collaboration between these two seemingly opposed disciplinary areas. In the area of eating disorders, sample neuroimaging has been providing insights into

[5] The human genome project was an international scientific research project carried out between 1990 and 2003, whose goal was to determine the base pairs that make up human DNA and identify, map, and sequence all the genes of the human genome from a physical and functional standpoint.

the neuropsychological pathways associated with certain aspects of EDs (McGuire & Matsumoto, 2004), while genome-wide association studies (GWAS) and pluripotent stem cells are helping to explain the role of genes in the etiology of anorexia nervosa (AN) (Stern & Bulik, 2020). These and other breakthroughs in genetic experimentation (such as the GLP-1 antagonists[6] *Ozempic* and *Wegovy*) have made a future without obesity, depression, anxiety, and indeed, any kind of morbidity seem possible. There are also benefits for relatives and sometimes patients themselves from being able to interpret their suffering as genetically or chemically based, rather than tied in with personal error or family dysfunction. So, is the "Brave New World"[7] of technological advancement the way out of human suffering?

The biotechnological approach is leading people to question the nature of their own bodies and minds in unprecedented ways. We have entered the age of biological and neurological citizenship, where neuroscientists are becoming the new experts in the management of human conduct (Rose & Abi-Rached, 2013). As neurobiology colonizes social and human sciences, it introduces the idea of a plastic, social brain, and a new way of managing the mind. Brain plasticity is seen as having enormous clinical potential for reversing disease, but, as Pitts-Taylor (2016) argues, this same science is also involved in the manufacture of pharmaceuticals, supplements, electrical stimulators, and military industries. It offers an alternative to biological determinism but also threatens the "freedom" of the body-subject through its technical governmentality. In everyday life, this new biology is already affecting how we conceive of our own identities. To be a morally acceptable citizen one now needs to monitor, evaluate, and work on oneself using expert knowledge from the "received facts" of science. In addition to the familiar biometrics upon which body shape and weight measurement norms are based, there are the various tests which allow practitioners to estimate a person's chances of inheriting

[6] Pharmaceutical drugs used to treat Type II Diabetes and now obesity, which mimic the action of the GLP-1, a hormone naturally produced in the stomach.

[7] The Brave New World analogy may seem far-fetched. Yet, as in Huxley's (1932) dystopian novel, these technologies hold the potential for hierarchical and highly selective social engineering. When Huxley wrote his book in 1931, history had yet to reveal the horrific implications of eugenics and selectivity based on hatred, discrimination, and racism.

particular diseases. This knowledge concerning the risks associated with lifestyle choices related to diet, exercise, and alcohol can prompt individuals to become "patients in waiting" (Rajan, 2006). The patient in waiting governs him/herself based on a medical paradigm that highlights the economic value of physical and mental health to the individual, to the health service, and to national productivity. They are bound by a science which is said to understand their brains and behavior far better than they can comprehend these things for themselves.

The relationship between food and technology has also been rapidly evolving. Keen to have their fingers in every pie, Tech giants, such *as Google*, have invested heavily in AI food technology, with Silicon Valley's lab food companies using inventive, but costly and bizarre ways, to replicate the products of animal husbandry. Unfortunately, as Steel (2021) points out, we are not that good at managing the food that we do produce. According to the United Nations Food and Agriculture Organization (FAO, 2024), globally farmers provide the daily equivalent of more than 2750 calories of food per person. While this should be more than enough to go round, since no ideal food systems exist, food distribution and consumption remain completely unequal. While around 850 million people worldwide live in hunger, more than double that are overweight or obese (Steel, 2020). Moreover, a fundamental mismatch exists between what global agriculture produces and what the world's population requires for a balanced diet as recommended by nutrition experts, with almost 40 percent consisting of starchy vegetables such as cassava and potatoes, which have an elevating effect on blood sugar (Kc et al., 2018).

As with psychiatry, biotechnology has not remained the province of experts. The past decades have witnessed the rise of the "quantified self" as we utilize self-tracking tools attached to our bodies to proactively monitor our mental and physical health and diets with a view to potentially acting on this (Swan, 2013). Courtesy of the big tech companies, self-trackers have become fashion and status accessories, making them indispensable items for tech-savvy consumers with disposable income. DNA testing, often done for personal amusement purposes, allows for the surveillance and monitoring of bodies on a vast scale. The collection, trading, and analysis of health-related big data, assisted by the rise of machine learning and AI, further enhances the ability of companies to advertise and sell their products to a digitally connected public. This emphasis on the quantitative aspects of bodies exists side-by-side with the illusion spread by neoliberalism and its allies—healthism, positive psychology, and now neurobiology—that science can enable us to be our "best version of self," whatever that shape or personality turns out to be. Neoliberal ideology has always assumed that if individuals only took responsibility for their own care, then providing expensive healthcare services could be largely avoided (Rose, 1998). Biometric technology has amplified the capacity to identify individuals who deviate from medical norms and subject them to systems of "care." The advent of neuroscience, biometrics, and artificial intelligence (AI) has allowed for the global tracking and monitoring of people's behaviors for political, economic, and medical purposes (Zuboff, 2015, 2019). Facial recognition is frequently highlighted as a cutting-edge surveillance tool while biometric measurements can identify numerous aspects of bodies. Nonetheless, not all individuals are subjected to the same levels of surveillance; those categorized as belonging to an outlier group and/or having a physical or mental health disorder face heightened monitoring, ostensibly for their own or others' safety and well-being. Many surveillance tools still exhibit racial biases, while history illustrates the sinister uses to which science and technology can be put in relation to the tracking and reconfiguration of categories of persons deemed to be deviant, disgustful, or lacking in health and intelligence.

Final Reflections

Some of the discussion in this book may seem removed from the everyday problems and sufferings of those experiencing an eating disorder and its impact on their own or their family's lives. The reservations expressed around such things as neuroscience may disappoint those who seek concrete answers to the complex and sometimes agonizing mental distress many people face daily. However as argued throughout the book, eating disorders cannot be fully understood without considering the social context in which they arise. The construction of disordered eating transcends individual concerns, having developed through the collective efforts of biomedical, psychiatric, legal, pharmaceutical, media, marketing, and consumer interest groups. Arguments surrounding the pros and cons of employing specific psychiatric labels hinge on a fundamental debate: whether mental disorders, including eating disorders, exist independently of diagnostic categories or are products of a reductionist medical profession. Some argue that these disorders are real phenomena, identifiable and treatable through established psychiatric frameworks. This view is reinforced by the fact that many psychiatric categories seem to align with observable patterns in the modern world, and a significant portion of the public readily adopts these labels, applying acronyms like ADHD, PTSD, and BED to their own experiences in everyday conversation. This widespread acceptance raises the question: should the proliferation of diagnoses be seen as a sign of social progress, reflecting a growing awareness and willingness to address mental health issues? Another possibility, and one not necessarily at odds with the first, is that we are now conditioned to interpret our experiences through a psychiatric lens. As more aspects of life become subject to psychiatric diagnosis, there is a growing risk that people will be encouraged to see their problems as requiring medical treatment rather than social or political solutions.

A society schooled to think in the language of psychiatry has implications for how we choose to speak about and view the sufferings of everyday life. As Brinkmann (2016) reminds us, other explanations rooted in esoteric, religious, or moral frameworks—such as concepts of sin or karma—still resonate with many people. This might suggest that psychiatry's dominance over our inner lives is not as universal as some critics attest. However, psychiatry is not a standalone science or ideology, its expansion is both instrumental in, and reflective of, biopower's focus on an incontestable governance of our inner lives. Most modern health systems include checks and balances, such that a person's medical and social care is seldom decided by a single individual. Nevertheless, we should not underestimate the power of a psychiatric label to reshape a person's life and liberty, and their perception of themselves and others in virtually every way. Those who can sum up others' sufferings and differences in the space of few words or an acronym hold an authority over the subject's mind and body, which may be impossible to contest on medical or legal grounds.

A further argument suggesting the need to pull back on psychiatry's expansion is the risk of pathologizing behaviors and experiences that were previously considered within the range of normalcy. If society continues to accept the binary categorization of people as either "normal" or "deficient," it inevitably faces the challenge of managing those deemed deficient. This management approach, rooted in diagnostic culture, risks overshadowing other, potentially more holistic ways of understanding and addressing human suffering. As psychiatry forces more people into treatment, it reinforces a view of these individuals as deficient or deviant (Dellwing & Harbusch, 2023). People who are diagnosed with mental health conditions are often seen as "other," reinforcing social divisions and potentially leading to discrimination and exclusion. This is particularly problematic when psychiatric labels are applied to behaviors or experiences that are culturally specific or context dependent. For instance, certain cultural practices or expressions of distress, such as sense of alienation or grief, may be misunderstood or misinterpreted through a western psychiatric lens, leading to inappropriate diagnoses and treatment.

This overuse of psychiatric categories raises ethical concerns about the overreach of psychiatry into areas of life that were once considered the domain of personal or moral judgment. As argued in the book, the pathologization of behaviors related to eating, such as binge eating or restrictive eating, may well have led to an increase in the number of people now labeled with eating disorders. While detection can raise awareness and lead to treatment for those who need it, it can also result in the stigmatization of behaviors that might otherwise be considered within the spectrum of normal human variation. When pointed out to them by medics and others, individuals are more likely to view themselves as sick or defective, reinforcing negative self-perceptions and exacerbating the very issues that psychiatric intervention aims to alleviate. This individualistic focus also tends to depoliticize mental health by framing it as a purely personal issue rather than a reflection of broader societal problems. When mental health is viewed solely through the lens of individual pathology, the structural inequalities, economic hardships, and social injustices that contribute to psychological distress are often overlooked. This can lead to a situation where the burden of mental health is placed entirely on the individual, obscuring the need for collective action to address the root causes of distress. The expansion of psychiatric categories may well be leading to a medicalization of everyday life, where normal emotional responses to life's challenges are increasingly viewed as symptoms of mental illness. This medicalization not only pathologizes normal human experiences but creates a dependency on psychiatric interventions, often in the form of medication.

Individualism tends to divert attention and resources away from community-based approaches that address mental health in a more holistic manner. Community interventions that focus on improving social support networks and fostering a sense of belonging and purpose have shown themselves to be effective in promoting mental well-being (Fixsen et al., 2020b). These approaches still receive less attention and funding compared to medicalized treatments, which are more aligned with the interests of the pharmaceutical industry and the healthcare system. This imbalance perpetuates a cycle where mental health issues are treated in isolation from the social conditions that contribute to them, leading to incomplete and often ineffective solutions. An example of this is that of obesity prevention. During decades of a war waged on fat, policies tackling obesity remained primarily focused on individual behavioral change, an approach which has yet to reverse childhood obesity or adult trends linked with chronic metabolic disease. Tackling the obesogenic environment requires comprehensive and multi-sectoral strategies that address the various factors contributing to unhealthy behaviors, and environments that promote obesity. Tactics suggested by activists include the lobbying of food manufacturers, imposing financial penalties on companies for harmful marketing practices, the provision of healthy meals and snacks in schools, providing easy to access recreational areas, parks, and gardens in densely populated areas, creating safe areas for exercise, and encouraging local communities to engage in activities together. Above and beyond this is the need for radical change to the political and economic systems, which have for generations ensured that the health chances of different communities, even in localities near to one another, can be grossly unequal.

Finally, there are major structural problems with the present agricultural and food systems, with the worst affected being those living in Africa, Asia, and Latin America (FAO, 2024). Corporate involvement in food production has undoubtedly increased food availability in rich countries. Arguably we have the most efficient food production and distribution system in human history, freeing up most peoples' time to spend on other activities. Yet the modern food system has also created significant environmental, social, and health damage, as well as poverty and hunger. According to the FAO and UN agencies, food prices that increased post Covid had yet to fall in 2024. With healthy diets remaining unaffordable for a third of the world's population (FAO, 2024), there is an urgent need for society to reevaluate its relationship with food sources. We need to recognize the intrinsic value of food and the broader implications of mass food production on global issues like climate change, water pollution, soil erosion, and antibiotic resistance (Li, 2017; Steel, 2020). These environmental challenges are inextricably linked to the health of humanity and must be addressed to ensure a sustainable future. The ecology of food and the rights of people to define their own food systems—deciding what food is produced, how it is produced, and how it is distributed—are central to reshaping our attitudes toward food and eating. Addressing these challenges requires a concerted effort to prioritize sustainability, equity, and health over short-term profit. This might include promoting organic and regenerative farming practices, supporting local and small-scale farmers, and advocating for fair trade practices that ensure fair wages and conditions for workers. Only by reimagining the way food is produced and distributed—and ensuring that people of all backgrounds are fairly treated—can we envisage a future where both people and the planet can thrive.

References

Ali, K., Farrer, L., Fassnacht, D. B., Gulliver, A., Bauer, S., & Griffiths, K. M. (2017). Perceived barriers and facilitators towards help-seeking for eating disorders: A systematic review. *International Journal of Eating Disorders, 50*(1), 9–21.

American Psychiatric Association Publishing. (2022, August 6). *DSM5-TR-diagnostic statistical manual of mental disorders.* https://www.appi.org/products/dsm

American Society of Plastic Surgeons. (2018, March 18). *New statistics reveal the shape of plastic surgery.* Retrieved November 26, 2024, from https://www.plasticsurgery.org/news/press-releases/new-statistics-reveal-the-shape-of-plastic-surgery

BEAT. (2023). *How many people have an eating disorder in the UK?* Retrieved August 24, 2024, from https://www.beateatingdisorders.org.uk/get-information-and-support/about-eating-disorders/how-many-people-eating-disorder-uk/

Berardi, J. (2019). *Change maker: Turn your passion for health and fitness into a powerful purpose and a wildly successful career.* BenBella Books.

Blackburn, M. R., & Hogg, R. C. (2024). # ForYou? The impact of pro-ana TikTok content on body image dissatisfaction and internalisation of societal beauty standards. *PloS One, 19*(8), e0307597.

Bordo, S. (1994). Feminism, Foucault, and the politics of the body. In *Reconstructing Foucault* (pp. 219–243). Brill.

Bordo, S. (1996). Hunger is ideology. In C. Luke (Ed.), *Feminisms and pedagogies of everyday life.* SUNY Press.

Brandt, A. M. (1978). Racism and research: The case of the Tuskegee Syphilis Study. *Hastings center report,* 21–29.

Bray, B., Bray, C., Bradley, R., & Zwickey, H. (2022). Binge Eating Disorder is a social justice issue: A cross-sectional mixed-methods study of Binge Eating Disorder experts' opinions. *International Journal of Environmental Research and Public Health, 19*(10), 6243.

Brinkmann, S. (2016). *Diagnostic cultures: A cultural approach to the pathologization of modern life.* Routledge.

Bruch, H. (1979). *The Golden Cage: The enigma of anorexia nervosa.* Vintage.

Chekhovska, L. (2017). Fitness industry: state and prospects of development in the countries of the world. *Slobozhanskyi herald of science and sport, 2*(58), 19–24.

Children's Commissioner. (2024). *Major conditions strategy consultation response.* Retrieved August 24, 2024, from https://assets.childrenscommissioner.gov.uk/wpuploads/2023/07/Major-Conditions-Strategy-response_final.pdf

Claudino, A. M., Pike, K. M., Hay, P., Keeley, J. W., Evans, S. C., Rebello, T. J., et al. (2019). The classification of feeding and eating disorders in the ICD-11 results of a field study comparing proposed ICD-11 guidelines with existing ICD-10 guidelines. *BMC Medicine, 17,* 1–17.

Clausen, L. (2020). Perspectives on involuntary treatment of anorexia nervosa. *Frontiers in Psychiatry, 11,* 533288.

Clausen, L., Larsen, J. T., Bulik, C. M., & Petersen, L. (2018). A Danish register-based study on involuntary treatment in anorexia nervosa. *International Journal of Eating Disorders, 51*(11), 1213–1222.
Cohen, S. (1972/2011). *Folk devils and moral panics*. Routledge.
Cohen, B. M. Z. (2016). *Psychiatric hegemony: A Marxist theory on mental illness*. Palgrave Macmillan.
Cooper, C. (2021). *Fat activism: A radical social movement*. Intellect.
Cox, N., & Webb, L. (2015). Poles apart: Does the export of mental health expertise from the Global North to the Global South represent a neutral relocation of knowledge and practice? *Sociology of Health & Illness, 37*(5), 683–697.
Crawford, R. (1980). Healthism and the medicalization of everyday life. *International Journal of Health Services, 10*(3), 365–388.
De Clercq, B., Abel, T., Moor, I., Elgar, F. J., Lievens, J., Sioen, I., et al. (2017). Social inequality in adolescents' healthy food intake: The interplay between economic, social and cultural capital. *The European Journal of Public Health, 27*(2), 279–286.
Dellwing, M., & Harbusch, M. (2023). Conclusion. In M. Harbusch (Ed.), *Troubled Persons Industries: The expansion of psychiatric categories beyond psychiatry*. Springer International Publishing.
DiNicola, V. F. (1990). Anorexia Multiforme: Self-starvation in historical and cultural context: Part II: Anorexia Nervosa as a Culture-Reactive Syndrome. *Transcultural Psychiatric Research Review, 27*(4), 245–286.
Fairplay. (2022). *Designing for Disorder: Instagram's Pro-eating Disorder Bubble*. Fairplay. Retrieved August 22, 2024, from https://fairplayforkids.org/wp-content/uploads/2022/04/designing_for_disorder.pd
Farber, S. K. (2013). Eating disorders in women's prisons: An under-reported phenomenon? *Advances in Eating Disorders, 1*(1), 39–50.
Fixsen, A., Cheshire, A., & Berry, M. (2020a). The social construction of a concept—Orthorexia Nervosa: Morality narratives and psycho-politics. *Qualitative Health Research, 30*(7), 1101–1113.
Fixsen, A., Seers, H., Polley, M., & Robins, J. (2020b). Applying critical systems thinking to social prescribing: A relational model of stakeholder "buy-in". *BMC Health Services Research, 20*, 1–13.
Fixsen, A., Ridge, D., Ponsford, O., Holder, M., & Saran, G. (2023). Battles over 'unruly bodies': Practitioners' interpretations of eating disorders and the utility of psychiatric labeling. *Sociology of Health & Illness, 45*(3), 560–579.

Food, Farming, and Countryside, Commission. (2024, November 15). The False Economy of Big Food. Retrieved November 23, from https://ffcc.co.uk/publications/the-false-economy-of-big-food

Food and Agriculture Organization of the United Nations (FAO). (2024, August 16). *Statistics*. Retrieved August 22, 2024, from https://www.fao.org/statistics/en

Fukuyama, F. (2003). *Our posthuman future: Consequences of the biotechnology revolution*. Farrar, Straus and Giroux.

Gao, Y., Bagheri, N., & Furuya-Kanamori, L. (2022). Has the COVID-19 pandemic lockdown worsened eating disorders symptoms among patients with eating disorders? A systematic review. *Journal of Public Health, 30*(11), 2743–2752.

Giddens, A. (1991). *Modernity and self-identity. Self in society in the modern age*. Polity.

Gill, R. (2017). The affective, cultural and psychic life of post feminism. A post-feminist sensibility 10 years on. *European Journal of Cultural Studies 20*(6), 606–626.

Giordano, S. (2005). *Understanding eating disorders: Conceptual and ethical issues in the treatment of anorexia and bulimia nervosa*. Oxford University Press.

Glass, R. (2024). *How stressed are teachers compare to other professions?* Schools Week. Retrieved August 22, 2024, from https://schoolsweek.co.uk/how-stressed-are-teachers-compared-with-other-professions/

Guarda, A. S., Pinto, A. M., Coughlin, J. W., Hussain, S., Haug, N. A., & Heinberg, L. J. (2007). Perceived coercion and change in perceived need for admission in patients hospitalized for eating disorders. *American Journal of Psychiatry, 164*(1), 108–114.

Gutteridge, N. (2024). *Mental health culture has gone too far says Mel Stride*. The Telegraph. Retrieved August 22, 2024, from https://www.telegraph.co.uk/politics/2024/03/20/mental-health-culture-has-gone-too-far-says-mel-stride/

Harbusch, M. (2022). Introduction: Are we all mad here? The normalization of trouble in everyday life. In M. Harbusch (Ed.), *Troubled Persons Industries: The expansion of psychiatric categories beyond psychiatry*. Springer International Publishing.

Hatch, A. R., Sternlieb, S., & Gordon, J. (2019). Sugar ecologies: Their metabolic and racial effects. *Food, Culture, & Society, 22*(5), 595–607.

Hay, P. (2020). Current approach to eating disorders: A clinical update. *Internal Medicine Journal, 50*(1), 24–29.

Hepworth, J., & Griffin, C. (1995). Conflicting opinions? 'Anorexia nervosa', medicine and feminism. In S. Wilkinson & C. Kitzinger (Eds.), *Feminism and discourse: Psychological perspectives*. Sage.

Heyes, C. J. (2007). Normalisation and the psychic life of cosmetic surgery. *Australian Feminist Studies, 22*(52), 55–71.

Holmes, S., Malson, H., & Semlyen, J. (2021). Regulating "untrustworthy patients": Constructions of "trust" and "distrust" in accounts of inpatient treatment for anorexia. *Feminism & Psychology, 31*(1), 41–61.

Huryk, K. M., Drury, C. R., & Loeb, K. L. (2021). Diseases of affluence? A systematic review of the literature on socioeconomic diversity in eating disorders. *Eating Behaviors, 43*, 101548.

Huxley, A. (1932). *Brave New World*. Chatto & Windous.

IPPR. (2022, December 7). *Revealed. Mental Health problems 'most common condition' among the sick forced out of UK workforce*. Retrieved August 22, 2024, from https://www.ippr.org/media-office/revealed-mental-health-problems-most-common-condition-among-the-sick-forced-out-of-uk-workforce

Jennings Mathis, K., Anaya, C., Rambur, B., Bodell, L. P., Graham, A. K., Forney, K. J., et al. (2020). Workforce diversity in eating disorders: A multi-methods study. *Western Journal of Nursing Research, 42*(12), 1068–1077.

Jönsson, K. (2009). Fysisk fostran och föraktet för svaghet: En kritisk analys av hälsodiskursens moraliska imperativ. *Educare, 1*, 7–20.

Kc, K. B., Dias, G. M., Veeramani, A., Swanton, C. J., Fraser, D., Steinke, D., et al. (2018). When too much isn't enough: Does current food production meet global nutritional needs? *PloS One, 13*(10), e0205683.

Keene, A. R. (2024). *Mental capacity Law and policy*. Retrieved August 22, 2024, from https://www.mentalcapacitylawandpolicy.org.uk/. Accessed 7 August 2024.

Kessler, R. C., Berglund, P. A., Chiu, W. T., Deitz, A. C., Hudson, J. I., Shahly, V., ... & Xavier, M. (2013). The prevalence and correlates of binge eating disorder in the World Health Organization World Mental Health Surveys. *Biological Psychiatry, 73*(9), 904–914.

Kestens, Y., & Daniel, M. (2010). Social inequalities in food exposure around schools in an urban area. *American Journal of Preventive Medicine, 39*(1), 33–40.

Kristensen, D. B., Lim, M., & Askegaard, S. (2016). Healthism in Denmark. *Health, 20*(5), 485–504.

Krug, I., Fuller-Tyszkiewicz, M., Hughes, E. K., & Roncero, M. (2022). What do we know about Other Specified Feeding or Eating Disorders, Unspecified

Feeding and Eating Disorder and the Other EXIAs (eg, Orthorexia, Bigorexia, Drunkorexia, Pregorexia etc.)? *Frontiers in Psychology, 13*, 953402.

Lee, S. (2001). From diversity to unity: The classification of mental disorders in 21st-century China. *Psychiatric Clinics of North America, 24*(3), 421–431.

Li, A. M. (2017). Ecological determinants of health: Food and environment on human health. *Environmental Science and Pollution Research International, 24*(10), 9002–9015.

Luckhurst, P. (2015, February 23). *The holy kale. Beyoncé wants London to full crazy in love with her new nutrition plan*. The Standard. Retrieved August 22 2024, from https://www.standard.co.uk/going-out/foodanddrink/the-holy-kale-beyonce-wants-london-to-fall-crazy-in-love-with-her-new-nutrition-plan-10064170.html

Lyons, D., & O'Malley, A. (2002). The labelling of dissent–politics and psychiatry behind the Great Wall. *Psychiatric Bulletin, 26*(12), 443–444.

Magrach, A., & Sanz, M. J. (2020). Environmental and social consequences of the increase in the demand for 'superfoods' world-wide. *People and Nature, 2*(2), 267–278.

Mathieu-Bolh, N., & Wendner, R. (2020). We are what we eat: Obesity, income, and social comparisons. *European Economic Review, 128*, 103495.

McBride, R.-S. (2022). Carceral psychiatry. In M. Harbusch (Ed.), *Troubled Persons Industries: The expansion of psychiatric categories beyond psychiatry*. Springer International Publishing.

McCuen-Wurst, C., Ruggieri, M., & Allison, K. C. (2018). Disordered eating and obesity: Associations between binge-eating disorder night-eating syndrome, and weight-related comorbidities. *Annals of the New York Academy of Sciences, 1411*(1), 96–105.

McGuire, P. K., & Matsumoto, K. (2004). Functional neuroimaging in mental disorders. *World Psychiatry, 3*(1), 6.

McPhail, D. (2013). Resisting biopedagogies of obesity in a problem population: Understandings of healthy eating and healthy weight in a Newfoundland and Labrador community. *Critical Public Health, 23*, 289–303.

Mehanna, H. M., Moledina, J., & Travis, J. (2008). Refeeding syndrome: What it is, and how to prevent and treat it. *British Medical Journal, 336*(7659), 1495–1498.

Miller, I. (2016). *A history of force feeding: Hunger strikes, prisons and medical ethics, 1909–1974* (p. 267). Springer Nature.

Mind. (2013, October 9). *Work is the biggest cause of stress in peoples' lives.* Retrieved August 24, 2024, from https://www.mind.org.uk/news-campaigns/news/work-is-biggest-cause-of-stress-in-people-s-lives/

Mitchison, D., Hay, P., Slewa-Younan, S., & Mond, J. (2014). The changing demographic profile of eating disorder behaviors in the community. *BMC Public Health, 14*, 1–9.

Moreno, R., Buckelew, S. M., Accurso, E. C., & Raymond-Flesch, M. (2023). Disparities in access to eating disorders treatment for publicly-insured youth and youth of color: A retrospective cohort study. *Journal of Eating Disorders, 11*(1), 10.

National Institute for Clinical Excellence (NICE). (2021, December 16). *Eating disorders recognition and treatment.* Retrieved August 22, 2024, from https://www.nice.org.uk/guidance/ng69/chapter/Recommendation

NHS Business Services Authority. (2023, July 6). *Medicines used in mental health- England-2015/16 to 2022/23.* Retrieved August 24, 2024, from https://www.nhsbsa.nhs.uk/statistical-collections/medicines-used-mental-health-england/medicines-used-mental-health-england-201516-202223

NHS England. (2021, October 15). *Hospital for admissions for eating disorders, 2015–2021.* https://digital.nhs.uk/supplementary-information/2021/hospital-admissions-for-eating-disorders-2015-2021

NHS England Digital. (2022, October 27). *Mental health statistics, annual figures, 2021 to 22.* Retrieved 26 November 2024, from https://digital.nhs.uk/data-and-information/publications/statistical/mental-health-act-statistics-annual-figures/2021-22-annual-figures

Nuckolls, C. W. (2022). Mental health categories and the construction of cultural identities in the United States and New Zealand. In M. Harbusch (Ed.), *Troubled Persons Industries: The expansion of psychiatric categories beyond psychiatry*. Springer International Publishing.

Office of the Surgeon General (OSG). (2021). Protecting Youth Mental Health: The U.S. In *Surgeon General's Advisory [Internet]*. US Department of Health and Human Services.

Orbach, S. (1978). *Fat is a feminist issue: The anti-diet guide to permanent weight loss*. Paddington Press.

Orbach, S. (1986). *Hunger strike: The anorectic's struggle as a metaphor for our age.* Faber & Faber.

Orbach, S. (2019). *Bodies*. Profile books.

Paris, J. (2020). *Overdiagnosis in psychiatry: How modern psychiatry lost its way while creating a diagnosis for almost all of life's misfortunes*. Oxford University Press.

Pitts-Taylor, V. (2016). *The brain's body: Neuroscience and corporeal politics*. Duke University Press.

Rajan, K. S. (2006). *Bio capital: The constitution of post-genomic life*. Duke University Press.

Rose, N. (1998). *Inventing ourselves: Psychology, power and personhood*. Cambridge University Press.

Rose, N., & Abi-Rached, J. (2013). *Neuro: The new brain sciences and the management of the mind*. Princeton University Press.

Royal College of Psychiatrists. (2024). *It's time to tackle the trap of inequality and mental illness*. Retrieved August 24, from https://www.rcpsych.ac.uk/news-and-features/latest-news/detail/2024/01/25/it-s-time-to-tackle-the-trap-of-inequality-and-mental-illness

Santomauro, D. F., Melen, S., Mitchison, D., Vos, T., Whiteford, H., & Ferrari, A. J. (2021). The hidden burden of eating disorders: An extension of estimates from the Global Burden of Disease Study 2019. *The Lancet Psychiatry, 8*(4), 320–328.

Sarwer, D. B. (2019). Body image, cosmetic surgery, and minimally invasive treatments. *Body Image, 31*, 302–308.

Scanlan, S. J., Cooper Stoll, L., & Lumm, K. (2008). Starving for change: The hunger strike and nonviolent action, 1906–2004. In *Research in social movements, conflicts and change* (pp. 275–323). Emerald Group Publishing Limited.

Seed, T., Fox, J., & Berry, K. (2016). Experiences of detention under the mental health act for adults with anorexia nervosa. *Clinical Psychology & Psychotherapy, 23*(4), 352–362.

Shilling, C. (2016). The rise of body studies and the embodiment of society: A review of the field. *Horizons in Humanities and Social Sciences: An International Refereed Journal, 2*(1), 1–14.

Soulliard, Z. A., Layland, E. K., Smith, J. C., Kipke, M. D., & Bray, B. C. (2022). Body image concerns, correlates, and community connection among Black and Latinx sexual minority cisgender men and transgender/gender nonconforming young adults. *LGBT health, 9*(2), 122–130.

Steel, C. (2020). *Sitopia: How food can save the world*. Random House.

Steel, C. (2021). *How food can save the world*. issuu. Retrieved August 22, 2024, from https://issuu.com/landscape-institute/docs/12421_landscape_issue_1-2021_v8a_issuu/s/11604694.

Stern, S. A., & Bulik, C. M. (2020). Alternative frameworks for advancing the study of eating disorders. *Trends in Neurosciences, 43*(12), 951–959.

Stice, E., Rohde, P., & Shaw, H. (2013). *The body project: A dissonance-based eating disorder prevention intervention*. Oxford University Press.

Summerfield, D. (2001). The invention of post-traumatic stress disorder and the social usefulness of a psychiatric category. *BMJ, 322*(7278), 95–98.

Summerfield, D. (2008). How scientifically valid is the knowledge base of global mental health? *BMJ, 336*(7651), 992–994.

Summerfield, D. (2012). Afterword: Against "global mental health". *Transcultural Psychiatry, 49*(3–4), 519–530.

Swan, M. (2013). The quantified self: Fundamental disruption in big data science and biological discovery. *Big Data, 1*(2), 85–99.

Tapsfield, J. (2024, March 22). *Tory deputy chair warns Brits are being incentivized to report mental health issues saying it is 'normal, not feel happy all the time'- amid fears over rising numbers being signed off sick.* Daily Mail. Retrieved August 24, 2024, from https://www.dailymail.co.uk/news/article-13227191/Tory-deputy-chair-Maclean-Brits-incentivised-mental-health-issues-life-hard.html

Thomas, S. B., & Casper, E. (2019). The burdens of race and history on Black people's health 400 years after Jamestown. *American Journal of Public Health, 109*(10), 1346–1347.

Thomas, J. J., Hartmann, A. S., & Killgore, W. D. (2013). Non-fat-phobic eating disorders: Why we need to investigate implicit associations and neural correlates. *International Journal of Eating Disorders, 46*(5).

Tompkins, K. W. (2009). Sylvester Graham's imperial dietetics. *Gastronomica, 9*(1), 50–60.

Tragantzopoulou, P., Fixsen, A., Cheshire, A., & Ridge, D. (2024). 'You are not alone, we've got you': Powerplays, devotion and punishment on healthy eating and pro-eating disorder websites. *Qualitative Health Research*. https://doi.org/10.1177/10497323241238628

Turner, B. S. (2008). *The body & society: Explorations in social theory* (3rd ed.). Sage.

Tyler, M., & Wilkinson, A. (2007). The tyranny of corporate slenderness: 'corporate anorexia' as a metaphor for our age. *Work, Employment and Society, 21*(3), 537–549.

Tyler, N., Miles, H. L., Karadag, B., & Rogers, G. (2019). An updated picture of the mental health needs of male and female prisoners in the UK: Prevalence, comorbidity, and gender differences. *Social Psychiatry and Psychiatric Epidemiology, 54*, 1143–1152.

UK Parliament. (2024, August 14). *Preparedness for online safety regulation*. Retrieved August 23, 2024, from, https://publications.parliament.uk/pa/cm5804/cmselect/cmpubacc/73/report.html

Umezulike, C. C. (2020). *The meaning-centred anorexic body: A human rights-based approach to involuntary treatment.* Doctoral thesis, Birkbeck, University of London.

van Voren, R. (2010). Political abuse of psychiatry—An historical overview. *Schizophrenia Bulletin, 36*(1), 33–35.

van Voren, R. (2016). Ending political abuse of psychiatry: Where we are at and what needs to be done. *BJPsych Bulletin, 40*(1), 30–33.

Verité. (2012). *Research on indicators of force labour in the supply chain of sugar in the Dominican Republic*. Retrieved August 23, 2024, from https://respect.international/research-on-indicators-of-forced-labor-in-the-supply-chain-of-sugar-in-the-dominican-republic/

Waldman, A. (2014, July 9). Eating disorders in women grossly under reported. *Humane exposures blog*. Retrieved August 23, 2024, from http://humaneexposures.com/blog/eating-disorders-in-womens-prisons-are-grossly-under-reported.html

Wildeman, S. (2013). Protecting rights and building capacities: Challenges to global mental health policy in light of the convention on the rights of persons with disabilities. *Journal of Law, Medicine & Ethics, 41*(1), 48–73.

Wooldridge, T., & Lytle, P. (2012). An overview of anorexia nervosa in males. *Eating Disorders, 20*(5), 368–378.

World Health Organization (WHO). (2019). *International Classification of Diseases 10th revision*: Ch. 5 Mental and behavioural disorders. Retrieved August 22, 2024, from https://icd.who.int/browse10/2019/en#/F50.0

Zhao, Q. (2022). *From the health professionals' perspective, how do social and cultural factors influence the development and treatment of eating disorders in China? A qualitative study*. Unpublished master's thesis, University of Westminster.

Zuboff, S. (2015). Big other: Surveillance capitalism and the prospects of an information civilization. *Journal of Information Technology, 30*, 75–89.

Zuboff, S. (2019). Surveillance capitalism and the challenge of collective action. *New Labor Forum, 28*(1), 10–29.

Index[1]

[1] Note: Page numbers followed by 'n' refer to notes.

A. Fixsen, *The Construction of Eating Disorders*, The Politics of Mental Health and Illness, https://doi.org/10.1007/978-3-031-70318-8

The manufacturer's authorised representative in the EU is Springer Nature Customer Service Centre GmbH, Europaplatz 3, 69115 Heidelberg, Germany. If you have any concerns regarding our products, please contact ProductSafety@springernature.com

Printed and bound by CPI Group (UK) Ltd, Croydon, CR0 4YY
23/09/2026
02221551-0004